Metabolic Features and Nutritional Interventions in Chronic Diseases

Metabolic Features and Nutritional Interventions in Chronic Diseases

Guest Editors

Yongting Luo
Junjie Luo
Peng An

MDPI

Basel • Beijing • Wuhan • Barcelona • Belgrade • Novi Sad • Cluj • Manchester

Guest Editors
Yongting Luo
Department of Nutrition and Health
China Agricultural University
Beijing
China

Junjie Luo
Department of Nutrition and Health
China Agricultural University
Beijing
China

Peng An
Department of Nutrition and Health
China Agricultural University
Beijing
China

Editorial Office
MDPI AG
Grosspeteranlage 5
4052 Basel, Switzerland

This is a reprint of the Special Issue, published open access by the journal *Nutrients* (ISSN 2072-6643), freely accessible at: https://www.mdpi.com/journal/nutrients/special_issues/TF0IR7GS48.

For citation purposes, cite each article independently as indicated on the article page online and as indicated below:

Lastname, A.A.; Lastname, B.B. Article Title. *Journal Name* **Year**, *Volume Number*, Page Range.

ISBN 978-3-7258-4919-2 (Hbk)
ISBN 978-3-7258-4920-8 (PDF)
https://doi.org/10.3390/books978-3-7258-4920-8

Contents

About the Editors vii

Yongting Luo, Peng An and Junjie Luo
Metabolic Features and Nutritional Interventions in Chronic Diseases
Reprinted from: *Nutrients* **2025**, *17*, 1826, https://doi.org/10.3390/nu17111826 1

Shucheng Zhang, Zhengwu Cui, Hao Zhang, Pengjie Wang, Fuqing Wang and Jian Zhang
Pea Albumin Extracted from Pea (*Pisum sativum* L.) Seeds Ameliorates High-Fat-Diet-Induced Non-Alcoholic Fatty Liver Disease by Regulating Lipogenesis and Lipolysis Pathways
Reprinted from: *Nutrients* **2024**, *16*, 2232, https://doi.org/10.3390/nu16142232 5

Tianyu Wang, Dawei Wang, Yinghui Ding, He Xu, Yue Sun, Jumin Hou and Yanrong Zhang
Targeting Non-Alcoholic Fatty Liver Disease with Hawthorn Ethanol Extract (HEE): A Comprehensive Examination of Hepatic Lipid Reduction and Gut Microbiota Modulation
Reprinted from: *Nutrients* **2024**, *16*, 1335, https://doi.org/10.3390/nu16091335 24

Jiaxin Shi, Yitong Cheng, Chenxuan Wang, Min Liu, Mingxuan Qu, Shuaishuai Zhou, et al.
Effects of Celastrol-Enriched Peanuts on Metabolic Health and the Development of Atherosclerosis
Reprinted from: *Nutrients* **2025**, *17*, 1418, https://doi.org/10.3390/nu17091418 39

Xinsheng Zhang, Peng Zhang, Yinghua Liu, Zhao Liu, Qing Xu, Yong Zhang, et al.
Effects of Caprylic Acid and Eicosapentaenoic Acid on Lipids, Inflammatory Levels, and the JAK2/STAT3 Pathway in ABCA1-Deficient Mice and ABCA1 Knock-Down RAW264.7 Cells
Reprinted from: *Nutrients* **2023**, *15*, 1296, https://doi.org/10.3390/nu15051296 60

Oliwia Gawlik-Kotelnicka, Jakub Rogalski, Karolina H. Czarnecka-Chrebelska, Jacek Burzyński, Paulina Jakubowska, Anna Skowrońska and Dominik Strzelecki
The Interplay Between Depression, Probiotics, Diet, Immunometabolic Health, the Gut, and the Liver—A Secondary Analysis of the Pro-Demet Randomized Clinical Trial
Reprinted from: *Nutrients* **2024**, *16*, 4024, https://doi.org/10.3390/nu16234024 75

Marta Potrykus, Sylwia Czaja-Stolc, Marta Stankiewicz, Michał Szymański, Igor Łoniewski, Łukasz Kaska and Monika Proczko-Stepaniak
Preoperative Multistrain Probiotic Supplementation Does Not Affect Body Weight Changes or Cardiometabolic Risk Factors in Bariatrics: Randomized, Double-Blind, Placebo-Controlled Clinical Trial
Reprinted from: *Nutrients* **2024**, *16*, 2055, https://doi.org/10.3390/nu16132055 89

Lin Zhu, Peng An, Wenting Zhao, Yi Xia, Jingyi Qi, Junjie Luo and Yongting Luo
Low Zinc Alleviates the Progression of Thoracic Aortic Dissection by Inhibiting Inflammation
Reprinted from: *Nutrients* **2023**, *15*, 1640, https://doi.org/10.3390/nu15071640 104

Lu Liu, Hang Yu, Jingmin Bai, Qing Xu, Yong Zhang, Xinsheng Zhang, et al.
Positive Association of Serum Vitamin B6 Levels with Intrapulmonary Lymph Node and/or Localized Pleural Metastases in Non-Small Cell Lung Cancer: A Retrospective Study
Reprinted from: *Nutrients* **2023**, *15*, 2340, https://doi.org/10.3390/nu15102340 118

Junzhou Chen, Conghui Yin, Yilong Zhang, Xin Lai, Chen Liu, Yuheng Luo, et al.
EGCG Alleviates DSS-Induced Colitis by Inhibiting Ferroptosis Through the Activation of the Nrf2-GPX4 Pathway and Enhancing Iron Metabolism
Reprinted from: *Nutrients* **2025**, *17*, 547, https://doi.org/10.3390/nu17030547 134

Yongpan An, Qian Wang, Panshuang Qiao, Jihan Liu, Ang Ma, Yutong Chen, et al.
Unveiling the Anti-Aging Potential of 3HB: Lifespan Extension and Cellular Senescence Delay
Reprinted from: *Nutrients* **2025**, *17*, 1647, https://doi.org/10.3390/nu17101647 . . . . **150**

About the Editors

Yongting Luo

Yongting Luo graduated with a Ph.D. degree in cell biology from the Institute of Biophysics, Chinese Academy of Sciences in 2012. Yongting Luo is an Associate Professor at the Department of Nutrition and Health of the China Agricultural University. Dr. Luo has received 10 scientific awards and participated in 21 scientific projects, being the coordinator for nine projects. His current research interests focus on the pathogenesis and nutritional intervention of cardiovascular diseases, including atherosclerosis, aortic dissection, and heart failure. To date, Dr. Luo has contributed to 68 scientific publications in international journals with referees.

Junjie Luo

Junjie Luo graduated with a Ph.D. degree in Biochemistry and Molecular biology from China Agricultural University in 2013. Dr. Luo is an associate professor and doctoral supervisor of the Department of Nutrition and Health, China Agricultural University. He has published 50 academic papers in internationally renowned journals such as European Heart Journal, Blood, Cell Research, Nucleic Acids Research, Science Bulletin, Advanced Science, and Cell Death & Disease, and American Journal of Clinical Nutrition. His current research interests focus on mitochondria and chronic diseases, molecular nutrition, and health-related topics.

Peng An

Dr. Peng An is an associate professor at the Department of Nutrition and Health of the China Agricultural University. He focuses on the mechanisms of micronutrient metabolism and the impacts on health and diseases using epidemiological study and molecular biology. His research interests include iron metabolism and related disorders; the mechanism of micronutrient metabolism; and the impact of micronutrients on metabolic diseases.

nutrients

Editorial

Metabolic Features and Nutritional Interventions in Chronic Diseases

Yongting Luo, Peng An and Junjie Luo *

Department of Nutrition and Health, China Agricultural University, Beijing 100193, China;
luo.yongting@cau.edu.cn (Y.L.); an-peng@cau.edu.cn (P.A.)
* Correspondence: luojj@cau.edu.cn

Metabolic dysfunction is closely linked to the pathogenesis and progression of various chronic diseases [1], including aging, cancer, and disorders of the cardiovascular system, liver, skin, and gut. Nutritional interventions, utilizing bioactive compounds or tailored dietary regimens, have emerged as effective strategies to modulate metabolic dysfunctions [2], thereby mitigating disease progression and reducing incidence rates. This Special Issue of *Nutrients*, entitled *"Metabolic Features and Nutritional Interventions in Chronic Diseases"*, serves as an interdisciplinary platform to compile research on metabolic characterization in chronic diseases and the development of novel nutritional interventions aimed at improving disease outcomes through metabolic regulation.

This Special Issue comprises ten papers, including seven research articles, one clinical trial, one secondary analysis of a clinical trial, and one retrospective study. The topics covered include the following: the potential association of serum vitamin B6 levels with preoperative non-small-cell lung cancer (NSCLC) upstaging (one paper); a clinical trial on preoperative multistrain probiotic supplementation on bariatric treatment outcomes (one paper); the therapeutic effect of Epigallocatechin-3-gallate (EGCG), a tea-derived antioxidant, on DSS-induced colitis and its underlying metabolic mechanisms (one paper); exploring the potential of a naturally occurring metabolite, 3-hydroxybutyrate (3HB), as an anti-aging intervention in two aging models (one paper); the experimental evaluation of caprylic acid and eicosapentaenoic acid on lipids and inflammatory levels, as well as their underlying mechanisms (one paper); the identification of a low-zinc diet as a potential nutritional intervention approach for the prevention of thoracic aortic dissection (TAD) through the modulation of aortic inflammation (one paper); exploring celastrol-enriched peanuts in reducing atherosclerosis and obesity (one paper); the potential beneficial effect of probiotics in reducing cardiovascular risk and depression (one paper); and nutritional interventions for non-alcoholic fatty liver disease (NAFLD) using either pea albumin or hawthorn ethanol extract (two papers).

NAFLD is a major liver disease worldwide, with a global adult prevalence of nearly 30% [3]. It is characterized by excessive lipid deposition in hepatocytes and can progress from simple fat accumulation to steatohepatitis, fibrosis, cirrhosis, and even hepatocellular carcinoma [4]. Multiple factors contribute to the pathogenesis of NAFLD [5], such as excessive dietary fat intake, abnormal hepatic lipid metabolism, and imbalanced gut microbiota. For this reason, identifying potential nutritional interventions that regulate the altered lipid metabolism in the liver is crucial for the prevention and management of NAFLD. In this Special Issue, Shucheng Zhang et al. reported that the oral administration of pea albumin (PA), the major protein extracted from pea (*Pisum sativum* L.) seeds, effectively ameliorated high-fat-diet-induced NAFLD in mice (Contribution 1). The intervention with PA lowered

 https://doi.org/10.3390/nu17111826

serum cholesterols, reduced hepatic steatosis and lipid accumulation, with concomitant improved insulin resistance, and reduced hepatic oxidative stress and inflammatory responses. In a second study on NAFLD within this Special Issue, Tianyu Wang et al. demonstrated that hawthorn ethanol extract (HEE) could effectively diminish hepatic lipid accumulation through facilitating triglyceride breakdown and suppressing fatty acid synthesis while also reducing blood lipids and liver inflammation (Contribution 2). The two studies highlight PA and HEE as promising dietary supplements for NAFLD management.

Besides NAFLD, metabolism dysfunction is also observed in many cardiovascular diseases [6], including atherosclerosis and aortic dissection. Alteration in lipid metabolism results in hyperlipidemia, an important contributor to atherosclerosis. Atherosclerosis has been considered a non-resolving autoinflammatory disease of the arterial walls [7]. As the main contributor of atherosclerotic cardiovascular disease (ASCVD), such as myocardial infarction and stroke, atherosclerosis is one of the leading causes of death worldwide [8]. Nutritional intervention has been considered a promising strategy for atherosclerosis [9]. In this Special Issue, Jiaxin Shi et al. innovatively developed a novel peanut cultivar enriched with celastrol (cel-peanut), a pentacyclic triterpenoid active component, and evaluated the anti-atherosclerosis effects (Contribution 3). They demonstrated that celastrol-enriched peanuts effectively normalized blood lipid profile, alleviated aortic plaque burden, reduced body weight, and promoted intestinal health in high-fat-diet-induced ApoE$^{-/-}$ mice. These beneficial effects of celastrol-enriched peanuts might result from the anti-inflammatory, antioxidant, and immunomodulatory properties of celastrol. In parallel with this study, another study in this Special Issue evaluated the effect of fatty acids on the development of atherosclerosis. Xinsheng Zhang et al. investigated the effects of caprylic acid (C8:0) and eicosapentaenoic acid (EPA) on lipids, inflammatory levels, and the JAK2/STAT3 pathway in ABCA1-deficient mice and macrophages (Contribution 4). They observed that EPA had better effects than C8:0 on inhibiting inflammation and improving blood lipids in the absence of ABCA1, and upregulation of the ABCA1 expression pathway by functional nutrients may provide potential targets for the prevention and treatment of atherosclerosis. On the other hand, by performing a secondary analysis of a randomized clinical trial, Oliwia Gawlik-Kotelnicka et al. demonstrated that probiotics used along with a healthy diet may provide additional benefits by reducing cardiovascular risk (Contribution 5). However, Marta Potrykus et al. reported a randomized, double-blind, placebo-controlled clinical trial, where they observed that preoperative multistrain probiotic supplementation showed no apparent effect on body weight changes or cardiometabolic risk factors in bariatrics (a surgical treatment of obesity) (Contribution 6). Therefore, although microbiota plays a crucial role in the development of and therapeutic options in obesity, the role of probiotic supplementation as a nutritional intervention in bariatric surgery requires further investigation. In addition to atherosclerosis, nutritional intervention also shows promise in the management of aortic dissection, a life-threatening condition caused by a tear in the intimal layer of the aortic wall. By employing a classical-aminopropionitrile monofumarate (BAPN)-induced aortic dissection model in mice, Lin Zhu et al. demonstrated that low zinc could improve aortic dissection and rupture and reduce mortality through attenuating aortic inflammation and suppressing the phenotype switch of aortic smooth muscle cells from contractile to synthetic types (Contribution 7). This study suggested that low zinc may serve as a potential nutritional intervention approach for the prevention of aortic dissection.

Nutritional intervention also shows promise in fighting other diseases or disease complications, such as cancer [10], tissue inflammation [11], and aging [12]. In this Special Issue, Lu Liu et al. evaluated a possible relationship between vitamin B levels and the development and progression of lung cancer (Contribution 8). Their retrospective study established a positive association of serum vitamin B6 levels with the intrapulmonary lymph node and/or local pleural metastases of non-small-cell lung cancer, and this association was stronger in females, current smokers, current drinkers, and those with a family history of cancer. Furthermore, Junzhou Chen et al. found that supplementation with a tea-derived antioxidant called EGCG could effectively alleviate DSS-induced colitis in mice by inhibiting ferroptosis and reducing oxidative damage in colonic epithelial cells (Contribution 9). Finally, Yongpan An et al. found that the supplementation of 3-hydroxybutyrate (3HB), an endogenous metabolite with established safety, effectively delayed cellular senescence and extended lifespan in both yeast and mice via metabolic reprogramming (Contribution 10). This study highlights 3HB as a potential anti-aging nutritional intervention.

In summary, chronic diseases exhibit distinct metabolic dysfunctions, and nutritional interventions—whether through bioactive nutrients or dietary modifications—offer promising avenues for disease management. The studies in this Special Issue underscore the therapeutic potential of nutritional strategies in modulating metabolic pathways, oxidative stress, and immune responses. These findings reinforce the paradigm of "food as medicine" and highlight the need for the further clinical exploration of these nutritional interventions.

Author Contributions: Y.L., P.A. and J.L. wrote and revised the manuscript. All authors have read and agreed to the published version of the manuscript.

Funding: This work was supported by the National Key R&D Program of China (2024YFF1105604), the National Natural Science Foundation of China (82470442, 82170429), the State Key Laboratory of Cardiovascular Disease, Fuwai Hospital, Chinese Academy of Medical Sciences (2024GZkf-05), the Pinduoduo-China Agricultural University Research Fund (PC2023B01014), the 111 project from the Education Ministry of China (B18053), and the 2115 Talent Development Program of China Agricultural University.

Conflicts of Interest: The authors declare no conflicts of interest.

List of Contributions:

1. Zhang, S.; Cui, Z.; Zhang, H.; Wang, P.; Wang, F.; Zhang, J. Pea Albumin Extracted from Pea (*Pisum sativum* L.) Seeds Ameliorates High-Fat-Diet-Induced Non-Alcoholic Fatty Liver Disease by Regulating Lipogenesis and Lipolysis Pathways. *Nutrients* **2024**, *16*, 2232. https://doi.org/10.3390/nu16142232.
2. Wang, T.; Wang, D.; Ding, Y.; Xu, H.; Sun, Y.; Hou, J.; Zhang, Y. Targeting Non-Alcoholic Fatty Liver Disease with Hawthorn Ethanol Extract (HEE): A Comprehensive Examination of Hepatic Lipid Reduction and Gut Microbiota Modulation. *Nutrients* **2024**, *16*, 1335. https://doi.org/10.3390/nu16091335.
3. Shi, J.; Cheng, Y.; Wang, C.; Liu, M.; Qu, M.; Zhou, S.; Chen, L.; Li, X.; Luo, J.; Luo, Y.; et al. Effects of Celastrol-Enriched Peanuts on Metabolic Health and the Development of Atherosclerosis. *Nutrients* **2025**, *17*, 1418. https://doi.org/10.3390/nu17091418.
4. Zhang, X.; Zhang, P.; Liu, Y.; Liu, Z.; Xu, Q.; Zhang, Y.; Liu, L.; Yang, X.; Li, L.; Xue, C. Effects of Caprylic Acid and Eicosapentaenoic Acid on Lipids, Inflammatory Levels, and the JAK2/STAT3 Pathway in ABCA1-Deficient Mice and ABCA1 Knock-Down RAW264.7 Cells. *Nutrients* **2023**, *15*, 1296. https://doi.org/10.3390/nu15051296.
5. Gawlik-Kotelnicka, O.; Rogalski, J.; Czarnecka-Chrebelska, K.H.; Burzyński, J.; Jakubowska, P.; Skowrońska, A.; Strzelecki, D. The Interplay Between Depression, Probiotics, Diet, Immunometabolic Health, the Gut, and the Liver—A Secondary Analysis of the Pro-Demet Randomized Clinical Trial. *Nutrients* **2024**, *16*, 4024. https://doi.org/10.3390/nu16234024.
6. Potrykus, M.; Czaja-Stolc, S.; Stankiewicz, M.; Szymański, M.; Łoniewski, I.; Kaska, Ł.; Proczko-Stepaniak, M. Preoperative Multistrain Probiotic Supplementation Does Not Affect Body Weight Changes or Cardiometabolic Risk Factors in Bariatrics: Randomized, Double-Blind, Placebo-Controlled Clinical Trial. *Nutrients* **2024**, *16*, 2055. https://doi.org/10.3390/nu16132055.

7. Zhu, L.; An, P.; Zhao, W.; Xia, Y.; Qi, J.; Luo, J.; Luo, Y. Low Zinc Alleviates the Progression of Thoracic Aortic Dissection by Inhibiting Inflammation. *Nutrients* **2023**, *15*, 1640. https://doi.org/10.3390/nu15071640.
8. Liu, L.; Yu, H.; Bai, J.; Xu, Q.; Zhang, Y.; Zhang, X.; Yu, Z.; Liu, Y. Positive Association of Serum Vitamin B6 Levels with Intrapulmonary Lymph Node and/or Localized Pleural Metastases in Non-Small Cell Lung Cancer: A Retrospective Study. *Nutrients* **2023**, *15*, 2340. https://doi.org/10.3390/nu15102340.
9. Chen, J.; Yin, C.; Zhang, Y.; Lai, X.; Liu, C.; Luo, Y.; Luo, J.; He, J.; Yu, B.; Wang, Q.; et al. EGCG Alleviates DSS-Induced Colitis by Inhibiting Ferroptosis Through the Activation of the Nrf2-GPX4 Pathway and Enhancing Iron Metabolism. *Nutrients* **2025**, *17*, 547. https://doi.org/10.3390/nu17030547.
10. An, Y.; Wang, Q.; Qiao, P.; Liu, J.; Ma, A.; Chen, Y.; Yang, D.; Ying, Y.; Li, N.; Lu, F.; et al. Unveiling the Anti-Aging Potential of 3HB: Lifespan Extension and Cellular Senescence Delay. *Nutrients* **2025**, *17*, 1647. https://doi.org/10.3390/nu17101647.

References

1. Kivimäki, M.; Bartolomucci, A.; Kawachi, I. The multiple roles of life stress in metabolic disorders. *Nat. Rev. Endocrinol.* **2022**, *19*, 10–27. [CrossRef] [PubMed]
2. Han, T.; Wei, W.; Jiang, W.; Geng, Y.; Liu, Z.; Yang, R.; Jin, C.; Lei, Y.; Sun, X.; Xu, J.; et al. The Future Landscape and Framework of Precision Nutrition. *Engineering* **2024**, *42*, 15–25. [CrossRef]
3. Quek, J.; Chan, K.E.; Wong, Z.Y.; Tan, C.; Tan, B.; Lim, W.H.; Tan, D.J.H.; Tang, A.S.P.; Tay, P.; Xiao, J.; et al. Global prevalence of non-alcoholic fatty liver disease and non-alcoholic steatohepatitis in the overweight and obese population: A systematic review and meta-analysis. *Lancet Gastroenterol. Hepatol.* **2023**, *8*, 20–30. [CrossRef] [PubMed]
4. Leung, P.B.; Davis, A.M.; Kumar, S. Diagnosis and Management of Nonalcoholic Fatty Liver Disease. *JAMA* **2023**, *330*, 1687. [CrossRef] [PubMed]
5. Powell, E.E.; Wong, V.W.-S.; Rinella, M. Non-alcoholic fatty liver disease. *Lancet* **2021**, *397*, 2212–2224. [CrossRef] [PubMed]
6. Karlstaedt, A.; Moslehi, J.; de Boer, R.A. Cardio-onco-metabolism: Metabolic remodelling in cardiovascular disease and cancer. *Nat. Rev. Cardiol.* **2022**, *19*, 414–425. [CrossRef] [PubMed]
7. Fredman, G.; MacNamara, K.C. Atherosclerosis is a major human killer and non-resolving inflammation is a prime suspect. *Cardiovasc. Res.* **2021**, *117*, 2563–2574. [CrossRef] [PubMed]
8. Deng, X.; Wang, J.; Yu, S.; Tan, S.; Yu, T.; Xu, Q.; Chen, N.; Zhang, S.; Zhang, M.R.; Hu, K.; et al. Advances in the treatment of atherosclerosis with ligand-modified nanocarriers. *Exploration* **2023**, *4*. [CrossRef] [PubMed]
9. Vesnina, A.; Prosekov, A.; Atuchin, V.; Minina, V.; Ponasenko, A. Tackling Atherosclerosis via Selected Nutrition. *Int. J. Mol. Sci.* **2022**, *23*, 8233. [CrossRef] [PubMed]
10. Mercier, B.D.; Tizpa, E.; Philip, E.J.; Feng, Q.; Huang, Z.; Thomas, R.M.; Pal, S.K.; Dorff, T.B.; Li, Y.R. Dietary Interventions in Cancer Treatment and Response: A Comprehensive Review. *Cancers* **2022**, *14*, 5149. [CrossRef] [PubMed]
11. Sears, B.; Saha, A.K. Dietary Control of Inflammation and Resolution. *Front. Nutr.* **2021**, *8*, 709435. [CrossRef] [PubMed]
12. Shea, M.K.; Strath, L.; Kim, M.; Đoàn, L.N.; Booth, S.L.; Brinkley, T.E.; Kritchevsky, S.B. Perspective: Promoting Healthy Aging through Nutrition: A Research Centers Collaborative Network Workshop Report. *Adv. Nutr.* **2024**, *15*, 100199. [CrossRef] [PubMed]

nutrients

Article

Pea Albumin Extracted from Pea (*Pisum sativum* L.) Seeds Ameliorates High-Fat-Diet-Induced Non-Alcoholic Fatty Liver Disease by Regulating Lipogenesis and Lipolysis Pathways

Shucheng Zhang [1,2], Zhengwu Cui [2], Hao Zhang [1,2], Pengjie Wang [1,*], Fuqing Wang [3] and Jian Zhang [2,*]

1 College of Food Science and Nutritional Engineering, China Agricultural University, Beijing 100083, China; zhangshucheng120@sina.com (S.Z.); zhanghaocau@cau.edu.cn (H.Z.)
2 Department of Nutrition and Health, China Agricultural University, Beijing 100193, China; 16653221635@163.com
3 Tibet Tianhong Science and Technology Co., Ltd., Lhasa 850000, China; fq7963@163.com
* Correspondence: wpj1019@cau.edu.cn (P.W.); tsnpzhj@163.com (J.Z.)

Abstract: Non-alcoholic fatty liver disease (NAFLD) is now recognized as the most prevalent liver disease globally. Pea albumin (PA) has demonstrated positive impacts on reducing obesity and improving glucose metabolism. In this research, a mouse model of NAFLD induced by a high-fat diet (HFD) was employed to examine the impact of PA on NAFLD and explore its potential mechanisms. The findings revealed that mice subjected to a HFD developed pronounced fatty liver alterations. The intervention with PA significantly lowered serum TC by 26.81%, TG by 43.55%, and LDL-C by 57.79%. It also elevated HDL-C levels by 1.2 fold and reduced serum ALT by 37.94% and AST by 31.21% in mice fed a HFD. These changes contributed to the reduction in hepatic steatosis and lipid accumulation. Additionally, PA improved insulin resistance and inhibited hepatic oxidative stress and inflammatory responses. Mechanistic studies revealed that PA alleviated lipid accumulation in HFD-induced NAFLD by activating the phosphorylation of AMPKα and ACC, inhibiting the expression of SREBF1 and FASN to reduce hepatic lipogenesis, and increasing the expression of ATGL, PPARα, and PPARγ to promote lipolysis and fatty acid oxidation. These results indicate that PA could serve as a dietary supplement for alleviating NAFLD, offering a theoretical foundation for the rational intake of PA in NAFLD intervention.

Keywords: non-alcoholic fatty liver disease; pea albumin; high-fat diet; hepatic steatosis; lipogenesis; lipolysis

1. Introduction

Non-alcoholic fatty liver disease (NAFLD) is defined by steatosis occurring in over 5% of hepatocytes in the absence of significant alcohol consumption or other chronic liver diseases, ultimately leading to excessive lipid deposition [1]. The health risks associated with NAFLD extend beyond simple steatosis; it can progress from simple fat accumulation to steatohepatitis, fibrosis, cirrhosis, and even hepatocellular carcinoma [2]. NAFLD is a major liver disease worldwide, comparable to obesity and diabetes, with an estimated global adult prevalence of approximately 29.62% [3]. However, the pathogenesis of NAFLD is not yet widely agreed upon, involving multiple factors such as excessive dietary fat intake, impaired insulin signaling, disrupted hepatic lipid metabolism, and increased oxidative stress or inflammatory responses in hepatocytes [4,5]. Among the many pathogenesis mechanisms, the "two-hit" hypothesis is currently the most widely accepted. According to this hypothesis, lipid accumulation in the liver, insulin resistance, and oxidative stress are the primary factors leading to NAFLD [4]. Long-term intake of high sugar and high fat, along with insulin resistance, act as the "first hit", causing lipid accumulation in the liver and the formation of NAFLD. This increases the susceptibility to the "second hit" (including oxidative stress and inflammation), leading to liver damage, which can result in more severe conditions such as non-alcoholic steatohepatitis (NASH) and even fibrosis [6]. Given the complex etiology of NAFLD, recommended interventions mainly include surgical, pharmacological, and lifestyle interventions. Surgical treatment can improve hepatic steatosis, but carries the risk of exacerbating liver fibrosis and the potential for postoperative relapse [7]. Currently, no specific drugs have been approved for the treatment of NAFLD. Although some medications can be used for patients with NAFLD and related conditions, their safety remains controversial. Pioglitazone is a widely studied drug for treating NAFLD, but it has side effects such as weight gain and other risks, including a potential increase in the incidence of bladder cancer and heart failure [8,9]. GLP-1 receptor agonists, such as liraglutide and semaglutide, have been shown to treat NAFLD; however, they can cause gastrointestinal side effects, including nausea and vomiting [10,11]. Despite the ongoing development of various therapeutic drugs and targets, lifestyle changes, including diet and exercise, continue to be the main interventions. Research has found that dietary intake of natural products can alleviate NAFLD with relatively high safety for humans.

Based on the characteristics of high efficacy and low toxicity, numerous studies have found that plant bioactive substances can intervene in NAFLD. Currently, the reported natural products that regulate hepatic lipid metabolism mainly include alkaloids, phenolic compounds, proteins, vitamins, and other bioactive substances. These substances primarily regulate lipid metabolism by suppressing hepatic lipid synthesis and enhancing lipid oxidation and decomposition, ultimately improving NAFLD. Betaine can reduce fatty acid synthesis by regulating SREBF1 and FASN and promote fatty acid oxidation by regulating PPARα and CPT-1, thereby reducing lipid accumulation in the liver [12]. Curcumin also affects hepatic lipid synthesis pathways by inhibiting the expression of SREBF1 and FASN, thus reducing hepatic fat synthesis [13]. β-Conglycinin can modulate hepatic lipid homeostasis by downregulating SREBF1 and upregulating PPARα protein expression [14]. Although there are many reports on the improvement of NAFLD by natural products, there are still numerous issues to be addressed regarding their actual efficacy and safety for consumption. These issues include adverse effects of berberine on the digestive system [15], the allergenicity of β-conglycinin [16], and the low efficacy of curcumin [17]. Therefore, continuously seeking safer and more effective natural bioactive substances is crucial for improving NAFLD.

Pea protein is a superior plant-based protein characterized by its balanced amino acid profile. Pea albumin (PA), which constitutes about 18–25% of pea protein, is abundant in sulfur-containing amino acids and other essential amino acids [17–20]. Research has found that PA is involved in lipid metabolism regulation. Liu et al. discovered that PA can regulate lipid metabolism in adipose tissue, alleviating obesity and related diseases [21]. Ruiz et al. demonstrated, through in vitro experiments, that PA hydrolysates significantly reduced lipid accumulation in 3T3-L1 cells [22]. Additionally, PA has been shown to inhibit colonic inflammation and modulate gut microbiota diversity. Miszkiewicz et al. found that PA possesses high free radical scavenging activity [23]. Dun et al. discovered that PA1F can regulate glucose metabolism in type 2 diabetic mice [24]. Therefore, PA might have the potential to alleviate hepatic lipid accumulation by regulating glucose and lipid metabolisms, oxidative stresses, and inflammatory responses associated with NAFLD development. Based on this analysis, we hypothesize that increasing the intake of PA in the diet could serve as an efficacious approach for the prevention and treatment of NAFLD. However, the effects and mechanisms of PA intervention in NAFLD are not yet clear.

In summary, we employed an HFD-induced NAFLD mouse model and administered oral PA during the induction period to evaluate the ameliorative effects of PA on hepatic steatosis in mice. The impacts of PA on NAFLD were assessed by analyzing changes in liver pathology, serum biochemical markers, and insulin resistance levels in the mice. Additionally, the expression of key proteins implicated in hepatic lipogenesis and lipolysis pathways was examined to explore the mechanisms by which PA influences the hepatic lipid metabolism. The findings from this study will contribute additional evidence to supporting the role of PA intervention in alleviating NAFLD.

2. Materials and Methods

2.1. Materials

Pea seed (*Pisum sativum* L.) was supplied by Yantai Shuangta Food Co., Ltd. (Yantai, China). Normal diet (ND, 10% energy from fat, D12450J) and high-fat diet (HFD, 60% energy from fat, D12492) products were obtained from SPF (Beijing, China) Biotechnology Co., Ltd. (Beijing, China). Triglyceride (TG, A110-1-1), total cholesterol (TC, A111-1-1), high-density lipoprotein cholesterol (HDL-C, A112-1-1), low-density lipoprotein cholesterol (LDL-C, A113-1-1), alanine aminotransferase (ALT, C009-2-1), aspartate aminotransferase (AST, C010-2-1), and superoxide dismutase (SOD, A001-3-2) assay kits were procured from Nanjing Jiancheng Bioengineering Institute (Nanjing, China). Malondialdehyde (MDA, S0131S) and glutathione peroxidase (GSH-Px, S0056) assay kits were purchased from Beyotime Biotech. Inc. (Nantong, China). The enzyme-linked immunosorbent assay (ELISA) kits for interleukin-1β (IL-1β, EK201B/3), interleukin-6 (IL-6, EK206/3), and tumor necrosis factor α (TNF-α, EK282/4) were purchased from Multisciences (Lianke) Biotech Co., Ltd. (Hangzhou, China). The ELISA kit for insulin (MM-0579M2) was obtained from Jiangsu Meimian Industrial Co., Ltd. (Yancheng, China). The primary rabbit antibodies against phospho-AMP-activated protein kinase alpha (*p*-AMPKα, AA393), AMPKα (AF1627), phospho-acetyl-CoA carboxylase (*p*-ACC, AA110), ACC(AF1867), sterol regulatory element binding transcription factor 1 (SREBF1, AF8055), fatty acid synthase (FASN, AG1915), peroxisome proliferator activated receptor-α (PPARα, AF7794), PPARγ (AF7797), and glyceraldehyde-3-phosphate dehydrogenase (GAPDH, AF1186) were obtained from Beyotime Biotech. Inc. (Nantong, China). The primary antibodies against adipose triglyceride lipase (ATGL, 55190-1-AP) was obtained from Proteintech Group, Inc. (Rosemont, IL, USA). The HRP-labeled goat anti-rabbit IgG(H + L) secondary antibody (A0208), ECL chemiluminescence kit (P0018FS) were purchased from Beyotime Biotech. Inc. (Nantong, China). The bicinchoninic acid (BCA) protein assay kit, Hematoxylin-eosin dye solution, and Oil Red O dye were procured from Beijing Solarbio Science & Technology Co., Ltd. (Beijing, China). All other chemicals and solvents were purchased from Sigma-Aldrich (St. Louis, MO, USA), unless otherwise described.

2.2. Preparation of Pea Albumin (PA)

The pea albumin (PA) was prepared following a previously described method, with minor adjustments [19]. In brief, ground pea seeds were treated to lipid extraction using hexane (1:3 *w*/*v*), and were subsequently air-dried. Next, the defatted meal was extracted (1:10 *w*/*v*) with 0.2 mol L^{-1} borate buffer (pH 8) containing 0.5 mol L^{-1} NaCl. The solution was centrifuged at 11,000× *g* for 30 min at 4 °C. The supernatant obtained was then adjusted to pH 4.5 using glacial acetic acid, stirred for 30 min at 4 °C, and subjected to centrifugation at 11,000× *g* for 30 min at 4 °C. The supernatant was dialyzed against distilled water and centrifuged at 11,000× *g* for 30 min at 4 °C. The supernatant was treated with 608 g L^{-1} $(NH_4)_2SO_4$, stirred for 2 h at 4 °C, and centrifuged at 11,000× *g* for 30 min at 4 °C. The coacervate was collected and fully dissolved in water. After dialyzing against distilled water, the dialyzed extract (i.e., PA) was lyophilized and stored at −20 °C for further analysis. PA was characterized using SDS-PAGE to monitor the electrophoretic pattern. Specifically, a 15% separating gel and a 5% stacking gel were used to isolate PA. The electrophoresis conditions were set at 80 V for 40 min, followed by 120 V for 1 h. Finally, the gel was placed in R-250 staining solution for staining. After destaining, photographs were taken using a gel imaging system (ChemiScope 6100, Qinxiang, Shanghai, China). The protein concentration of PA was determined using the Kjeldahl method. The amino acid concentration in PA was analyzed using an amino acid analyzer (Biochrom 30+, BioChrom Ltd., Cambridge, UK).

2.3. Experimental Design and Animal Treatment

Forty male four-week-old C57BL/6N mice were obtained from Beijing Vital River Laboratory Animal Technology Co., Ltd. (Beijing, China). The mice were kept under standard conditions of ambient temperature (24 ± 2 °C) and relative humidity (50 ± 5%) with a 12 h light/dark cycle. After a one-week acclimatization period, mice were randomly divided into five groups (n = 8 per group): (1) normal diet (ND) group, fed with a normal diet and supplied with normal saline; (2) high-fat diet (HFD) group, fed with a high-fat diet and supplied with normal saline; (3) low-dose PA (PA-L) group, fed with a high-fat diet and supplied with 0.375 g/kg bw PA; (4) middle-dose PA (PA-M) group, fed with a high-fat diet and supplied with 0.75 g/kg bw PA; and the (5) high-dose PA (PA-H) group, fed with a high-fat diet and supplied with 1.5 g/kg bw PA. A detailed schedule of PA administration throughout the experiment period is shown in Figure 1A. The body weight of each group was recorded weekly over an 8-week trial. At the end of the 8-week intervention, the mice were sacrificed after an overnight fast. Blood samples were collected in test tubes. The serum was obtained using centrifugation (1000× g, 15 min, 4 °C) and stored at −80 °C for further study. Liver and white adipose tissue (including epididymal fat and subcutaneous fat) were collected and weighted. Parts of the liver tissues were fixed in 4% paraformaldehyde, while the remaining parts were quickly frozen in liquid nitrogen and stored at −80 °C until further processing. The experimental protocols were approved by the Institutional Animal Care and Use Committee of China Agricultural University (Approval Code: AW72303202-5-3).

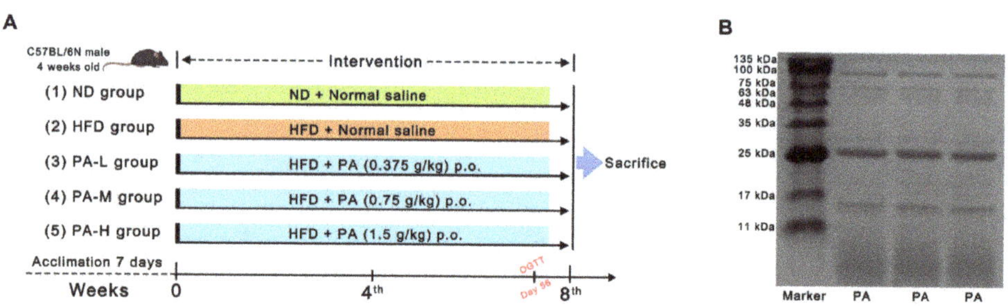

Figure 1. Experiment design and protein pattern of PA. (**A**) Detailed program of PA oral administration throughout the experiment period. (**B**) SDS-PAGE visualization for PA.

2.4. Body Composition Measures

In the 8th week, the body fat composition of mice was measured using a nuclear magnetic resonance (NMR) analyzer (MesoQMR23-060H-I, NIUMAG, Suzhou, China). First, the device magnet temperature was stabilized to 32 °C, followed by instrument calibration. A standard oil sample was placed into the mouse restraint tube and positioned at the designated spot in the probe coil for self-testing. The peak signal coefficient between 0.99 and 1.01 indicated that the instrument was functioning normally. The NMR body composition analysis system was used to measure the fat mass of the mice, and the body fat content was expressed as fat mass/body weight × 100% [25,26]. Additionally, coronal images of the mice were obtained using the NMR imaging system. Initial parameter adjustments were performed, including automatic tuning of the center frequency, electronic shimming, and locating the soft pulse amplitude. After pre-scanning, image parameters and sequence parameters were set to complete the sampling of mice coronal images.

2.5. Oral Glucose Tolerance Test (OGTT) and Indexes of Insulin Resistance

An oral glucose tolerance test (OGTT) was conducted in the 7th week of the experimental timeline [21]. Following a 12 h fast, mice were given a glucose solution orally at a dosage of 2 g/kg body weight. Blood samples were drawn from the mice's tail veins, and the glucose concentrations were determined at 0, 30, 60, 90, and 120 min after oral administration using the Yuwell 580 glucose meter (Yuwell Group, Danyang, China). After the test, the area under curve (AUC) for the blood glucose versus the time plot for each treatment group was calculated using integration. Following a 12 h fast at the conclusion of the 8th week, blood samples were taken from the tail vein to assess fasting blood glucose (FBG) concentration. Fasting insulin (FINS) was measured using an ELISA kit in accordance with the manufacturer's guidelines. Insulin resistance was assessed using the Homeostasis Model Assessment-Insulin Resistance (HOMA-IR), which was calculated as HOMA-IR = FBG × FINS/22.5.

2.6. Histopathological Analysis

For the histological analyses, liver tissues were fixed in 4% paraformaldehyde for 24 h and were subsequently embedded in paraffin. Finally, liver tissues were then sectioned into 4 μm thick slices and stained using H&E [27]. The structure of liver tissue was observed under the Leica DM6B microscope (Leica, Wetzlar, Germany). The NAFLD activity score (NAS) was calculated by summing the individual scores for steatosis (0–3), hepatocellular ballooning (0–2), and lobular inflammation (0–3). In addition, liver tissues were embedded in an optimal cutting temperature (OCT) compound at −80 °C and were subsequently stained with Oil Red O. Stained liver tissue was observed with a Leica DM6B microscope (Leica, Wetzlar, Germany), and quantitative analysis was performed using ImageJ software (vision 1.8.0).

2.7. Serum and Hepatic Biochemical Analysis

Blood was collected from eyeballs under terminal anesthesia, and serum was collected by centrifuging at 1000× *g* at 4 °C for 15 min. The serum concentrations of TG, TC, HDL-C, and LDL-C, as well as the activities of ALT, and AST were analyzed according to the assay kits' manufacturer's instructions. Subsequently, the levels of TG and TC in the liver were measured with commercially available kits.

2.8. Liver Oxidative Stress and Inflammation Analysis

The concentrations of MDA, SOD, and GSH-Px in liver tissues were assayed to evaluate antioxidant capacity using commercially available kits. Subsequently, the protein levels of IL-1β, IL-6, and TNF-α in liver tissue were detected using an ELISA kit by following the manufacturer's instructions.

2.9. Immunoblotting Analysis

Liver tissues were lysed using a RIPA buffer and were centrifuged to obtain the supernatant. The total protein concentrations were measured using a BCA protein assay kit. Protein samples with equivalent amounts were separated on 10% SDS-PAGE gels and were then transferred to PVDF membranes. The membranes were blocked using 5% BSA, followed by incubation with individual primary antibodies (*p*-AMPKα, AMPKα, *p*-ACC, ACC, SREBF1, FASN, PPARα, PPARγ, and ATGL) overnight at 4 °C. After washing, the membranes were then incubated with secondary antibodies at room temperature for 1 h. Following incubation, the PVDF membranes were washed. Finally, protein bands were visualized using an ECL kit. The protein expressions were quantified by using ImageJ vision 1.8.0 software with GAPDH for normalization.

2.10. Statistical Analysis

The analysis was conducted using the SPSS 23.0 software. Results were presented as mean ± SEM. The normality of the data were assessed using the Shapiro–Wilk test. Regarding the data with a normal distribution, statistical disparities between groups were analyzed with one-way analysis of variance (ANOVA) followed by an LSD post hoc test. For non-normally distributed data, the Kruskal–Wallis test was employed. $p < 0.05$ was considered to be statistically significant. Figures were created using GraphPad Prism 9.2.0.

3. Results

3.1. Characterization of Pea Albumin (PA)

The protein content of the PA prepared in this study was measured to be 92.65% using the Kjeldahl method. To determine the protein composition of PA, a SDS-PAGE analysis was conducted. The electrophoresis results are shown in Figure 1B, where four major bands can be clearly observed at 6, 16, 24, and 100 kDa. Among these, the protein bands with molecular weights of 6 kDa and 24 kDa accounted for the largest proportion. The four bands correspond to lipoxygenase (100 kDa), PA2 (24 kDa), trypsin inhibitor (16 kDa), and PA1 (6 kDa). Additionally, the amino acid composition of PA was analyzed, as presented in Table 1. The essential amino acids account for approximately 16.71%, glycine accounts for about 25.20%, and branched-chain amino acids (Leu, Val, Ile) account for about 7.34%.

Table 1. Protein content and amino acid composition of PA.

Items	Amount
Protein (%)	92.65 ± 0.66
Essential amino acids (%)	
Lysine	3.92 ± 0.01^{h}
Leucine	3.81 ± 0.02^{i}
Threonine	2.52 ± 0.01^{j}
Valine	2.26 ± 0.03^{k}
Phenylalanine	1.91 ± 0.01^{l}
Isoleucine	1.27 ± 0.02^{m}
Tryptophan	0.73 ± 0.02^{o}
Methionine	0.29 ± 0.02^{p}
Nonessential amino acids (%)	
Glycine	25.20 ± 0.05^{a}
Proline	15.89 ± 0.02^{b}
Alanine	11.14 ± 0.04^{c}
Glutamate	10.20 ± 0.02^{d}
Arginine	8.47 ± 0.01^{e}
Aspartate	6.09 ± 0.03^{f}
Serine	4.31 ± 0.01^{g}
Tyrosine	0.99 ± 0.01^{n}
Histidine	0.99 ± 0.04^{n}

Values are expressed as mean ± SD ($n = 3$). Different superscript letters indicate significant differences ($p < 0.05$) among the amino acid content.

3.2. PA Reduced HFD-Induced Weight Gain and Fat Accumulation in Mice

HFD induction is a common method for establishing a mouse model of NAFLD. Given the frequent association between obesity and NAFLD in patients, we evaluated the body weight, food intake, and body fat content of the mice. During the 8-week experiment period, the mice were weighed weekly. The results indicate that, in comparison to the ND group, the HFD group exhibited a significant increase in body weight (Figure 2A, $p < 0.05$). By the eighth week, the body weight of the HFD group had risen by 17.5% compared to the ND group. Treatment with PA significantly inhibited the HFD-induced weight gain in a dose-dependent manner ($p < 0.05$). In terms of food intake, the mice fed a ND had significantly higher intake compared to those fed a HFD (Figure 2B, $p < 0.05$). Additionally, there was no difference in food intake between the HFD group and those treated with PA (Figure 2B, $p > 0.05$). However, no significant difference in energy intake was observed among all the groups (Figure 2C, $p > 0.05$). Through the appearance of the mice (Figure 2D) and MRI images (Figure 2E), it was evident that the HFD increased body fat in the mice, while the PA treatment group showed less fat accumulation. The body composition assessment indicated that feeding with a HFD significantly elevated the percentage of body fat mass in mice (Figure 2F, $p < 0.05$). In contrast, different doses of PA significantly reduced the percentage of body fat mass in a dose-dependent manner ($p < 0.05$). The relative weights of subcutaneous fat and epididymal fat can serve as references for the body fat ratio [28]. The subcutaneous fat and epididymal fat indices of the HFD group were significantly higher compared to the ND group (Figure 2G,H, $p < 0.05$). Nevertheless, PA treatment notably decreased the subcutaneous fat and epididymal fat index ($p < 0.05$) in a dose-dependent manner. The results indicated that PA intervention can reduce HFD-induced weight gain by inhibiting body fat accumulation.

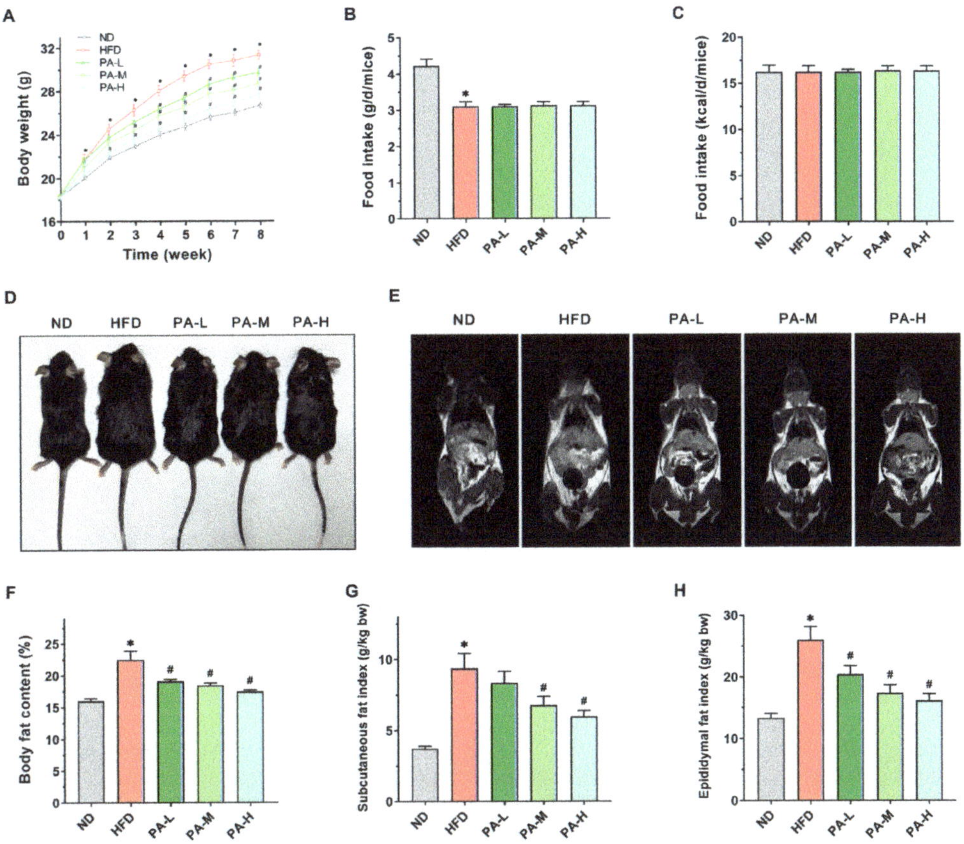

Figure 2. Effects of PA on body weight and fat accumulation in HFD-induced mice. (**A**) Body weight changes from week 0 to week 8. (**B**) Daily food intake per mouse in grams. (**C**) Daily energy intake per mouse. (**D**) Representative photos of the mice after 8 weeks. (**E**) Representative coronal sections of MRI studies. (**F**) Body fat percentage in mice. (**G**) Subcutaneous fat mass index. (**H**) Epididymal fat mass index. Results are expressed as mean ± SEM. $n = 8$ per group. * $p < 0.05$, HFD vs. ND; # $p < 0.05$, HFD vs. PA-L, PA-M, or PA-H.

3.3. PA Ameliorated Serum Lipid Profiles of HFD-Induced Mice

Disturbances in the lipid metabolism may result in lipid accumulation within the liver, promoting the progression of NAFLD [29]. To investigate the effects of PA on lipid metabolism in HFD-induced mice, we evaluated serum levels of TG, TC, HDL-C, and LDL-C, as well as the activities of AST and ALT. In the HFD group, serum TG levels were 2.26-fold higher compared to the ND group (Figure 3A), while serum TC levels showed a 1.45-fold increase relative to the ND group (Figure 3B). Additionally, serum LDL-C levels were 4.04 times higher in the HFD group than in the ND group (Figure 3D). However, PA intervention significantly reduced the serum levels of TG TC, and LDL-C in a concentration-dependent manner ($p < 0.05$). In the HFD group, serum HDL-C levels exhibited a significant reduction, decreasing by 18.33% compared to the ND group (Figure 3C, $p < 0.05$). After intervention with different doses of PA, the serum HDL-C levels increased by 7.41%, 10.85%, and 20.69% compared to the HFD group, respectively, although these changes were not statistically significant ($p > 0.05$). AST and ALT are typically used as biomarkers reflecting liver injury in NAFLD [30]. The serum ALT and AST activities in the HFD group were significantly elevated compared to those in the ND group (Figure 3E,F, $p < 0.05$). When orally administrated with PA, the serum ALT and AST activities reduced in a dose-dependent manner. The above data indicate that PA could effectively improve lipid metabolism abnormalities and liver injury induced by HFD, thereby alleviating the development of NAFLD.

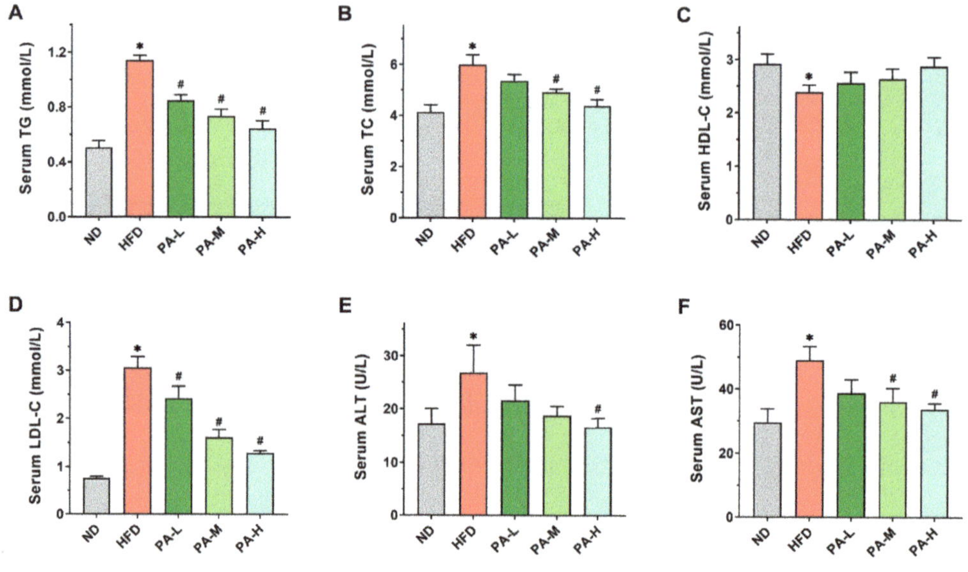

Figure 3. Effects of PA on serum lipid profiles in HFD-induced mice. (**A–D**) Serum TG, TC, HDL-C, and LDL-C levels. (**E**,**F**) Serum ALT and AST activities. Results are expressed as mean ± SEM. $n = 8$ per group. * $p < 0.05$, HFD vs. ND; # $p < 0.05$, HFD vs. PA-L, PA-M, or PA-H.

3.4. PA Attenuated Hepatic Steatosis of HFD-Induced NAFLD Mice

To assess the alleviating effects of PA on hepatic steatosis in NAFLD, we employed a HFD-induced NAFLD mice model. Liver weight, liver morphology, hepatic lipid profile, and liver tissue H&E and Oil Red O-stained sections were evaluated. As shown in Figure 4A, the liver index in the HFD group exhibited a significant 8.48% increase compared to the ND group ($p < 0.05$). However, PA intervention reduced the liver index, with the PA-M and PA-H groups showing significant reductions of 8.16% and 7.43%, respectively, compared to the HFD group ($p < 0.05$). Meanwhile, upon observing the liver morphology (Figure 4B), the livers of the ND group were reddish-brown with thin and smooth edges. In contrast, the livers of the HFD group mice appeared darker, with thickened and blunt edges, and were noticeably larger compared to the ND group. Following PA intervention, the liver color of the mice gradually returned from dark to a bright reddish-brown with increasing intervention doses, and the blunt edges diminished. Liver tissue lipid analysis showed that the TG and TC levels in the HFD group were significantly elevated compared to the ND group, increasing by 4.05 times and 2.79 times, respectively (Figure 4C,D, $p < 0.05$). PA intervention significantly reduced the liver levels of TG and TC in a concentration-dependent manner. These data indicate that PA could improve the hepatic lipid profile. Histopathological analysis of H&E stained liver sections showed that liver tissue structure in the ND group was normal, with no lesions (Figure 4G). In contrast, the HFD group exhibited steatosis, characterized by vacuolar degeneration, ballooning degeneration, and inflammatory infiltration. PA intervention effectively reduced the degree of hepatic steatosis, decreasing fat droplet accumulation, vacuolar degeneration, and inflammatory cell infiltration. Furthermore, high-dose PA intervention was the most effective in inhibiting hepatic steatosis. In the meantime, the NAS was significantly higher in the HFD group compared to the ND group (Figure 4E, $p < 0.05$). PA intervention resulted in a significant reduction in the NAS compared to the HFD group ($p < 0.05$). To further characterize hepatic steatosis, liver tissue was stained with Oil Red O. The results were similar to those observed with H&E staining. Significant lipid accumulation was observed in the liver of the HFD group, which markedly decreased with increasing doses of PA intervention (Figure 4H). Quantitative analysis of the Oil Red O-stained area in liver tissue indicated that the lipid droplet area in the HFD group was approximately 2.81 times larger than that in the ND group (Figure 4F, $p < 0.05$). After PA intervention, the lipid droplet area significantly decreased, reducing by approximately 11.73%, 44.43%, and 59.17% compared to the HFD group. In summary, the results indicated that PA intervention can significantly alleviate hepatic steatosis in NAFLD mice.

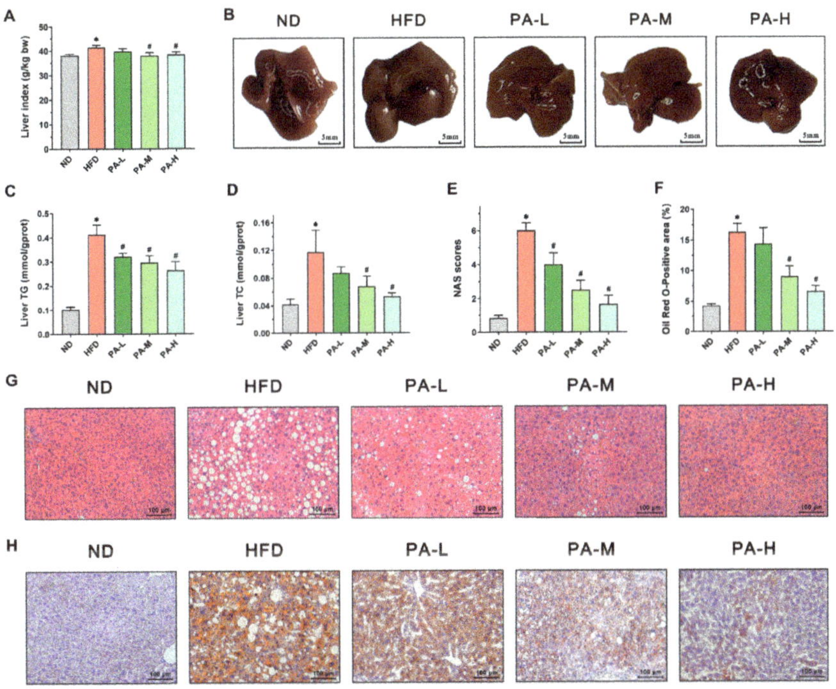

Figure 4. Effects of PA on hepatic steatosis in HFD-induced NAFLD mice. (**A**) Liver index. (**B**) Representative photos of livers. (**C**,**D**) Liver TG and TC levels. (**E**) NAFLD activity score of the liver. (**F**) Oil Red O-positive area of the liver. (**G**) Representative H&E stains of a liver section (Scale bar = 100 μm). (**H**) Representative Oil Red O stains of a liver section (Scale bar = 100 μm). Results are expressed as mean ± SEM. $n = 8$ per group. * $p < 0.05$, HFD vs. ND; $^{\#}$ $p < 0.05$, HFD vs. PA-L, PA-M, or PA-H.

3.5. PA Inhibits Hepatic Lipid Accumulation by Modulating Lipid Synthesis and Degradation Pathways

To further assess the mechanisms by which PA alleviates NAFLD, we measured the expression of lipid metabolism-related proteins in the liver using immunoblotting. Firstly, the expression of AMPKα, SREBF1, ACC, and FASN, which are related to lipogenesis, has been evaluated. The findings indicated that PA treatment markedly increased the phosphorylation levels of AMPKα and ACC in a manner dependent on the dosage (Figure 5B,D, $p < 0.05$). Furthermore, PA was found to decrease the elevated expression of SREBF1 and FASN proteins in the livers of NAFLD mice induced with a HFD (Figure 5C,E, $p < 0.05$). In addition, we examined the effects of PA on the expression levels of lipolysis-related proteins such as ATGL, PPARα, and PPARγ. The intervention of PA dose-dependently prevented the decrease in ATGL, PPARα, and PPARγ protein expression induced with HFD (Figure 5G–I, $p < 0.05$). These data demonstrate that PA can alleviate NAFLD by inhibiting HFD-induced lipid synthesis and promoting lipid degradation.

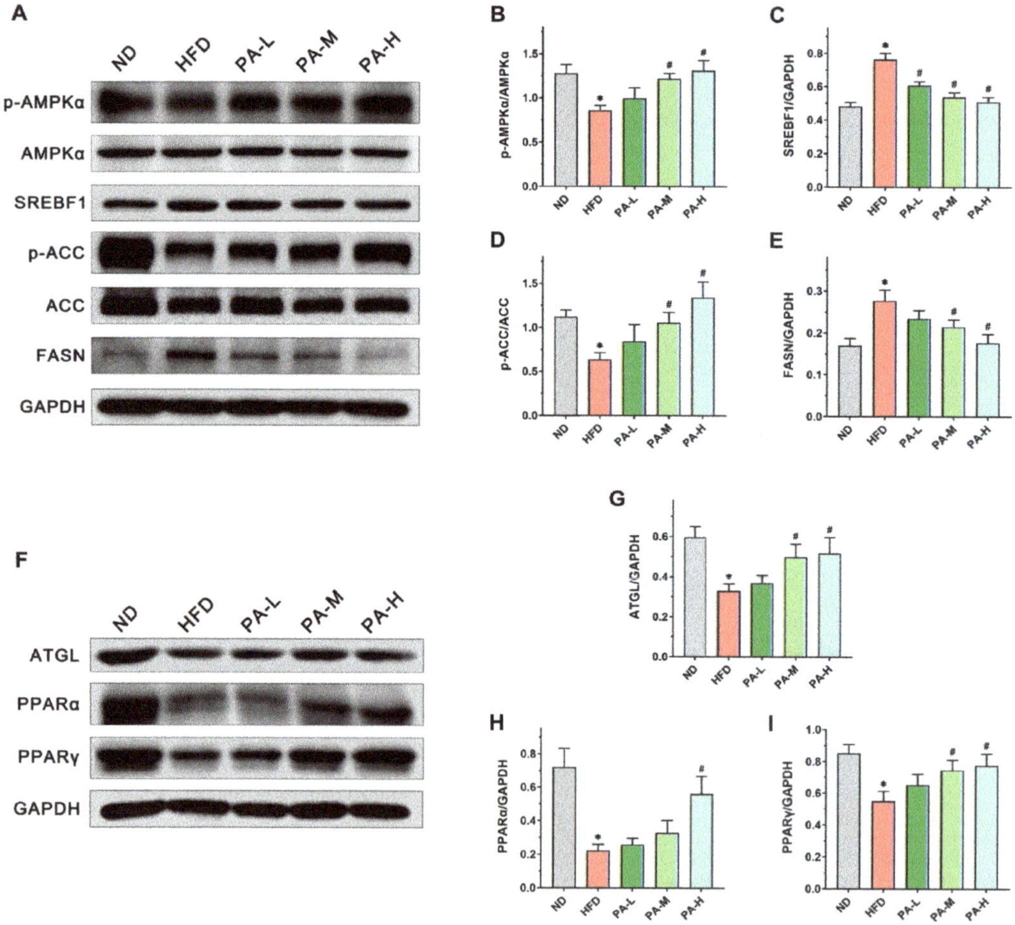

Figure 5. Effects of PA on the expression of lipid metabolism-related proteins in the liver of HFD-induced NAFLD mice. (**A**) Representative Western blots of markers for lipogenesis in the liver. (**B–E**) Quantification of protein expression of *p*-AMPKα/AMPKα, SREBF1, *p*-ACC/ACC, and FASN. (**F**) Representative Western blots of markers for lipolysis in the liver. (**G–I**) Quantification of protein expression of ATGL, PPARα, and PPARγ. Results are expressed as mean ± SEM. $n = 6$ per group. * $p < 0.05$, HFD vs. ND; # $p < 0.05$, HFD vs. PA-L, PA-M or PA-H.

3.6. PA Ameliorated Elevated Blood Glucose and Insulin Resistance of HFD-Induced Mice

Insulin resistance constitutes a significant pathogenic mechanism in NAFLD [31], with OGTT and HOMA-IR serving as crucial indicators for its assessment [32]. Figure 6A illustrates that mice in the HFD group consistently showed markedly higher serum glucose levels across all time points. In contrast, mice receiving the PA intervention showed enhanced glucose tolerance at all time points during OGTT. The AUC value of the OGTT in the HFD group was approximately 1.36 times that of the ND group, while the high-dose PA intervention significantly reduced the AUC value by approximately 19.71% compared to the HFD group (Figure 6B, $p < 0.05$). These findings demonstrated that the PA intervention markedly enhanced glucose tolerance in mice induced with HFD. Additionally, fasting blood glucose and serum insulin concentrations were notably elevated in the HFD group compared to the ND group (Figure 6C,D, $p < 0.05$). The HOMA-IR value in the HFD group was notably higher than that in the ND group (Figure 6E, $p < 0.05$). The PA intervention significantly mitigated the HFD-induced elevations in fasting blood glucose levels, serum insulin concentrations, and HOMA-IR values in a dose-dependent manner. The results indicated that PA intervention could significantly improve HFD-induced insulin resistance.

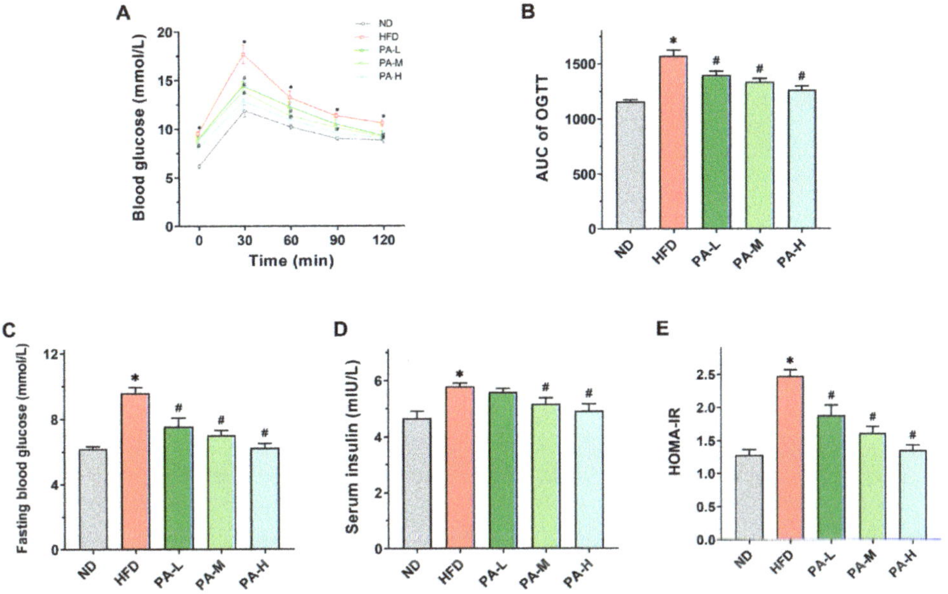

Figure 6. Effects of PA on glucose metabolism in HFD-induced mice. (**A**) Blood glucose profile of OGTT at week 7. (**B**) AUC measured during OGTT. (**C**) Fasting blood glucose levels in mice. (**D**) Serum insulin levels in mice. (**E**) HOMA-IR index in mice. Results are expressed as mean ± SEM. $n = 8$ per group. * $p < 0.05$, HFD vs. ND; # $p < 0.05$, HFD vs. PA-L, PA-M, or PA-H.

3.7. PA Attenuates Hepatic Oxidative Stress and Inflammatory Response of HFD-Induced Mice

Various studies have shown that the development of NAFLD is always accompanied by oxidative stress and inflammatory responses [33–35]. To evaluate hepatic oxidative stress, levels of MDA and activities of SOD and GSH-Px in the liver were measured. In comparison to the ND group, mice in the HFD group exhibited markedly elevated MDA levels (Figure 7A, $p < 0.05$) and significantly decreased activities of SOD and GSH-Px in the liver (Figure 7B,C, $p < 0.05$). The PA intervention markedly decreased hepatic MDA levels and substantially enhanced SOD and GSH-Px activities in a dose-dependent manner ($p < 0.05$), confirming the antioxidant effects of PA in the liver. Next, we evaluated the effect of PA on the hepatic levels of pro-inflammatory cytokines IL-1β, IL-6, and TNF-α.

The concentrations of hepatic IL-1β, IL-6, and TNF-α were significantly elevated in the HFD group compared to the ND group (Figure 7D–F, $p < 0.05$). However, high-dose PA intervention significantly reduced the hepatic levels of IL-1β, IL-6, and TNF-α ($p < 0.05$). These findings suggest that PA can effectively suppress HFD-induced hepatic inflammation.

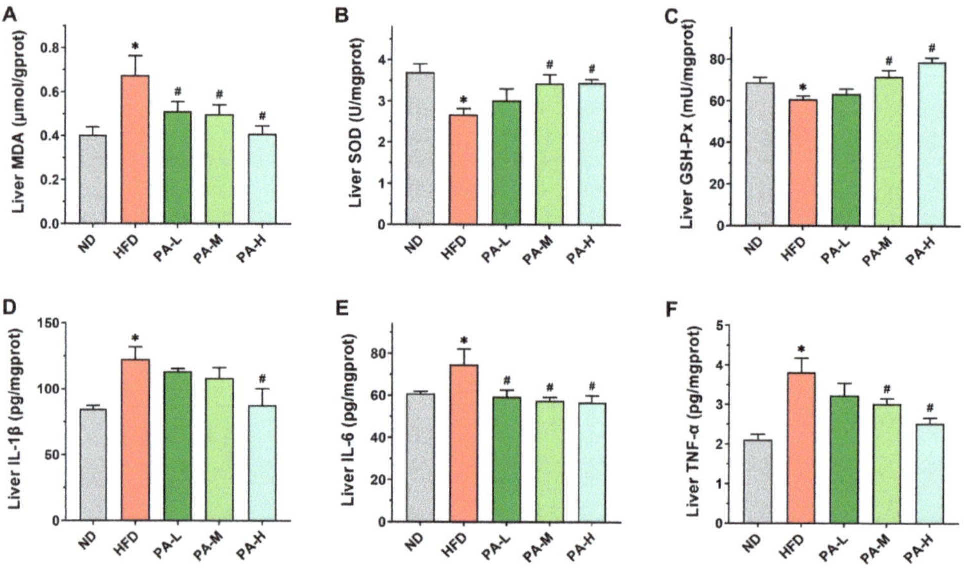

Figure 7. Effects of PA on hepatic oxidative stress and inflammatory response in HFD-induced mice. (**A–F**) Levels of MDA, SOD, GSH-Px, IL-1β, IL-6, and TNF-α in the liver of mice. Results are expressed as mean ± SEM. n = 8 per group. * $p < 0.05$, HFD vs. ND; # $p < 0.05$, HFD vs. PA-L, PA-M, or PA-H.

4. Discussion

NAFLD, the most prevalent metabolic liver disease globally, is characterized by hepatic steatosis [36]. Its pathogenesis is closely associated with insulin resistance, fatty acid synthesis, lipid peroxidation, oxidative stress, and gut microbiota dysbiosis. Currently, no specific drugs are available worldwide for the prevention or alleviation of NAFLD. The search for natural active substances to alleviate NAFLD is a potential intervention and treatment strategy. In our earlier studies, we showed that PA has beneficial effects in alleviating HFD-induced obesity [21]. Therefore, increasing the intake of PA in the diet could be an effective strategy for preventing and treating NAFLD. In this study, we determined the protein profile of PA using SDS-PAGE (Figure 1B). PA mainly consists of four proteins: lipoxygenase (100 kDa), PA2 (24 kDa), trypsin inhibitor (16 kDa), and PA1 (6 kDa), which are consistent with the composition reported in the literature [37]. It has been found that amino acid composition is related to the development of NAFLD. Glycine can alleviate NAFLD by promoting fatty acid β-oxidation and glutathione synthesis, while increased intake of branched-chain amino acids can significantly improve liver function [38]. Amino acid composition analysis of PA revealed that glycine accounts for approximately 25.20% and branched-chain amino acids account for approximately 7.34% of PA (Table 1). These results suggest that PA possesses material basis to alleviate NAFLD.

HFD induction is a common method for establishing an NAFLD mouse model. To evaluate the ameliorative effects of PA on NAFLD, we established an NAFLD mouse model induced with a HFD for 8 weeks. Mice in the HFD group exhibited significantly increased body weight, body fat percentage, serum lipid levels, serum transaminase levels, and insulin resistance. Additionally, lipid accumulation, steatosis, oxidative stress, and inflammatory damage were observed in the liver. According to the NAS assessment based on the criteria proposed by the NASH Clinical Research Network [39], the liver tissues of mice induced with a HFD were pathologically evaluated. In this study, the NAS of the HFD-induced mice reached 6, which is a diagnostic for NASH when the score exceeds 5. These comprehensive results indicated the successful establishment of the HFD-induced NAFLD mouse model, which is consistent with previously reported findings in the literature [40,41].

To investigate the effects and mechanisms of PA in alleviating NAFLD, we administered different doses of PA to the mice via gavage simultaneously with the induction of the NAFLD model. We found that PA can alleviate HFD-induced hepatic lipid accumulation by modulating serum lipid profiles, reducing insulin resistance, and enhancing antioxidant and anti-inflammatory capacities. The underlying mechanisms are likely mediated through the regulation of key proteins involved in hepatic lipogenesis, lipolysis, and fatty acid oxidation pathways. Currently, the most widely accepted pathogenesis mechanism of NAFLD is the "two-hit" hypothesis. The initial hit involves the accumulation of lipids, primarily triglycerides, in hepatocytes, leading to steatosis [4,42]. This study found that PA intervention substantially alleviated hepatic steatosis caused by the HFD. Specifically, morphological and histological examinations revealed that PA significantly reduced fat deposition in the liver. Compared to the HFD group, low, medium, and high doses of PA intervention reduced the area of red lipid droplets in Oil Red O staining of mice liver by 11.73%, 44.43%, and 59.17%, respectively. Additionally, the levels of TG and TC in the livers of PA-treated mice were markedly lower compared to those in the HFD group. These results suggest that PA significantly reduced hepatic lipid accumulation. Prolonged lipid retention in the liver frequently induces liver damage, potentially worsening NAFLD progression [5]. H&E staining and NAS results showed that PA intervention significantly reduced the number of hepatic fat vacuoles, ballooning degeneration, and inflammatory cell infiltration compared to the HFD group, with a significant decrease in NASs. While H&E staining and NAS are standard methods for pathological assessment, they depend on the subjective judgment of pathologists, potentially leading to inconsistencies in scoring. Consequently, we quantified the levels of commonly used biomarkers of liver function, specifically serum ALT and AST. When hepatocytes are in a pathological state of damage, they release ALT and AST into the bloodstream [43]. Therefore, increased levels of ALT and AST in the serum indicate a certain degree of liver damage. In this experiment, it was observed that PA intervention significantly reduced serum ALT and AST activities compared to the HFD group. The results demonstrated that PA mitigated HFD-induced liver damage. However, elevated levels of ALT and AST are typically observed when liver damage is already severe, making these biomarkers potentially unsuitable for the early detection or prediction of liver disease. Therefore, we also evaluated the effects of PA on the serum lipid profile, insulin resistance, oxidative stress, and inflammation levels to elucidate how PA intervention reduces hepatic steatosis and liver damage. The liver disease induced with a HFD in mice closely resembles the pathogenesis of human NAFLD. Ipsen et al. demonstrated that cereal proteins can improve lipid metabolism disorders and alleviate liver damage [44]. Lemus-Conejo et al. showed that lupin peptides can reduce AST and ALT related to liver damage, thereby alleviating HFD-induced NAFLD in mice [45]. Our study results also indicated that PA intervention can reduce HFD-induced hepatic steatosis and liver damage. Therefore, increasing PA intake as a dietary supplement might be an effective strategy for preventing and treating human NAFLD.

Disorders in the lipid metabolism can exacerbate the accumulation of fat in hepatocytes, contributing to the development and advancement of NAFLD and subsequently impairing liver function [46]. This study found that PA significantly enhanced the serum lipid profile by lowering serum levels of TG, TC, and LDL-C, while increasing the levels of HDL-C in mice. These findings align with prior research indicating that supplementation with pea protein can reduce serum cholesterol levels by modulating the microbiome [47]. Naik et al. found that cereal proteins can increase serum HDL concentrations [48]. Studies have shown that the phosphorylation of AMPK induces the phosphorylation of ACC, thereby reducing ACC activity and inhibiting TG formation. Therefore, PA may improve the serum lipid profile in mice by activating the AMPK pathway [49]. Given the critical role of lipid metabolism disorders in NAFLD pathogenesis, the improvement in serum lipid profile by PA intervention may have beneficial effects in alleviating NAFLD. Additionally, insulin resistance represents the predominant metabolic anomaly in NAFLD, with established research highlighting its close association with the initial pathogenic mechanisms of NAFLD [50,51]. The activation of the hepatic de novo lipogenesis pathway induced by insulin resistance contributes significantly to lipid accumulation in NAFLD [52]. Insulin resistance decreases the liver's ability to convert glucose into glycogen, leading to excessive synthesis of fatty acids from the surplus glucose, which are then esterified into TG, resulting in the excessive accumulation of TG in hepatocytes [53]. Research has shown that in NAFLD patients, metabolic disorders such as insulin resistance lead to a liver fat synthesis rate that is three times higher than in normal individuals [54]. Therefore, intervening in insulin resistance is an important approach to alleviate hepatic lipid accumulation. Ofosu et al.'s research indicates that grain bioactive peptides can alleviate metabolic syndrome, including type 2 diabetes and obesity [55]. This experiment found that PA could improve glucose tolerance, lower fasting blood glucose levels, and alleviate insulin resistance in NAFLD mice in a dose-dependent manner. Studies have shown that HFD feeding leads to increased phosphorylation of insulin receptor substrate 1 (IRS1), therefore inhibiting the IR/IRS-1 interaction and ultimately causing insulin resistance [56]. Liu et al. demonstrated that PA can inhibit IRS1 phosphorylation [21]. Therefore, in this study, PA may alleviate a HFD-induced insulin resistance by inhibiting the IRS1 phosphorylation pathway. These findings suggest that PA intervention can alleviate hepatic lipid accumulation in NAFLD by reducing insulin resistance and regulating lipid metabolism disorders induced with a HFD.

The "second hit" in NAFLD involves hepatic oxidative stress caused by excessive lipid accumulation, resulting in the production of significant ROS quantities [57]. When liver tissue is exposed to ROS, it triggers an inflammatory response, thereby accelerating the progression towards NASH [4]. Therefore, inhibiting oxidative stress and inflammatory responses represents a pivotal strategy for intervening in NAFLD. Under normal physiological conditions, cells can eliminate ROS and uphold cellular balance via internal antioxidant defense mechanisms like SOD and GSH-Px [58]. However, under oxidative stress in the liver, mitochondria become damaged, leading to the reduced metabolism of SOD and GSH-Px and an increase in MDA levels [59]. The findings from this research revealed a significant increase in liver MDA levels and a notable decrease in SOD and GSH-Px activities in the HFD group, indicating that HFD induced hepatic oxidative stress. In contrast, PA intervention significantly enhanced the activities of SOD and GSH-Px in the liver and reduced the MDA content, suggesting that PA intervention can alleviate HFD-induced oxidative stress in the liver. Research has shown that regulating the Nrf2 signaling pathway can modulate antioxidant enzymes such as NQO1, HO-1, providing protective effects against oxidative stress-induced cellular damage [60]. Specific upregulation of Nrf2 has been used to treat NAFLD induced by long-term HFD [61]. Ran et al. discovered that activation of the Nrf2/HO-1 signaling axis in the liver of HFD-fed mice can maintain antioxidant levels [33]. Zhu et al. found that activating the Nrf2/ARE pathway exerts antioxidant effects, thus preventing and treating NAFLD [40]. Therefore, PA may inhibit HFD-induced hepatic oxidative stress by modulating the Nrf2 signaling pathway. Studies have established that the development of NAFLD is also regulated by pro-inflammatory cytokines IL-1β, IL-6, and TNF-α [62]. Our study revealed significant elevation of IL-1β, IL-6, and TNF-α levels in the livers of HFD-induced NAFLD mice, whereas PA intervention markedly decreased these cytokine levels. Similarly, previous research has also found that PA can effectively inhibit the elevation of IL-1β, IL-6, and TNF-α levels in colitis [20]. The research confirmed that activation of TLR4 leads to the activation of NF-κB, promoting the release of pro-inflammatory cytokines and triggering liver inflammation [63]. Zhao et al. demonstrated that inhibiting the TLR4/NF-κB/NLRP3 signaling pathway can regulate the secretion of inflammatory factors to improve NAFLD [64]. Wang et al. found that the TLR4-NF-κB pathway is a key mechanism in mitigating inflammation damage in NAFLD [34]. Our earlier research also found that PA has the ability to block the NF-κB and STAT3 signaling pathways [20]. Based on these findings, we believe that the improvement of inflammatory response in NAFLD by PA is associated with the inhibition of the hepatic TLR-4/NF-κB pathway. The above results demonstrate that PA intervention can mitigate the "second hit" of HFD-induced NAFLD by suppressing oxidative stress and inflammatory responses.

Based on the above conclusions, we confirm that PA can alleviate HFD-induced NAFLD. Next, we investigated the mechanisms through which PA regulates hepatic lipid accumulation in NAFLD. Hepatic lipid metabolism primarily involves de novo lipogenesis, triglyceride synthesis, triglyceride hydrolysis, and fatty acid oxidation [65]. These hepatic lipid metabolism processes are regulated by various proteins. FASN and ACC serve as rate-limiting enzymes in fatty acid synthesis [66], while SREBF1 is a key transcription factor that regulates fatty acid synthesis by controlling the expression of crucial enzymes like FASN and ACC [67]. As a key energy sensor and regulator of the systemic metabolism, AMPK plays a vital role in maintaining lipid metabolism balance [68]. Phosphorylation of AMPK can inhibit the expression of SREBF1 while increasing the phosphorylation level of ACC, promoting the inactivation of ACC [69,70]. Lee et al. demonstrated that activating AMPK phosphorylation can enhance ACC phosphorylation, thereby inhibiting the expression of SREBF1 and FASN, reducing hepatic lipid accumulation [71]. Kawaguchi et al. indicated that wheat bran peptides can alleviate HFD-induced NAFLD in mice by upregulating the AMPK/ACC pathway [72]. ATGL serves as the rate-limiting enzyme in triglyceride hydrolysis, primarily functioning to convert triglycerides into free fatty acids and glycerol [73]. Research has shown that PPARα is crucial in the hepatic lipid metabolism by enhancing the transcription levels of various fatty acid oxidation proteins, thereby promoting mitochondrial fatty acid oxidation [74]. Additionally, ATGL deficiency can reduce the expression of the PPARα gene, leading to impaired mitochondrial fatty acid oxidation function [75]. Research has shown that the activation of PPARγ can reduce the transfer of fatty acids to the liver [76], decrease insulin resistance [77], and inhibit the expression of IL-6 and TNF-α [78]. In this research, HFD induction led to an upregulation of SREBF1 and FASN expression in the liver, a decrease in the phosphorylation of AMPKα and ACC, and a downregulation of ATGL, PPARα, and PPARγ expression. On the contrary, PA intervention can increase the phosphorylation of AMPKα and ACC, reduce the expression of SREBF1 and FASN, and enhance the expression of ATGL, PPARα, and PPARγ, thereby inhibiting de novo lipogenesis while promoting triglyceride hydrolysis and mitochondrial fatty acid oxidation. From these results, it can be concluded that PA alleviates hepatic steatosis by modulating the lipid metabolism, thereby mitigating the progression of NAFLD.

5. Conclusions

In conclusion, PA intervention can improve dyslipidemia, insulin resistance, oxidative stress, and inflammatory responses induced with a high-fat diet intake, thereby reducing hepatic steatosis, and alleviating the development of NAFLD. PA reduces hepatic lipid accumulation in mice by regulating the expression of proteins involved in hepatic lipogenesis and lipolysis (Figure 8). However, this study has some limitations, such as not determining the exact manner in which PA is absorbed in the intestines or the form in which PA is transported through the blood to ultimately target the liver. Therefore, further research is needed to isolate PA to identify the specific components within PA that regulate lipogenesis and lipolysis, in order to better understand its potential mechanisms of action. Overall, PA can serve as a natural dietary supplement to provide a new strategy for improving NAFLD.

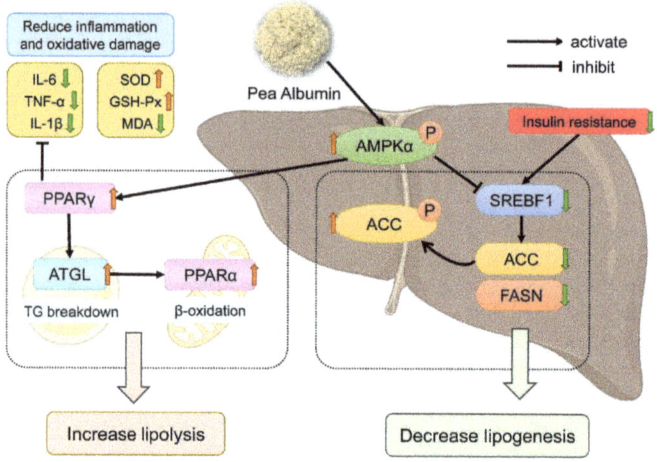

Figure 8. Schematic illustration of the mechanism of pea albumin in ameliorating HFD-induced NAFLD. The red upward arrows represent increase; the green downward arrows represent decrease.

Author Contributions: Conceptualization, J.Z. and P.W.; methodology, H.Z.; validation, S.Z. and H.Z.; formal analysis, S.Z. and Z.C.; investigation, S.Z. and Z.C.; resources, J.Z. and P.W.; data curation, F.W.; writing—original draft preparation, S.Z.; writing—review and editing, J.Z. and P.W.; visualization, F.W.; supervision, J.Z. and P.W.; funding acquisition, P.W. All authors have read and agreed to the published version of the manuscript.

Funding: This research was funded by the 111 project from the Education Ministry of China, grant number B18053.

Institutional Review Board Statement: The animal study protocol was approved by the Institutional Animal Care and Use Committee of China Agricultural University (protocol code AW72303202-5-3, approved on 27 March 2023).

Informed Consent Statement: Not applicable.

Data Availability Statement: The data presented in this study are available on request from the corresponding author. The data are not publicly available due to privacy and ethical reasons.

Acknowledgments: We thank the support of the experimental platform of Beijing Advanced Innovation Center for Food Nutrition and Human Health.

Conflicts of Interest: F.W. was employed by Tibet Tianhong Science and Technology Co., Ltd. The remaining authors declare that the research was conducted in the absence of any commercial or financial relationships that could be construed as a potential conflict of interest.

References

1. Brunt, E.M.; Wong, V.W.S.; Nobili, V.; Day, C.P.; Sookoian, S.; Maher, J.J.; Bugianesi, E.; Sirlin, C.B.; Neuschwander-Tetri, B.; Rinella, M.E. Nonalcoholic fatty liver disease. *Nat. Rev. Dis. Primers* **2015**, *1*, 15080. [CrossRef] [PubMed]
2. Paternostro, R.; Trauner, M. Current treatment of non-alcoholic fatty liver disease. *J. Intern. Med.* **2022**, *292*, 190–204. [CrossRef] [PubMed]
3. Younossi, Z.; Anstee, Q.M.; Marietti, M.; Hardy, T.; Henry, L.; Eslam, M.; George, J.; Bugianesi, E. Global burden of NAFLD and NASH: Trends, predictions, risk factors and prevention. *Nat. Rev. Gastroenterol. Hepatol.* **2018**, *15*, 11–20. [CrossRef] [PubMed]
4. Buzzetti, E.; Pinzani, M.; Tsochatzis, E.A. The multiple-hit pathogenesis of non-alcoholic fatty liver disease (NAFLD). *Metab. Clin. Exp.* **2016**, *65*, 1038–1048. [CrossRef] [PubMed]
5. Friedman, S.L.; Neuschwander-Tetri, B.A.; Rinella, M.; Sanyal, A.J. Mechanisms of NAFLD development and therapeutic strategies. *Nat. Med.* **2018**, *24*, 908–922. [CrossRef] [PubMed]
6. Chalasani, N.; Younossi, Z.; Lavine, J.E.; Charlton, M.; Cusi, K.; Rinella, M.; Harrison, S.A.; Brunt, E.M.; Sanyal, A.J. The diagnosis and management of nonalcoholic fatty liver disease: Practice guidance from the American association for the study of liver diseases. *Hepatology* **2018**, *67*, 328–357. [CrossRef] [PubMed]

7. Lassailly, G.; Caiazzo, R.; Buob, D.; Pigeyre, M.; Verkindt, H.; Labreuche, J.; Raverdy, V.; Leteurtre, E.; Dharancy, S.; Louvet, A.; et al. Bariatric surgery reduces features of nonalcoholic steatohepatitis in morbidly obese patients. *Gastroenterology* **2015**, *149*, 379–388. [CrossRef] [PubMed]
8. Cusi, K.; Orsak, B.; Bril, F.; Lomonaco, R.; Hecht, J.; Ortiz-Lopez, C.; Tio, F.; Hardies, J.; Darland, C.; Musi, N. Long-term pioglitazone treatment for patients with nonalcoholic steatohepatitis and prediabetes or type 2 diabetes mellitus: A randomized trial. *Ann. Intern. Med.* **2016**, *165*, 305–315. [CrossRef]
9. Yoneda, M.; Honda, Y.; Ogawa, Y.; Kessoku, T.; Kobayashi, T.; Imajo, K.; Ozaki, A.; Nogami, A.; Taguri, M.; Yamanaka, T. Comparing the effects of tofogliflozin and pioglitazone in non-alcoholic fatty liver disease patients with type 2 diabetes mellitus (ToPiND study): A randomized prospective open-label controlled trial. *BMJ Open Diabetes Res. Care* **2021**, *9*, e001990. [CrossRef]
10. Newsome, P.N.; Buchholtz, K.; Cusi, K.; Linder, M.; Okanoue, T.; Ratziu, V.; Sanyal, A.J.; Sejling, A.-S.; Harrison, S.A. A placebo-controlled trial of subcutaneous semaglutide in nonalcoholic steatohepatitis. *N. Engl. J. Med.* **2021**, *384*, 1113–1124. [CrossRef]
11. Armstrong, M.J.; Gaunt, P.; Aithal, G.P.; Barton, D.; Hull, D.; Parker, R.; Hazlehurst, J.M.; Guo, K.; Abouda, G.; Aldersley, M.A. Liraglutide safety and efficacy in patients with non-alcoholic steatohepatitis (lean): A multicentre, double-blind, randomised, placebo-controlled phase 2 study. *Lancet* **2016**, *387*, 679–690. [CrossRef] [PubMed]
12. Chen, W.; Zhang, X.; Xu, M.; Jiang, L.; Zhou, M.; Liu, W.; Chen, Z.; Wang, Y.; Zou, Q.; Wang, L. Betaine prevented high-fat diet-induced NAFLD by regulating the fgf10/ampk signaling pathway in $ApoE^{-/-}$ mice. *Eur. J. Nutr.* **2021**, *60*, 1655–1668. [CrossRef] [PubMed]
13. Maithilikarpagaselvi, N.; Sridhar, M.G.; Swaminathan, R.P.; Sripradha, R.; Badhe, B. Curcumin inhibits hyperlipidemia and hepatic fat accumulation in high-fructose-fed male wistar rats. *Pharm. Biol.* **2016**, *54*, 2857–2863. [CrossRef]
14. Li, D.; Ikaga, R.; Yamazaki, T. Soya protein β-conglycinin ameliorates fatty liver and obesity in diet-induced obese mice through the down-regulation of PPARγ. *Br. J. Nutr.* **2018**, *119*, 1220–1232. [CrossRef]
15. Yan, H.; Xia, M.; Wang, Y.; Chang, X.; Yao, X.; Rao, S.; Zeng, M.; Tu, Y.; Feng, R.; Jia, W.; et al. Efficacy of berberine in patients with non-alcoholic fatty liver disease. *PLoS ONE* **2015**, *10*, e0134172. [CrossRef] [PubMed]
16. Shan, D.; Yu, H.; Lyu, B.; Fu, H. Soybean β-conglycinin: Structure characteristic, allergenicity, plasma lipid-controlling, prevention of obesity and non-alcoholic fatty liver disease. *Curr. Protein Pept. Sci.* **2021**, *22*, 831–847. [CrossRef] [PubMed]
17. Panahi, Y.; Kianpour, P.; Mohtashami, R.; Jafari, R.; Simental-Mendia, L.E.; Sahebkar, A. Efficacy and safety of phytosomal curcumin in non-alcoholic fatty liver disease: A randomized controlled trial. *Drug Res.* **2017**, *67*, 244–251. [CrossRef]
18. Aranda-Olmedo, I.; Ruiz, R.; Jesus Peinado, M.; Rubio, L.A. A pea (*Pisum sativum* L.) seed albumin extract prevents colonic dss induced dysbiosis in mice. *J. Funct. Foods* **2017**, *35*, 279–294. [CrossRef]
19. Rubio, L.A.; Perez, A.; Ruiz, R.; Angeles Guzman, M.; Aranda-Olmedo, I.; Clemente, A. Characterization of pea (*Pisum sativum*) seed protein fractions. *J. Sci. Food Agric.* **2014**, *94*, 280–287. [CrossRef]
20. Zhang, S.; Jin, W.; Zhang, W.; Ren, F.; Wang, P.; Liu, N. Pea albumin attenuates dextran sulfate sodium-induced colitis by regulating NF-kappa B signaling and the intestinal microbiota in mice. *Nutrients* **2022**, *14*, 3611. [CrossRef]
21. Liu, N.; Song, Z.; Jin, W.; Yang, Y.; Sun, S.; Zhang, Y.; Zhang, S.; Liu, S.; Ren, F.; Wang, P. Pea albumin extracted from pea (*Pisum sativum* L.) seed protects mice from high fat diet-induced obesity by modulating lipid metabolism and gut microbiota. *J. Funct. Foods* **2022**, *97*, 105234. [CrossRef]
22. Ruiz, R.; Olias, R.; Clemente, A.; Rubio, L.A. A pea (*Pisum sativum* L.) seed vicilins hydrolysate exhibits PPARγ ligand activity and modulates adipocyte differentiation in a 3t3-l1 cell culture model. *Foods* **2020**, *9*, 793. [CrossRef] [PubMed]
23. Miszkiewicz, H.; Okrajni, J.; Bielecki, S. Changes in the content and anti-oxidative activity of polyphenols and albumins in pea during its fermentation in an sssr bioreactor. *Zywnosc-Nauka Technol. Jakosc* **2008**, *15*, 67–79.
24. Dun, X.; Li, F.; Wang, J.; Chen, Z. The effect of pea albumin 1f on glucose metabolism in mice. *Peptides* **2008**, *29*, 891–897. [CrossRef] [PubMed]
25. Heo, S.W.; Chung, K.S.; Yoon, Y.S.; Kim, S.Y.; Ahn, H.S.; Shin, Y.K.; Lee, S.H.; Lee, K.T. Standardized ethanol extract of *cassia mimosoides* var. *Nomame* makino ameliorates obesity via regulation of adipogenesis and lipogenesis in 3t3-l1 cells and high-fat diet-induced obese mice. *Nutrients* **2023**, *15*, 613. [CrossRef]
26. Radlinger, B.; Ress, C.; Folie, S.; Salzmann, K.; Lechuga, A.; Weiss, B.; Salvenmoser, W.; Graber, M.; Hirsch, J.; Holfeld, J.; et al. Empagliflozin protects mice against diet-induced obesity, insulin resistance and hepatic steatosis. *Diabetologia* **2022**, *66*, 754–767. [CrossRef] [PubMed]
27. Shan, S.; Zhou, J.; Yin, R.; Zhang, L.; Shi, J.; Qiao, Q.; Li, Z. Millet bran protein hydrolysate displays the anti-non-alcoholic fatty liver disease effect via activating peroxisome proliferator-activated receptor γ to restrain fatty acid uptake. *J. Agric. Food Chem.* **2023**, *71*, 1628–1642. [CrossRef] [PubMed]
28. Liu, Z.; Patil, I.Y.; Jiang, T.; Sancheti, H.; Walsh, J.P.; Stiles, B.L.; Yin, F.; Cadenas, E. High-fat diet induces hepatic insulin resistance and impairment of synaptic plasticity. *PLoS ONE* **2015**, *10*, e0128274. [CrossRef] [PubMed]
29. Zou, Y.; Zhong, L.; Hu, C.; Zhong, M.; Peng, N.; Sheng, G. LDL/HDL cholesterol ratio is associated with new-onset NAFLD in chinese non-obese people with normal lipids: A 5-year longitudinal cohort study. *Lipids Health Dis.* **2021**, *20*, 28. [CrossRef]
30. Bazick, J.; Donithan, M.; Neuschwander-Tetri, B.A.; Kleiner, D.E.; Brunt, E.; Wilson, L.; Doo, E.; Lavine, J.E.; Loomba, R. Clinical model for NASH or advanced fibrosis in patients with diabetes and NAFLD. *Gastroenterology* **2014**, *146*, S948. [CrossRef]

31. Ramanathan, R.; Ali, A.H.; Ibdah, J.A. Mitochondrial dysfunction plays central role in nonalcoholic fatty liver disease. *Int. J. Mol. Sci.* **2022**, *23*, 7280. [CrossRef] [PubMed]
32. Gutch, M.; Kumar, S.; Razi, S.M.; Gupta, K.K.; Gupta, A. Assessment of insulin sensitivity/resistance. *Indian J. Endocrinol. Metab.* **2015**, *19*, 160–164. [CrossRef] [PubMed]
33. Ran, X.; Hu, G.; He, F.; Li, K.; Li, F.; Xu, D.; Liu, J.; Fu, S. Phytic acid improves hepatic steatosis, inflammation, and oxidative stress in high-fat diet (HFD)-fed mice by modulating the gut–liver axis. *J. Agric. Food. Chem.* **2022**, *70*, 11401–11411. [CrossRef] [PubMed]
34. Wang, R.; Wang, L.; Wu, H.; Zhang, L.; Hu, X.; Li, C.; Liu, S. Noni (*Morinda citrifolia* L.) fruit phenolic extract supplementation ameliorates NAFLD by modulating insulin resistance, oxidative stress, inflammation, liver metabolism and gut microbiota. *Food Res. Int.* **2022**, *160*, 111732. [CrossRef] [PubMed]
35. Zhang, J.; Zhou, X.; Wang, X.; Zhang, J.; Yang, M.; Liu, Y.; Cao, J.; Cheng, G. Que zui tea ameliorates hepatic lipid accumulation and oxidative stress in high fat diet induced nonalcoholic fatty liver disease. *Food Res. Int.* **2022**, *156*, 111196. [CrossRef] [PubMed]
36. Cardoso, A.C.; de Figueiredo-Mendes, C.; Villela-Nogueira, C.A. Current management of NAFLD/NASH. *Liver Int.* **2021**, *41*, 89–94. [CrossRef] [PubMed]
37. Yang, S.; Li, X.; Hua, Y.; Chen, Y.; Kong, X.; Zhang, C. Selective complex coacervation of pea whey proteins with chitosan to purify main 2s albumins. *J. Agric. Food Chem.* **2020**, *68*, 1698–1706. [CrossRef] [PubMed]
38. Rom, O.; Liu, Y.; Liu, Z.; Zhao, Y.; Wu, J.; Ghrayeb, A.; Villacorta, L.; Fan, Y.; Chang, L.; Wang, L.; et al. Glycine-based treatment ameliorates NAFLD by modulating fatty acid oxidation, glutathione synthesis, and the gut microbiome. *Sci. Transl. Med.* **2020**, *12*, eaaz2841. [CrossRef] [PubMed]
39. Kleiner, D.E.; Brunt, E.M.; Van Natta, M.; Behling, C.; Contos, M.J.; Cummings, O.W.; Ferrell, L.D.; Liu, Y.C.; Torbenson, M.S.; Unalp-Arida, A. Design and validation of a histological scoring system for nonalcoholic fatty liver disease. *Hepatology* **2005**, *41*, 1313–1321. [CrossRef]
40. Zhu, L.; Xiao, M.; Luo, J.; Li, S.; Liu, W.; Wu, J.; Song, Z. Polysaccharides from *Ostrea rivularis* rebuild the balance of gut microbiota to ameliorate non-alcoholic fatty liver disease in $ApoE^{-/-}$ mice. *Int. J. Biol. Macromol.* **2023**, *235*, 123853. [CrossRef]
41. Zineldeen, D.H.; Tahoon, N.M.; Sarhan, N.I. Aicar ameliorates non-alcoholic fatty liver disease via modulation of the HGF/NF-κB/SNARK signaling pathway and restores mitochondrial and endoplasmic reticular impairments in high-fat diet-fed rats. *Int. J. Mol. Sci.* **2023**, *24*, 3367. [CrossRef] [PubMed]
42. Tilg, H.; Moschen, A.R. Evolution of inflammation in nonalcoholic fatty liver disease: The multiple parallel hits hypothesis. *Hepatology* **2010**, *52*, 1836–1846. [CrossRef] [PubMed]
43. Henao-Mejia, J.; Elinav, E.; Jin, C.; Hao, L.; Mehal, W.Z.; Strowig, T.; Thaiss, C.A.; Kau, A.L.; Eisenbarth, S.C.; Jurczak, M.J.; et al. Inflammasome-mediated dysbiosis regulates progression of NAFLD and obesity. *Nature* **2012**, *482*, 179–185. [CrossRef] [PubMed]
44. Ipsen, D.H.; Lykkesfeldt, J.; Tveden-Nyborg, P. Molecular mechanisms of hepatic lipid accumulation in non-alcoholic fatty liver disease. *Cell. Mol. Life Sci.* **2018**, *75*, 3313–3327. [CrossRef] [PubMed]
45. Lemus-Conejo, A.; Grao-Cruces, E.; Toscano, R.; Varela, L.M.; Claro, C.; Pedroche, J.; Millan, F.; Millan-Linares, M.C.; Montserrat-de la Paz, S. A lupine (*Lupinus angustifolious* L.) peptide prevents non-alcoholic fatty liver disease in high-fat-diet-induced obese mice. *Food Funct.* **2020**, *11*, 2943–2952. [CrossRef] [PubMed]
46. Mato, J.M.; Alonso, C.; Noureddin, M.; Lu, S.C. Biomarkers and subtypes of deranged lipid metabolism in non-alcoholic fatty liver disease. *World J. Gastroenterol.* **2019**, *25*, 3009–3020. [CrossRef] [PubMed]
47. Tong, L.; Xiao, T.; Wang, L.; Lu, C.; Liu, L.; Zhou, X.; Wang, A.; Qin, W.; Wang, F. Plant protein reduces serum cholesterol levels in hypercholesterolemia hamsters by modulating the compositions of gut microbiota and metabolites. *Iscience* **2021**, *24*, 103435. [CrossRef] [PubMed]
48. Naik, H.S.; Srilatha, C.; Sujatha, K.; Sreedevi, B.; Prasad, T.N.V.K.V. Supplementation of whole grain flaxseeds (*Linum usitatissimum*) along with high cholesterol diet and its effect on hyperlipidemia and initiated atherosclerosis in wistar albino male rats. *Vet. World* **2018**, *11*, 1433–1439. [CrossRef] [PubMed]
49. Xi, Y.; Wu, M.; Li, H.; Dong, S.; Luo, E.; Gu, M.; Shen, X.; Jiang, Y.; Liu, Y.; Liu, H. Baicalin attenuates high fat diet-induced obesity and liver dysfunction: Dose-response and potential role of CaMKKβ/AMPK/ACC pathway. *Cell Physiol. Biochem.* **2015**, *35*, 2349–2359. [CrossRef]
50. Hannah, W.N., Jr.; Harrison, S.A. Lifestyle and dietary interventions in the management of nonalcoholic fatty liver disease. *Dig. Dis. Sci.* **2016**, *61*, 1365–1374. [CrossRef]
51. Rachakonda, V.; Wills, R.; DeLany, J.P.; Kershaw, E.E.; Behari, J. Differential impact of weight loss on nonalcoholic fatty liver resolution in a north American cohort with obesity. *Obesity* **2017**, *25*, 1360–1368. [CrossRef] [PubMed]
52. Chen, M.; Guo, W.; Li, Q.; Xu, J.; Cao, Y.; Liu, B.; Yu, X.; Rao, P.; Ni, L.; Lv, X. The protective mechanism of *lactobacillus plantarum* fzu3013 against non-alcoholic fatty liver associated with hyperlipidemia in mice fed a high-fat diet. *Food Funct.* **2020**, *11*, 3316–3331. [CrossRef] [PubMed]
53. Aragones, G.; Gonzalez-Garcia, S.; Aguilar, C.; Richart, C.; Auguet, T. Gut microbiota-derived mediators as potential markers in nonalcoholic fatty liver disease. *BioMed Res. Int.* **2019**, *2019*, 8507583. [CrossRef] [PubMed]
54. Musso, G.; Gambino, R.; Cassader, M. Recent insights into hepatic lipid metabolism in non-alcoholic fatty liver disease (NAFLD). *Prog. Lipid Res.* **2009**, *48*, 1–26. [CrossRef] [PubMed]

55. Ofosu, F.K.; Mensah, D.-J.F.; Daliri, E.B.-M.; Oh, D.-H. Exploring molecular insights of cereal peptidic antioxidants in metabolic syndrome prevention. *Antioxidants* **2021**, *10*, 518. [CrossRef] [PubMed]
56. Werner, E.D.; Lee, J.; Hansen, L.; Yuan, M.; Shoelson, S.E. Insulin resistance due to phosphorylation of insulin receptor substrate-1 at serine 302. *J. Biol. Chem.* **2004**, *279*, 35298–35305. [CrossRef] [PubMed]
57. Rolo, A.P.; Teodoro, J.S.; Palmeira, C.M. Role of oxidative stress in the pathogenesis of nonalcoholic steatohepatitis. *Free Radic. Biol. Med.* **2012**, *52*, 59–69. [CrossRef] [PubMed]
58. Abdelmegeed, M.A.; Banerjee, A.; Yoo, S.-H.; Jang, S.; Gonzalez, F.J.; Song, B.-J. Critical role of cytochrome p450 2e1 (cyp2e1) in the development of high fat-induced non-alcoholic steatohepatitis. *J. Hepatol.* **2012**, *57*, 860–866. [CrossRef] [PubMed]
59. Liao, M.; Sun, C.; Li, R.; Li, W.; Ge, Z.; Adu-Frimpong, M.; Xu, X.; Yu, J. Amelioration action of gastrodigenin rhamno-pyranoside from moringa seeds on non-alcoholic fatty liver disease. *Food Chem.* **2022**, *379*, 132087. [CrossRef]
60. Zhai, K.F.; Duan, H.; Khan, G.J.; Xu, H.; Han, F.K.; Cao, W.G.; Gao, G.Z.; Shan, L.L.; Wei, Z.J. Salicin from *alangium chinense* ameliorates rheumatoid arthritis by modulating the Nrf2-HO-1-ROS pathways. *J. Agric. Food. Chem.* **2018**, *66*, 6073–6082. [CrossRef]
61. Qiu, M.; Xiao, F.; Wang, T.; Piao, S.; Zhao, W.; Shao, S.; Yan, M.; Zhao, D. Protective effect of hedansanqi tiaozhi tang against non-alcoholic fatty liver disease in vitro and in vivo through activating Nrf2/HO-1 antioxidant signaling pathway. *Phytomedicine* **2020**, *67*, 153140. [CrossRef] [PubMed]
62. Schroeder, T.; Kucharczyk, D.; Baer, F.; Pagel, R.; Derer, S.; Jendrek, S.T.; Suenderhauf, A.; Brethack, A.-K.; Hirose, M.; Moeller, S.; et al. Mitochondrial gene polymorphisms alter hepatic cellular energy metabolism and aggravate diet-induced non-alcoholic steatohepatitis. *Mol. Metab.* **2016**, *5*, 283–295. [CrossRef]
63. Andresen, L.; Jorgensen, V.L.; Perner, A.; Hansen, A.; Eugen-Olsen, J.; Rask-Madsen, J. Activation of nuclear factor κB in colonic mucosa from patients with collagenous and ulcerative colitis. *Gut* **2005**, *54*, 503–509. [CrossRef] [PubMed]
64. Zhao, H.; Gao, X.; Liu, Z.; Zhang, L.; Fang, X.; Sun, J.; Zhang, Z.; Sun, Y. Sodium alginate prevents non-alcoholic fatty liver disease by modulating the gut–liver axis in high-fat diet-fed rats. *Nutrients* **2022**, *14*, 4846. [CrossRef]
65. Tang, C.; Zhou, W.; Shan, M.; Lu, Z.; Lu, Y. Yogurt-derived *lactobacillus plantarum* q16 alleviated high-fat diet-induced non-alcoholic fatty liver disease in mice. *Food Sci. Hum. Wellness* **2022**, *11*, 1428–1439. [CrossRef]
66. Horton, J.D.; Goldstein, J.L.; Brown, M.S. Srebps: Activators of the complete program of cholesterol and fatty acid synthesis in the liver. *J. Clin. Investig.* **2002**, *109*, 1125–1131. [CrossRef]
67. Wang, H.; Peng, H.; Chien, Y.; Chen, Y.; Lu, N.; Yang, S. Effects of fish oil on lipid metabolism and its molecular biological regulators in chronic ethanol-fed rats. *Nutrients* **2018**, *10*, 802. [CrossRef] [PubMed]
68. Ruderman, N.; Prentki, M. Amp kinase and malonyl-coa: Targets for therapy of the metabolic syndrome. *Nat. Rev. Drug Discov.* **2004**, *3*, 340–351. [CrossRef]
69. Li, Y.; Xu, S.; Mihaylova, M.M.; Zheng, B.; Hou, X.; Jiang, B.; Park, O.; Luo, Z.; Lefai, E.; Shyy, J.Y.J.; et al. AMPK phosphorylates and inhibits srebp activity to attenuate hepatic steatosis and atherosclerosis in diet-induced insulin-resistant mice. *Cell Metab.* **2011**, *13*, 376–388. [CrossRef]
70. Yuan, E.; Duan, X.; Xiang, L.; Ren, J.; Lai, X.; Li, Q.; Sun, L.; Sun, S. Aged oolong tea reduces high-fat diet-induced fat accumulation and dyslipidemia by regulating the AMPK/ACC signaling pathway. *Nutrients* **2018**, *10*, 187. [CrossRef]
71. Lee, J.H.; Woo, K.J.; Hong, J.; Han, K.I.; Kim, H.S.; Kim, T.J. Heat-killed enterococcus faecalis inhibit fl83b hepatic lipid accumulation and high fat diet-induced fatty liver damage in rats by activating lipolysis through the regulation the AMPK signaling pathway. *Int. J. Mol. Sci.* **2023**, *24*, 4486. [CrossRef] [PubMed]
72. Kawaguchi, T.; Ueno, T.; Nogata, Y.; Hayakawa, M.; Koga, H.; Torimura, T. Wheat-bran autolytic peptides containing a branched-chain amino acid attenuate non-alcoholic steatohepatitis via the suppression of oxidative stress and the upregulation of AMPK/ACC in high-fat diet-fed mice. *Int. J. Mol. Med.* **2017**, *39*, 407–414. [CrossRef] [PubMed]
73. Ong, K.T.; Mashek, M.T.; Bu, S.Y.; Greenberg, A.S.; Mashek, D.G. Adipose triglyceride lipase is a major hepatic lipase that regulates triacylglycerol turnover and fatty acid signaling and partitioning. *Hepatology* **2011**, *53*, 116–126. [CrossRef] [PubMed]
74. Venalainen, T.; Molnar, F.; Oostenbrink, C.; Carlberg, C.; Perakyla, M. Molecular mechanism of allosteric communication in the human PPARα-RXRα heterodimer. *Proteins Struct. Funct. Bioinf.* **2010**, *78*, 873–887. [CrossRef] [PubMed]
75. Wu, Q.; Wang, Q.; Fu, J.; Ren, R. Polysaccharides derived from natural sources regulate triglyceride and cholesterol metabolism: A review of the mechanisms. *Food Funct.* **2019**, *10*, 2330–2339. [CrossRef] [PubMed]
76. Lalloyer, F.; Staels, B. Fibrates, glitazones, and peroxisome proliferator-activated receptors. *Arterioscler. Thromb. Vasc. Biol.* **2010**, *30*, 894–899. [CrossRef] [PubMed]
77. Maeda, N.; Takahashi, M.; Funahashi, T.; Kihara, S.; Nishizawa, H.; Kishida, K.; Nagaretani, H.; Matsuda, M.; Komuro, R.; Ouchi, N.; et al. PPARγ ligands increase expression and plasma concentrations of adiponectin, an adipose-derived protein. *Diabetes* **2001**, *50*, 2094–2099. [CrossRef]
78. Jiang, F.; Zhang, Z.; Zhang, Y.; Wu, J.; Yu, L.; Liu, S. L-carnitine ameliorates the liver inflammatory response by regulating carnitine palmitoyltransferase i-dependent PPARγ signaling. *Mol. Med. Rep.* **2016**, *13*, 1320–1328. [CrossRef]

nutrients

MDPI

Article

Targeting Non-Alcoholic Fatty Liver Disease with Hawthorn Ethanol Extract (HEE): A Comprehensive Examination of Hepatic Lipid Reduction and Gut Microbiota Modulation

Tianyu Wang [1], Dawei Wang [2], Yinghui Ding [1], He Xu [1], Yue Sun [1], Jumin Hou [1] and Yanrong Zhang [2,*]

[1] College of Food Science and Engineering, Changchun University, Changchun 130022, China; wangty84@ccu.edu.cn (T.W.); dyh15585679977102З@163.com (Y.D.); xh1796293949@163.com (H.X.); 15844448981@163.com (Y.S.); houjm@ccu.edu.cn (J.H.)

[2] School of Food Science and Engineering, Jilin Agricultural University, Changchun 130118, China; wangdawei@jlau.edu.cn

* Correspondence: zhangyanrong@jlau.edu.cn

Abstract: Recent studies have highlighted the lipid-lowering ability of hawthorn ethanol extract (HEE) and the role played by gut flora in the efficacy of HEE. Our study sought to explore the effects of HEE on non-alcoholic fatty liver disease (NAFLD) in normal flora and pseudo germ-free mice. The results showed that HEE effectively diminished hepatic lipid accumulation, ameliorated liver function, reduced inflammatory cytokine levels and blood lipid profiles, and regulated blood glucose levels. HEE facilitated triglyceride breakdown, suppressed fatty acid synthesis, and enhanced intestinal health by modulating the diversity of the gut microbiota and the production of short-chain fatty acids in the gut. In addition, HEE apparently helps to increase the presence of beneficial genera of bacteria, thereby influencing the composition of the gut microbiota, and the absence of gut flora affects the efficacy of HEE. These findings reveal the potential of hawthorn for the prevention and treatment of NAFLD and provide new perspectives on the study of functional plants to improve liver health.

Keywords: nonalcoholic fatty liver disease; hawthorn ethanol extract; gut microbiota; high-fat diet; short-chain fatty acids

1. Introduction

The clinicopathologic manifestation of nonalcoholic fatty liver disease (NAFLD) is an atypical accumulation of triglycerides in the hepatocytes without or with a minimal history of alcohol consumption. As of now, there is no specialized medication proven to effectively prevent or manage NAFLD [1]. Hence, studying the underlying mechanisms of NAFLD and identifying potential targets for intervention is crucial in the prevention and management of NAFLD. The disease's emergence is thought to be multifactorial, with recent studies demonstrating imbalanced gut microbiota playing a role in NAFLD and contributing to its progression by influencing metabolic outputs, the metabolism of sugars and fats, immunological activities, and inflammatory processes [2,3].

A high-fat diet (HFD) induces ecological dysregulation of the gut microbiota and leads to increased intestinal permeability in mice. Gut microbiota imbalance can lead to inflammatory responses and is closely linked to NAFLD and cancer [4–6]. Several gut microbiota and their metabolites play a crucial role in maintaining liver and intestinal health, such as short-chain fatty acids (SCFAs) in the gut, which are closely associated with inflammation, as well as glucose and lipid metabolism [7]. As metabolic byproducts of microbes, SCFAs are not only the preferred energy substrates for the intestinal epithelial cells, but are also crucial components in regulating antioxidants and the balance of the gut microbiota [8]. Therefore, the significance of microorganisms that generate SCFAs is increasingly recognized. The adjustment of the proportions of intestinal microbial communities can be optimized through prebiotics provided in food or dietary supplements.

Previous research has indicated that probiotics have diverse effects on the gut microbiota of mice with NAFLD, including improvements in the metabolism of related metabolites such as SCFAs, bile acids, and digestive enzymes. These functional metabolites can restore liver function, blood lipid levels, and cytokine levels in mice with NAFLD [9,10]. Currently, supplementation with probiotics and prebiotics is the mainstay of improving the balance of the gut microbiota, thereby becoming a potential therapeutic direction for the treatment of NAFLD [11,12]. Recent pharmacological studies have indicated that certain food–medicine dual-purpose items can treat NAFLD by modulating the gut microbiota. Saponins found in ginseng have been shown to suppress inflammatory responses in rats with a model of NAFLD, regulate lipid metabolism, and alleviate liver damage [13]. Ganoderma lucidum polysaccharides are capable of modulating bile acid levels and metabolites of the gut microbiota, and ameliorating NAFLD by altering gut microbiota composition [14,15]. These research findings indicate that herbs act as prebiotics in the gastrointestinal tract when consumed as dietary supplements.

The fruit of the hawthorn (Crataegus pinnatifida), which is extensively utilized in traditional herbal practices for lipid reduction, has been the focus of recent research. Studies indicate that extracts enriched with hawthorn fruit polyphenols can counteract dysfunction in pancreatic β-cells due to high fructose intake by alleviating oxidative stress in the endoplasmic reticulum. The active ingredients include compounds from flavonoids and triterpenes [16]. As a functional food, its extract also protects the vascular endothelium, restores endothelial dysfunction, and promotes endothelial relaxation [17]. Furthermore, hawthorn extract can modulate immune responses and regulate lymphocyte subsets. Additionally, studies have shown that hawthorn extract has a protective effect against microcystin-induced liver injury [18].

Although the abundant flavonoid compounds in extracts have a wide range of pharmacological applications, their poor water solubility often results in low oral bioavailability [19,20]. This indicates that the intake of these extracts through gavage might engage the gut microbiota, subsequently promoting health improvements. The exact mechanism of hawthorn extracts' effect on lipid metabolism by altering the gut microbiota is still to be fully understood. In this study, we investigated the therapeutic effect of HEE on NAFLD in mice and the contribution of gut microbiota to the regulation of lipid metabolism in HEE by using a HFD that induces NAFLD and a pseudo-bacteria-free mouse model caused by antibiotics, thus laying the foundation for future clinical studies.

2. Materials and Methods

2.1. Preparation of Hawthorn Ethanol Extract (HEE)

Initially, fresh hawthorn fruits were carefully broken and ground before undergoing drying at a controlled temperature of 45 °C until a fine powder was obtained. Subsequently, the dried powder was subjected to extraction with water at 50 °C, followed by concentration and another drying process. To further refine the extract, it underwent an additional three rounds of extraction using 95% ethanol, resulting in the final product known as HEE. The main active ingredients were detected by HPLC-MS as organic acids and flavonoids, with 252.4 μg of citric acid, 61.5 μg of hawthorn acid, 79.3 μg of caffeic acid, 1,225 μg of catechins, 145.5 μg of quercetin, 34.5 μg of hyperoside, and 14.2 μg of apigenin8-C-glucoside per gram of fresh fruit.

2.2. Animal Experiments

Male 5-week-old SPF-grade C57BL/6/J mice were purchased from Vital River Laboratories located in Beijing, China. Mice were randomized into normal dietary control groups after the acclimatization period. After an acclimatization period, mice were randomly divided into a normal-flora control group (NFNDC, TP 23300, Trophic Animal Feed High-Tech Co., Ltd., Nantong, China. The composition of high-fat feed is shown in

Table S1) and four high-fat diet model groups (NFHFD, normal flora model. NFHFDHEE, normal flora HEE. PGHFD, pseudo germ-free model. PGHFDHEE, pseudo germ-free HEE. 60% fat diet TP 23302, Trophic Animal Feed High-Tech Co., Ltd., China) of six mice each and fed for 16 weeks. The dose of HEE was set at 150 mg/kg, a dosage proven to have minimal side effects, thus selected as the optimal dose for the experiment. HEE was dissolved in 0.5% carboxymethyl cellulose (CMC; National Medicines Corporation Chemical Reagent Co., Ltd., Shanghai, China) to prepare the gavage solution. Two of the high-fat diet groups (PGHFD and PGHFDHEE groups) underwent antibiotic treatment for two weeks, during which the PGHFDHEE group and NFHFDHEE group were orally administered 150 mg/kg HEE daily for 4 consecutive weeks, following the antibiotic treatment. The other two groups of mice (NFHFD group and PGHFD group) and the NFNDC group received an equivalent dose of 0.5% CMC. Food consumption, body weight, and fasting blood glucose levels were measured weekly. At week 16, the mice were euthanized, and mouse feces were collected the day before. In a controlled environment, mouse blood was drawn under dim light conditions and allowed to clot for 60 min at 25 °C. The blood was then centrifuged at $3000\times g$ for 10 min. Subsequently, the serum was separated and stored in a deep-freeze reservoir at a temperature of −80 °C for subsequent analyses. Liver and epididymal fat weights were recorded. Fecal and tissue samples were stored at −80 °C for further analysis. All animal experimental protocols in this study were reviewed by the Animal Ethics Committee and accurately implemented during use, and the entire experimental process was carried out with animal ethics in mind.

2.3. Pseudo-Germfree Mice (PG) Treated with Antibiotics

After a 10-week period on an HFD, two groups of mice from the HFD regimen (PGHFD and PGHFDHEE) were exposed to antibiotic therapy involving a combination of vancomycin (3.125 g), ampicillin (6.25 g), metronidazole (6.25 g), and neomycin (6.25 g) dissolved in 500 mL of saline, delivered via gavage at a dosage of 10 mg per mouse daily [21]. Throughout this intervention, changes in body weight and food consumption were carefully monitored, and fecal specimens were obtained. Following a two-week period post-antibiotic treatment, the PGHFDHEE and NFHFDHEE groups were subjected to a 4-week intervention with HEE extract.

2.4. Histopathological Analysis of Animals

Some fresh epididymal fat was fixed by a 4% solution of paraformaldehyde with phosphate-buffered saline, maintained at 4 °C for a period ranging from 2 to 4 h, before being encased in paraffin, after which it was cut into 10 μm sections. The sections were then subjected to staining procedures using hematoxylin and eosin (H&E) for histological examination. Liver tissues were immediately frozen in liquid nitrogen for further oil red O staining. These cryosections were then cut into 10-micron slices at low temperatures and stained with oil red O to assess lipid accumulation. The imagery of the stained tissue sections was captured employing a digital slide scanning system, and the subsequent analysis was conducted using ImagePro Plus v6.0 software to quantify and evaluate the staining results.

2.5. Mouse Serum Indicator Assay

The concentrations of serum biochemical markers, including TG, TC, LDL-c, HDL-c, ALT, and AST, alkaline phosphatase (ALP), and cholinesterase (CHE), were quantified utilizing an automated biochemical analysis device (Mindray BS-480; Mindray, Shenzhen, China). Serum cytokines were obtained according to the appropriate kit instructions.

Serum levels of TNF-α, IL-6, LBP, and LPS were measured using ELISA kits (SenBeiJia Biological Technology Co., Ltd., Nanjing, China) according to the kit instructions.

2.6. Quantitative Reverse Transcription–Polymerase Chain Reaction (qRT-PCR) Analysis

Total RNA was extracted from colon and liver tissues using TRIzol reagent (Invitrogen, Carlsbad, CA, USA). Subsequent to the isolation, RNA integrity was assessed, ensuring that each RNA sample (1 μg) met the requisite purity and concentration criteria for further processing. Then, these samples were reverse-transcribed into complementary DNA (cDNA) using HiScript III-RT SuperMix (+gDNA wiper; Vazyme, Nanjing, China). For a qualitative assessment of gene expression, the polymerase chain reaction (PCR) was employed alongside agarose gel electrophoresis. This step provided a visual confirmation of the specific amplification and integrity of the target transcripts. The gel electrophoresis enabled the verification of the expected size of PCR products, serving as a preliminary validation of the amplification specificity and efficiency.

Advancing to quantitative analysis, quantitative PCR (qPCR) was executed on a CFX Connect real-time PCR detection system (Bio-Rad, Hercules, CA, USA). The qPCR assay was optimized to ensure specificity, efficiency, and reproducibility, employing SYBR Green or TaqMan probes for the detection of the amplification products. Gene expression was quantified using the $2^{-\Delta\Delta Ct}$ method, thus providing a relative expression level of the gene of interest. Primer sequences for qPCR are shown in Supplementary Table S2.

2.7. Gut Microbiota Analysis

The MP Stool Genomic DNA Extraction Kit was used to extract total DNA from mouse feces. PCR amplification of the 16S rDNA V3-V4 heavy region was performed according to the instructions, in 50 μL of reaction mixture (including 25 μL of 2× TaqMasterMix solution, 1 μL of each primer, 1 μL of template, and 22 μL of ddH_2O (BasalMedia Co., Ltd., Shanghai, China)), using this DNA as a template with the universal primer 341F/806R. The PCR products were purified using nucleic acid gel electrophoresis and a DNA Gel Purification Kit. The concentration of purified products was measured with the Qubit™ dsDNA BR Assay Kit, and libraries were prepared using the TruSeq DNA LT Sample Preparation Kit for sequencing on the Illumina MiSeq system. Data analysis was conducted using the QIIME2 platform with the DADA2 plugin, and by annotating species using the q2-feature-classifier plugin with the Silva database reference. Microbial diversity was assessed using the q2-diversity plugin, with alpha diversity indicated by observed OTUs and Faith's PD indices, and beta diversity analyzed through PCoA based on Bray–Curtis distances among samples [22,23] (all the kits were purchased from Enzyme Exemption Industry Co., Ltd., Yancheng, Jiangsu, China).

2.8. Analysis of Short-Chain Fatty Acids

Intestinal content samples were freeze-dried to eliminate moisture. Approximately 50 mg of the dried material was mixed with 500 μL of saturated NaCl and 20 μL of 15.84 mmol/L 2-ethylbutyric acid, shaken after a 30 min soak for full dissolution. The mixture was then acidified with 40 μL of 10% sulfuric acid and vortexed for even blending, followed by the addition of 1 mL pre-chilled ether, and vortexed again. After centrifugation at 10,000× *g* at 4 °C for 15 min, the supernatant was transferred to a new tube. Moisture was removed with 0.25 g of anhydrous sodium sulfate, and the sample was centrifuged again. The aliquot of the clear supernatant was prepared for GC-MS analysis. Samples were analyzed using a GC-MS system (QP2010 Ultra, SHIMADZU, Kyoto, Japan) with an Rtx-Wax column. The setup involved an inlet temperature of 240 °C, an oven starting at 100 °C, helium as the carrier gas, and specific pressures and flow rates to ensure accurate readings. The temperature was gradually increased from 100 °C to 200 °C following a specific program. Various SCFAs were detected using a selected ion monitoring mode in the mass spectrometer, set between 2 and 100 (m/z) [24].

2.9. Statistical Analysis

The data were reported as mean values accompanied by standard deviations. An analysis of the data obtained from the animal experiments was conducted utilizing one-way analysis of variance (ANOVA). Post hoc multiple comparisons among the groups were carried out employing Dunnett's test. In all statistical analyses, a significance level with a confidence interval of 95% or $p < 0.05$ was used as the critical value for determining statistical significance.

3. Results

3.1. The Mitigating Effect of HEE on HFD-Induced NAFLD in Mice

We evaluated the impact of HEE on mice suffering from NAFLD induced by HFD. The daily food intake, body weight, liver mass, and blood glucose levels of five mouse groups were monitored (Figure 1). No significant pattern changes were observed in food consumption among the groups (Figure 1B). However, both body and liver weights decreased after HEE treatment, regardless of whether in a normal microbiota environment or under antibiotic treatment (Figure 1C,F). By comparing the weight gain, it can be seen that the model mice gained significantly more weight than the control mice, and in the HEE intervention, mice gained significantly less weight than the model mice (Figure 1C,D). Similar ameliorative effects were observed for the liver-to-body weight ratio and fasting blood glucose levels (Figure 1G,H). Nonetheless, the regulatory effects were not significant in the antibiotic-treated groups, predicting that the disruption of the intestinal flora by antibiotics might have affected the efficacy of HEE.

Figure 2A,B show sections of the liver with oil red-O staining and epididymal fat H&E, which indicated that lipid accumulation in the liver and epididymal fat were significantly reduced in the HEE group compared with the non-HEE group. Serum biochemical markers indicated that HEE improved liver function, significantly decreased ALT and AST levels in the NFHFD and PGHFD groups, and helped to regulate alkaline phosphatase (ALP) levels in the NFHFD group, although it did not significantly improve cholinesterase (CHE) levels (Figure 2C–F). Therefore, HEE effectively modulates lipid accumulation and liver function in HFD mice.

3.2. Modulation of Lipid Profile and Inflammation-Related Cytokines by HEE in HFD Mice

A high-fat diet causes dyslipidemia and inflammatory responses in the organism, so we further investigated the modulatory effects of HEE on serum lipids and inflammation-associated cytokines in HFD mice. Our findings reveal that, in comparison to the high-fat diet group, HEE significantly reduces the levels of serum TG, TC, and LDL-c, irrespective of the presence of a normal microbiota or an antibiotic-treated environment. Additionally, HEE notably increased the level of HDL-c in the NFHFDHEE group. This indicates HEE's potential in modulating lipid profiles and inflammatory responses in the context of dietary-induced hyperlipidemia (Figure 3A–D).

Systemic inflammation in NAFLD mice and the therapeutic effect of HEE were investigated by detecting cytokines in serum (Figure 3E–H). We observed that HEE effectively modulated the levels of tumor necrosis factors α (TNFα), endotoxin lipopolysaccharide (LPS), and lipopolysaccharide binding protein (LBP) in the NFHFDHEE group, while significantly alleviating the levels of LPS and interleukin-6 (IL-6) in the PGHFD group. Consequently, HEE has shown its beneficial effects by reducing the inflammatory response induced by a high-fat diet, thereby decreasing the liver's susceptibility to the effects of endotoxins. This underscores HEE's therapeutic potential in ameliorating diet-induced hepatic inflammation.

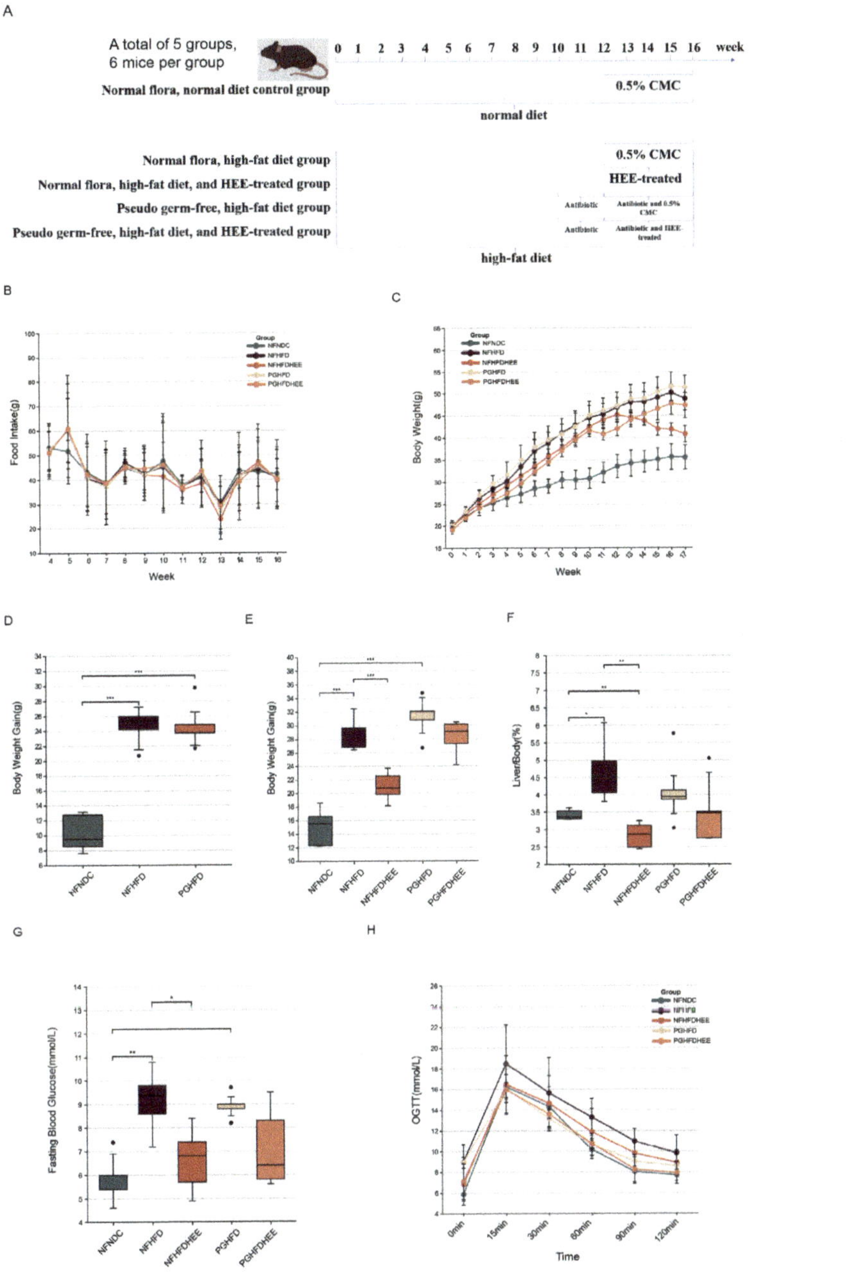

Figure 1. Effects of HEE on appetite, body weight, and blood glucose in high-fat-diet mice. (**A**) Animal experiment process. (**B**) Food intake in mice aged 4 to 16 weeks. (**C**) The body weights of mice in each group were recorded weekly from 0 to 16 weeks. (**D**) Establishment of a model for mouse food intake from 0 to 10 weeks. (**E**) Body weight gain during the intervention. (**F**) Liver-to-body weight ratio (100%). (**G**) Fasting blood glucose in mice at week 16. (**H**) Oral glucose tolerance of mice in each group. Data are shown as mean ± SD. (For each group, n = 5, * $p < 0.05$; ** $p < 0.01$; *** $p < 0.001$). The black dots in the graph indicate the values detected for each sample.

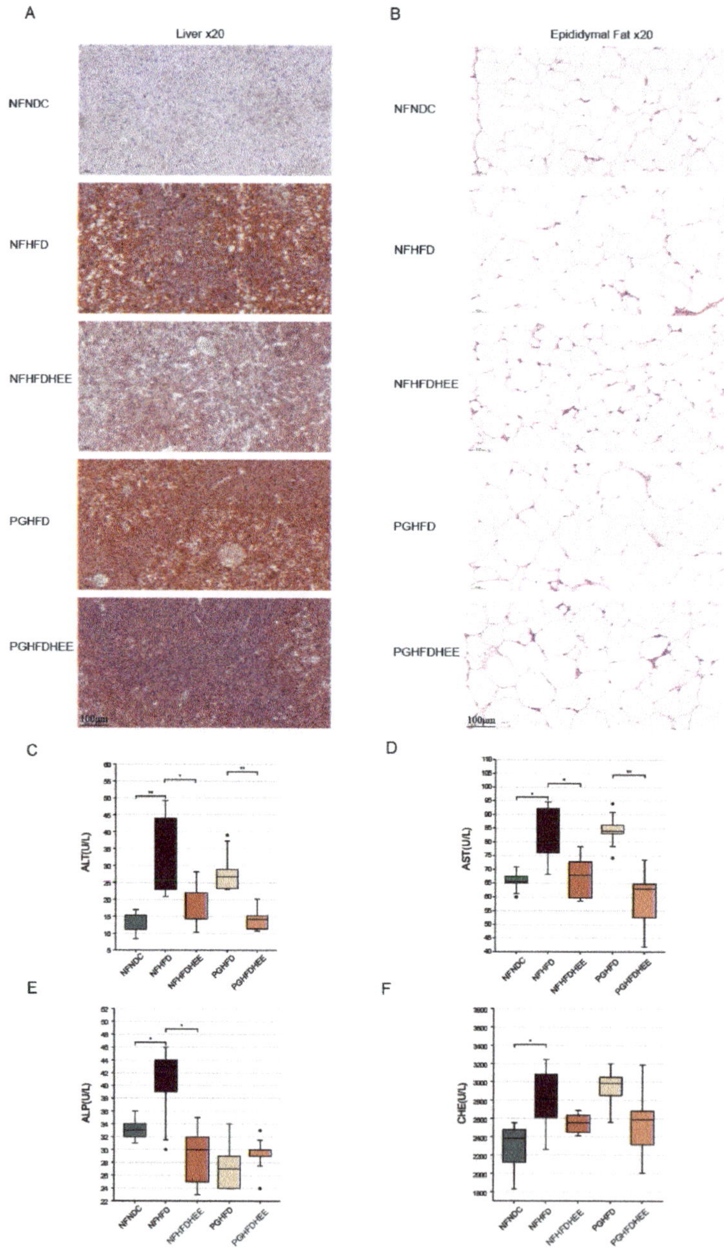

Figure 2. The effects of HEE on the liver function of high-fat-diet mice. (**A**) Oil red O-stained sections of the liver of mice in each group. (**B**) H&E-stained sections of epididymal fat from various groups of mice. (**C–F**) Serum biochemical indices in mice: alanine aminotransferase (ALT), glutamine aminotransferase (AST), alkaline phosphatase (ALP), and cholinesterase (CHE). Data are shown as mean ± SD. (For each group, n = 5, * $p < 0.05$; ** $p < 0.01$). The black dots in the graph indicate the values detected for each sample.

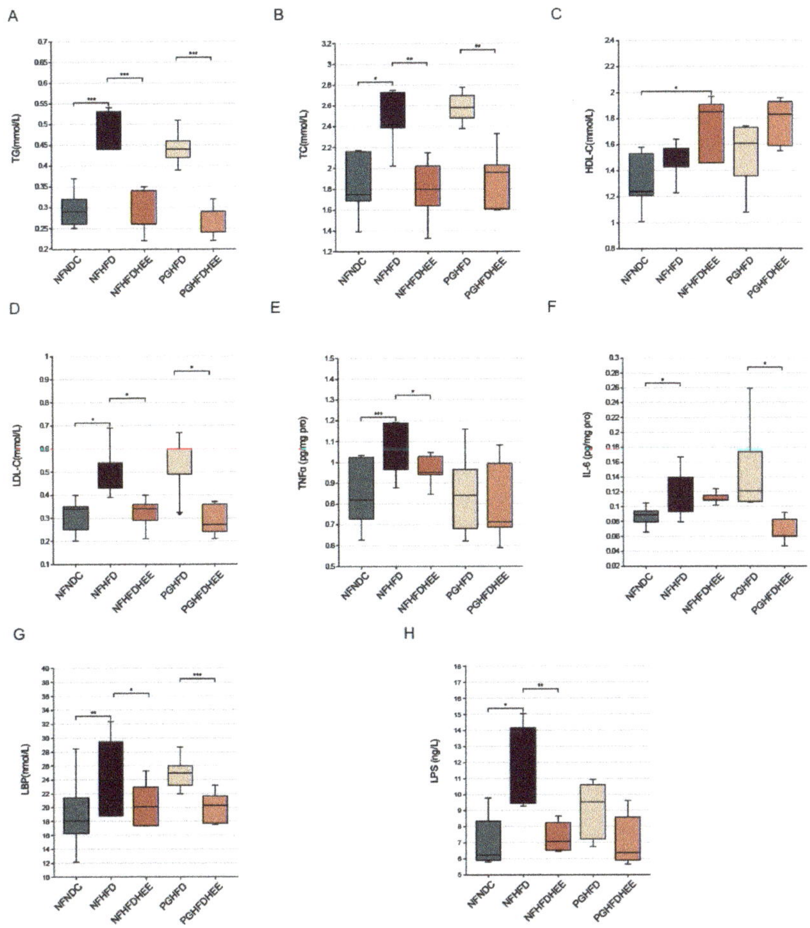

Figure 3. Effects of HEE on blood lipid levels and inflammation levels in mice. (**A–D**) Serum triglycerides (TG), serum total cholesterol (TC), high-density lipoprotein (HDL-c), and low-density lipoprotein (LDL-c) levels in all groups of mice. (**E–H**) Cytokine levels in mice of all groups: tumor necrosis factors α, interleukin-6, endotoxin lipopolysaccharide, and lipopolysaccharide binding protein. Data are shown as mean ± SD. (For each group, n = 5, * $p < 0.05$; ** $p < 0.01$; *** $p < 0.001$).

3.3. Effects of HEE on the Expression of Genes Related to Intestinal SCFAs and Hepatic Lipid Metabolism in Mice

Studies indicated that HFD alters the gut microbiome in the cecum and colon, increasing concentrations of SCFAs, such as propionate in the cecum and isovalerate and valerate in the colon. However, the concentration of SCFAs dropped significantly after antibiotic treatment, highlighting the crucial role of the gut microbiome (Figure 4A,C).

Through significant changes in liver and adipose tissue slices and glycerol triacylglycerol indicators, we further investigated the metabolic status of triglycerides in the liver. We selected key enzymes in the lipolytic process, such as adipose triglyceride lipase (ATGL), hormone-sensitive lipase (HSL), and monoacylglycerol lipase (MGL) in adipose tissue. Our results showed that ATGL and HSL gene expression was significantly activated in the NFHFDHEE group compared with the high-fat model group, whereas no significant changes were observed in the PG group. Interestingly, HEE similarly affected the activation of MGL in the PGHFDHEE group, promoting lipolysis (Figure 4B,D–F).

Thus, HEE promotes lipolysis in the liver and plays an important role in regulating hepatic lipid metabolism.

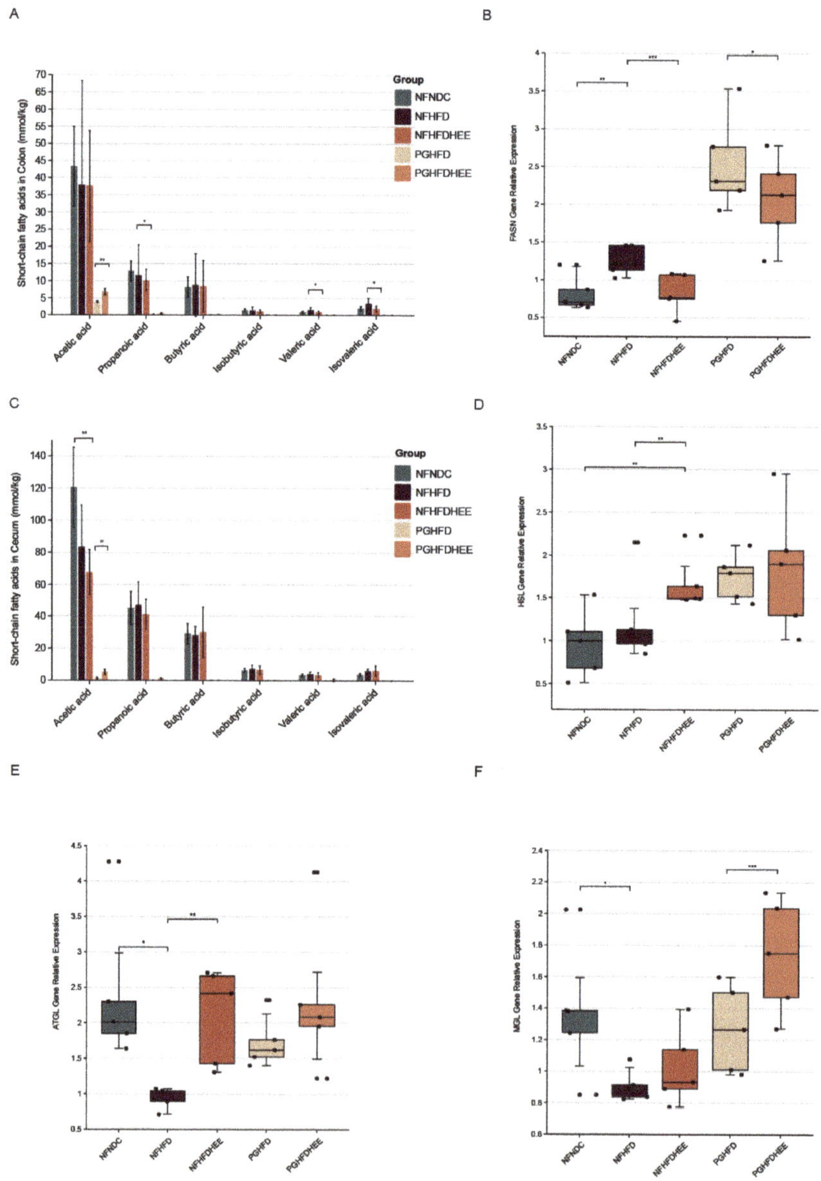

Figure 4. Regulation of short-chain fatty acids and hepatic lipid metabolism-related genes in the mouse intestine by HEE. (**A**) SCFAs in the colon. (**B**) FASN gene expression in liver. (**C**) SCFAs in the cecum. (**D**) HSL gene expression in liver. (**E**) ATGL gene expression in the liver. (**F**) MGL gene expression in the liver. Data are shown as mean ± SD. (For each group, n = 5, * $p < 0.05$; ** $p < 0.01$; *** $p < 0.001$). The black dots in the graph indicate the values detected for each sample.

3.4. HEE Modulates the Gut Microbiota in HFD Mice

To investigate the modulatory effects of HEE on the gut microbiota of high-fat-diet-fed mice, we assessed changes in fecal microbial community structure after the administration of HEE using 16S rRNA analysis. The treatment notably adjusted the prevalence of Bacteroidetes and Firmicutes within the NFHFDHEE group, elevating *Bacteroidetes* quantities to similar levels as those observed in the control group, as illustrated in Figure 5A,B. This adjustment is further reflected by the *Bacteroidetes*-to-*Firmicutes* ratio. Among the antibiotic-treated cohort, *Verrucomicrobia* dominance was observed, which was marked by reduced microbial diversity and lower abundance.

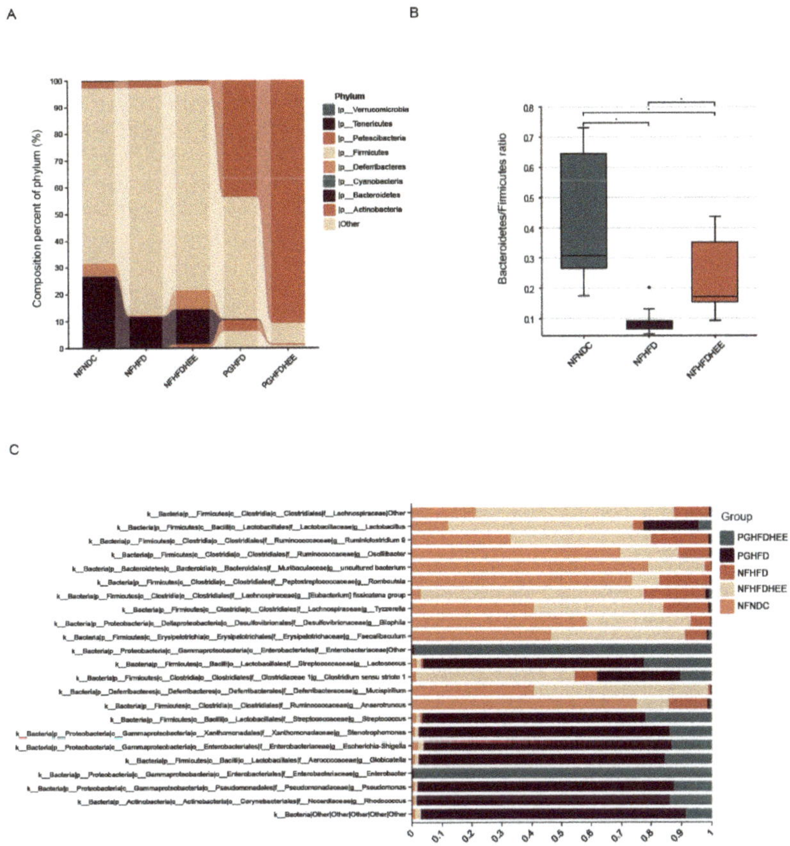

Figure 5. Regulatory effects of HEE on the gut microbiota of mice subjected to a high-fat diet. (**A**) The impact of HEE on the phylum level of gut microbiota in high-fat-diet mice. (**B**) The effects of HEE on *Bacteroidetes* and *Firmicutes* in the intestines. (**C**) Effect of HEE on the diversity of intestinal flora of mice at the genus level. Data are shown as mean ± SD. (For each group, n = 5, * $p < 0.05$).

We further delved into the alterations at the genus level within the gut microbiota, as depicted in Figure 5C, showcasing the proportional distribution of dominant bacterial genera across five groups. The gut microbiota composition of SPF-maintained normal mice starkly contrasted with that of pseudo-germ-free mice treated with antibiotics (PG). Notably, in the NFHFDHEE group, genera such as unidentified *Lachnospiraceae*, *Lactobacillus*, the *[Eubacterium] fissicatena group*, *Ruminiclostridium 9*, and *Romboutsia* predominated, suggesting their pivotal physiological roles—a trend similarly observed in the NFNDC group. Conversely, the PG group harbored various potentially pathogenic genera like *Streptococcus*,

Stenotrophomonas, *Enterobacter*, *Enterobacteriaceae*, and *Escherichia-Shigella*. This phenomenon hints at the vulnerability of the gut microbial environment after antibiotic treatment and emphasizes the critical role of microbial diversity in maintaining the integrity of the gut barrier.

In summary, HEE possesses the ability to modulate the composition of the gut microbiota by promoting the prevalence of beneficial genera.

We investigated the recovery after antibiotic treatment, the lipid-lowering effect of microorganisms, and the modulation of gut flora by HEE through a comprehensive analysis of the diversity of gut flora. This was achieved through a principal coordinates analysis (PCoA) of intestinal samples from various mouse groups (Figure 6A). The results revealed that NFNDC and NFHFD groups displayed slight separation along the PCO3 axis in PCoA, while NFHFDHEE showed significant divergence, indicating the efficacy of HEE in modulating gut microbiota diversity. Post-antibiotic treatment, the PGHFD group significantly diverged from the normal group along the PCO2 axis, indicating a significant change in the gut microbiota of the PG group due to the antibiotic. Principal component analysis (PCA) further highlighted distinctions between NFNDC and NFHFD groups along PC2, signifying the non-negligible effect of the HFD on the gut microbiota of mice (Figure 6B). Moreover, samples from the NFHFDHEE group showed differentiation from NFHFD along PC1, predicting the effects of the diet and HEE treatments on microbial community structure.

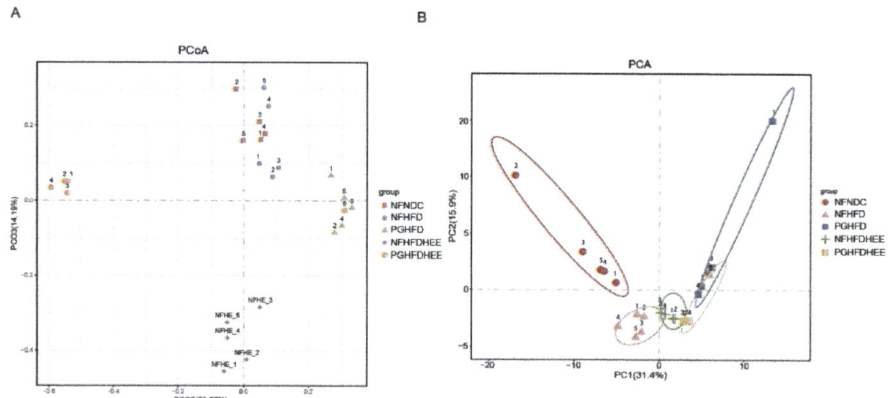

Figure 6. Modulation of intestinal species diversity in mice by HEE. (**A**) Principal co-ordinates analysis (PCoA) in the intestines of each group of mice. (**B**) PCA (principal component analysis) is applied in various groups of mouse intestines.

Finally, we utilized a heatmap for cluster analysis and inter-group differential comparison (Supplementary Figure S1), identifying bacterial genera with relatively higher abundance in the intestinal microbiota of different mouse groups, aiming to discern patterns. In the heatmap, the central yellow section highlights significant bacterial genera in the PG group, including previously mentioned genera such as *Streptococcus*, *Stenotrophomonas*, *Enterobacter*, *Enterobacteriaceae*, and *Escherichia-Shigella*. These genera cluster together, forming a large group. Similarly, the elevated yellow section in the top-left corner represents the NF group post-HEE intervention, where genera like unidentified *Lachnospiraceae*, *Lactobacillus*, the *[Eubacterium] fissicatena* group, *Ruminiclostridium 9*, and *Romboutsia* also cluster into a large group. The distance between these two clusters is notably significant. The impacts of a high-fat diet, interventions by HEE, and antibiotic treatments have evidently contributed to the diverse composition of gut microbiota among different groups. HEE has been found to promote an increase in the abundance of beneficial microorganisms.

4. Discussion

The results for food intake and body weight (Figure 1) indicate that after 11–12 weeks of antibiotic treatment, the mice experienced a slowdown in weight gain, which then resumed after week 13 in the PGHFD group. This may be related to the use of high-dose quad antibiotics in the short term. Although there was a downward trend in weight gain, liver-to-body weight ratio, and blood glucose levels in the PGHFDHEE group, it was not significant. The difference between PGHFDHEE and NFHFDHEE was solely the involvement of the gut microbiota, revealing the potential impact of the gut microbiota on the weight loss and blood sugar reduction effects of HEE. Studies have shown a strong relationship between gut flora and obesity and blood sugar, and gut flora management has emerged as a new way to treat obesity [25]. Understanding the causal relationship between the gut microbiome and metabolic risk may help us to identify susceptible individuals for early, targeted intervention [26].

Liver and epididymal fat sections, along with liver function indicators (Figure 2), show that while HEE has a certain alleviating effect on the liver of HFD mice in the PG group, the effect is not significant, aligning closely with the observations mentioned earlier. Regarding lipid profiles and inflammatory markers, HEE contributes similarly across groups, effectively regulating blood lipids and suppressing inflammation to some extent (Figure 3). However, there are differences in emphasis between the NF and PG groups in terms of indicators; in the PG group, after HEE intervention, acetic acid levels rise while other fatty acid concentrations remain low, likely due to the antibiotic-induced depletion of the gut microbiota [27].

Several studies have reported that numerous acetic acid-producing bacteria have the potential to prevent the development of NAFLD [28]. In contrast, the NF group exhibited a decreasing trend in the levels of acetic and propionic acids in the cecum and colon, with concentrations in the cecum being 2–3 times higher than those in the colon. Additionally, significant changes in the levels of valeric acid and isovaleric acid were observed. In the cecum, the level of valeric acid was relatively high, and the promotional effect of HEE on valeric acid production could likely be due to an increased relative abundance of acid-producing bacterial populations. Studies have shown that *Lactobacillus acidophilus* can inhibit hepatocellular carcinoma associated with NAFLD by producing valeric acid [29].

In terms of regulating the gut microbiota, HEE adjusted the proportions of the *Bacteroidetes* and *Firmicutes* phyla and also modulated the abundance at the genus level (Figures 5 and 6). It significantly increased the abundance of beneficial bacterial genera, including *Lactobacillus*, *Lachnospiraceae*, the *[Eubacterium] fissicatena* group, *Ruminiclostridium 9*, and *Romboutsia*. Conversely, some potentially harmful bacteria were also identified in the PG group, including *Streptococcus*, *Stenotrophomonas*, *Enterobacter*, *Enterobacteriaceae*, and *Escherichia-Shigella*. *Lactobacillus plantarum* offers protective benefits for HFD mice with NAFLD [30]. *Lactobacillus* rhamnosus regulates blood lipid levels and alleviates fatty liver by modulating a high-fat, high-cholesterol diet [31]. *Romboutsia* has the capability to modulate lipid metabolic functions in obese rats [32]. The *Lachnospiraceae* belongs to the phylum Firmicutes and is an important part of the intestinal microbial community. Members of this family are known for producing SCFAs, particularly butyrate and acetate, which are crucial for the host's gut health and immune system function [33]. *Ruminiclostridium* species, including *Ruminiclostridium 9*, are recognized for their capacity to ferment dietary fibers and other indigestible carbohydrates, resulting in an increased production of intestinal SCFAs, such as butyrate, acetate, and propionate. In contrast, HEE had no significant effect on the intestinal flora of PG mice, which may be attributed to the strong destructive effect of antibiotics on the intestinal flora, masking the effect of HEE on the intestinal flora, and the harmful bacterial genera became dominant in the fragile intestines of the PG mice. A species within the genus *Streptococcus* has been reported as a potential risk factor for NAFLD. This indicates a significant link between certain bacterial species and the development or exacerbation of NAFLD [34]. *Stenotrophomonas* is a Gram-negative bacteria that includes a spectrum of species, from those commonly found in soil and plants to opportunistic human pathogens like *Stenotrophomonas maltophilia*. However, certain strains of *S. maltophilia* are known to be pathogenic to humans, presenting challenges due to their multidrug-resistant profiles [35]. *Enterobacter* can induce liver inflammation and exacerbate lipid accumulation [36,37]. At the same time, *Enterobacteriaceae* also acts as a trigger for endotoxins in NAFLD [38]. HEE interventions prevented the wild growth of these harmful genera, increased the abundance of beneficial genera, and increased the diversity of the flora. Overall, HEE modulates the intestinal flora, which translates into a pattern that benefits the alleviation of non-alcoholic fatty liver. Meanwhile HEE's own effects still cannot be ignored. When the gut flora is disrupted, HEE is still able to alleviate NAFLD, although it is not as effective as when the gut flora is not disrupted.

5. Conclusions

In conclusion, our study demonstrated that HEE could effectively alleviate hepatic lipid accumulation, reduce blood lipids, and decrease the level of inflammation in both normal colony and pseudo sterile mice. HEE was able to regulate key enzymes involved in triglyceride catabolism to promote lipid metabolism, as well as inhibit the expression of fatty acid synthase and change the lipid metabolism pattern in the liver. Our study also highlights the effectiveness of HEE when the gut flora is disrupted and the potentiating effect of HEE modulation of the gut flora in normal flora for the treatment of NAFLD with HEE. HEE was found to affect the diversity of intestinal bacteria, improve the structure of the intestinal microbiota in mice, increase the level of beneficial bacterial species, and regulate the concentration of SCFAs in the intestinal tract. These beneficial effects were significantly reduced in PG mice. This study provides valuable insights into the efficacy and possible pathways of hawthorn in the treatment of NAFLD, which has a wide range of application scenarios as a common food ingredient. Future studies should focus on the exact components of hawthorn that alter the gut flora as well as the specific genera of gut flora with beneficial effects.

Supplementary Materials: The following supporting information can be downloaded at https://www.mdpi.com/article/10.3390/nu16091335/s1, Figure S1: Heatmap of cluster analysis for each asample; Table S1: Composition of diets; Table S2: Primer sequences used for real-time quantitative PCR.

Author Contributions: Conceptualization and methodology, T.W.; software and data curation, Y.D., H.X. and Y.S.; writing, J.H.; project administration, D.W.; supervision, Y.Z. All authors have read and agreed to the published version of the manuscript.

Funding: This research was funded by the Science and Technology Projects of Jilin Provincial Department of Education (JJKH20210617KJ) and the Science and Technology Development Project Foundation of Jilin Province (20210203179SF).

Institutional Review Board Statement: The animal study protocol was approved by the Animal Care Ethics Committee of the Changchun University of Traditional Chinese Medicine (protocol code 2021506 on 16 November 2021).

Informed Consent Statement: Not applicable.

Data Availability Statement: All data presented in this study are available in the main body of the manuscript.

Conflicts of Interest: This work has not been published previously and the authors declare no conflicts of interest.

References

1. Friedman, S.L.; Neuschwander-Tetri, B.A.; Rinella, M.; Sanyal, A.J. Mechanisms of NAFLD development and therapeutic strategies. *Nat. Med.* **2018**, *24*, 908–922. [CrossRef]
2. Aron-Wisnewsky, J.; Vigliotti, C.; Witjes, J.; Le, P.; Holleboom, A.G.; Verheij, J.; Nieuwdorp, M.; Clément, K. Gut microbiota and human NAFLD: Disentangling microbial signatures from metabolic disorders. *Nat. Rev. Gastroenterol. Hepatol.* **2020**, *17*, 279–297. [CrossRef]

3. Hrncir, T.; Hrncirova, L.; Kverka, M.; Hromadka, R.; Machova, V.; Trckova, E.; Kostovcikova, K.; Kralickova, P.; Krejsek, J.; Tlaskalova-Hogenova, H. Gut microbiota and NAFLD: Pathogenetic mechanisms, microbiota signatures, and therapeutic interventions. *Microorganisms* **2021**, *9*, 957. [CrossRef] [PubMed]
4. Yang, J.; Wei, H.; Zhou, Y.; Szeto, C.-H.; Li, C.; Lin, Y.; Coker, O.O.; Lau, H.C.H.; Chan, A.W.; Sung, J.J. High-fat diet promotes colorectal tumorigenesis through modulating gut microbiota and metabolites. *Gastroenterology* **2022**, *162*, 135–149.e2. [CrossRef]
5. Velázquez, K.T.; Enos, R.T.; Bader, J.E.; Sougiannis, A.T.; Carson, M.S.; Chatzistamou, I.; Carson, J.A.; Nagarkatti, P.S.; Nagarkatti, M.; Murphy, E.A. Prolonged high-fat-diet feeding promotes non-alcoholic fatty liver disease and alters gut microbiota in mice. *World J. Hepatol.* **2019**, *11*, 619. [CrossRef] [PubMed]
6. Kang, H.; You, H.J.; Lee, G.; Lee, S.H.; Yoo, T.; Choi, M.; Joo, S.K.; Park, J.H.; Chang, M.S.; Lee, D.H. Interaction effect between NAFLD severity and high carbohydrate diet on gut microbiome alteration and hepatic de novo lipogenesis. *Gut Microbes* **2022**, *14*, 2078612. [CrossRef] [PubMed]
7. He, J.; Zhang, P.; Shen, L.; Niu, L.; Tan, Y.; Chen, L.; Zhao, Y.; Bai, L.; Hao, X.; Li, X. Short-chain fatty acids and their association with signalling pathways in inflammation, glucose and lipid metabolism. *Int. J. Mol. Sci.* **2020**, *21*, 6356. [CrossRef] [PubMed]
8. Ma, J.; Piao, X.; Mahfuz, S.; Long, S.; Wang, J. The interaction among gut microbes, the intestinal barrier and short chain fatty acids. *Anim. Nutr.* **2022**, *9*, 159–174. [CrossRef]
9. Perumpail, B.J.; Li, A.A.; John, N.; Sallam, S.; Shah, N.D.; Kwong, W.; Cholankeril, G.; Kim, D.; Ahmed, A. The therapeutic implications of the gut microbiome and probiotics in patients with NAFLD. *Diseases* **2019**, *7*, 27. [CrossRef]
10. Carpi, R.Z.; Barbalho, S.M.; Sloan, K.P.; Laurindo, L.F.; Gonzaga, H.F.; Grippa, P.C.; Zutin, T.L.M.; Girio, R.J.; Repetti, C.S.F.; Detregiachi, C.R.P. The effects of probiotics, prebiotics and synbiotics in non-alcoholic fat liver disease (NAFLD) and non-alcoholic steatohepatitis (NASH): A systematic review. *Int. J. Mol. Sci.* **2022**, *23*, 8805. [CrossRef]
11. Ferolla, S.M.; de Almeida Armiliato, G.N.; Couto, C.A.; Ferrari, T.C.A. Probiotics as a complementary therapeutic approach in nonalcoholic fatty liver disease. *World J. Hepatol.* **2015**, *7*, 559. [CrossRef]
12. Elshaghabee, F.M.; Rokana, N.; Panwar, H.; Heller, K.J.; Schrezenmeir, J. Probiotics for dietary management of non-alcoholic fatty liver disease. *Environ. Chem. Lett.* **2019**, *17*, 1553–1563. [CrossRef]
13. Hou, Y.; Gu, D.; Peng, J.; Jiang, K.; Li, Z.; Shi, J.; Yang, S.; Li, S.; Fan, X. Ginsenoside Rg1 regulates liver lipid factor metabolism in NAFLD model rats. *ACS Omega* **2020**, *5*, 10878–10890. [CrossRef]
14. Zhong, D.; Xie, Z.; Huang, B.; Zhu, S.; Wang, G.; Zhou, H.; Lin, S.; Lin, Z.; Yang, B. Ganoderma lucidum polysaccharide peptide alleviates hepatoteatosis via modulating bile acid metabolism dependent on FXR-SHP/FGF. *Cell. Physiol. Biochem.* **2018**, *49*, 1204–1220. [CrossRef]
15. Fontes, A.; Ramalho-Santos, J.; Zischka, H.; Azul, A.M. Mushrooms on the plate: Trends towards NAFLD treatment, health improvement and sustainable diets. *Eur. J. Clin. Investig.* **2022**, *52*, e13667. [CrossRef] [PubMed]
16. Lien, H.-M.; Lin, H.-T.; Huang, S.-H.; Chen, Y.-R.; Huang, C.-L.; Chen, C.-C.; Chyau, C.-C. Protective Effect of Hawthorn Fruit Extract against High Fructose-Induced Oxidative Stress and Endoplasmic Reticulum Stress in Pancreatic β-Cells. *Foods* **2023**, *12*, 1130. [CrossRef] [PubMed]
17. Lu, M.; Zhang, L.; Pan, J.; Shi, H.; Zhang, M.; Li, C. Advances in the study of vascular protective effects and molecular mechanisms of hawthorn (*Crataegus anamesa* Sarg.) extracts in cardiovascular diseases. *Food Funct.* **2023**, *14*, 5870–5890. [CrossRef]
18. Wang, Y.; Guo, Y.; Liu, H.; Du, X.; Shi, L.; Wang, W.; Zhang, S. Hawthorn fruit extract protect against MC-LR-induced hepatotoxicity by attenuating oxidative stress and apoptosis. *Environ. Toxicol.* **2023**, *38*, 1239–1250. [CrossRef] [PubMed]
19. Zhang, M.; Zhu, S.; Yang, W.; Huang, Q.; Ho, C.-T. The biological fate and bioefficacy of citrus flavonoids: Bioavailability, biotransformation, and delivery systems. *Food Funct.* **2021**, *12*, 3307–3323. [CrossRef]
20. Zhao, J.; Yang, J.; Xie, Y. Improvement strategies for the oral bioavailability of poorly water-soluble flavonoids: An overview. *Int. J. Pharm.* **2019**, *570*, 118642. [CrossRef]
21. Zuo, F.; Nakamura, N.; Akao, T.; Hattori, M. Pharmacokinetics of berberine and its main metabolites in conventional and pseudo germ-free rats determined by liquid chromatography/ion trap mass spectrometry. *Drug Metab. Dispos.* **2006**, *34*, 2064–2072. [CrossRef]
22. Bolyen, E.; Rideout, J.R.; Dillon, M.R.; Bokulich, N.A.; Abnet, C.C.; Al-Ghalith, G.A.; Alexander, H.; Alm, E.J.; Arumugam, M.; Asnicar, F. Reproducible, interactive, scalable and extensible microbiome data science using QIIME 2. *Nat. Biotechnol.* **2019**, *37*, 852–857. [CrossRef]
23. Estaki, M.; Jiang, L.; Bokulich, N.A.; McDonald, D.; González, A.; Kosciolek, T.; Martino, C.; Zhu, Q.; Birmingham, A.; Vázquez-Baeza, Y. QIIME 2 enables comprehensive end-to-end analysis of diverse microbiome data and comparative studies with publicly available data. *Curr. Protoc. Bioinform.* **2020**, *70*, e100. [CrossRef]
24. Wang, B.; Kong, Q.; Li, X.; Zhao, J.; Zhang, H.; Chen, W.; Wang, G. A high-fat diet increases gut microbiota biodiversity and energy expenditure due to nutrient difference. *Nutrients* **2020**, *12*, 3197. [CrossRef]
25. Bianchi, F.; Duque, A.L.R.F.; Saad, S.M.I.; Sivieri, K. Gut microbiome approaches to treat obesity in humans. *Appl. Microbiol. Biotechnol.* **2019**, *103*, 1081–1094. [CrossRef] [PubMed]
26. Cunningham, A.; Stephens, J.; Harris, D. Gut microbiota influence in type 2 diabetes mellitus (T2DM). *Gut Pathog.* **2021**, *13*, 50. [CrossRef] [PubMed]
27. Crotti, E.; Rizzi, A.; Chouaia, B.; Ricci, I.; Favia, G.; Alma, A.; Sacchi, L.; Bourtzis, K.; Mandrioli, M.; Cherif, A. Acetic acid bacteria, newly emerging symbionts of insects. *Appl. Environ. Microbiol.* **2010**, *76*, 6963–6970. [CrossRef] [PubMed]

28. Hong, Y.; Sheng, L.; Zhong, J.; Tao, X.; Zhu, W.; Ma, J.; Yan, J.; Zhao, A.; Zheng, X.; Wu, G. Desulfovibrio vulgaris, a potent acetic acid-producing bacterium, attenuates nonalcoholic fatty liver disease in mice. *Gut Microbes* **2021**, *13*, 1930874.
29. Lau, H.C.-H.; Zhang, X.; Ji, F.; Lin, Y.; Liang, W.; Li, Q.; Chen, D.; Fong, W.; Kang, X.; Liu, W. *Lactobacillus acidophilus* suppresses non-alcoholic fatty liver disease-associated hepatocellular carcinoma through producing valeric acid. *eBioMedicine* **2024**, *100*, 104952. [CrossRef]
30. Chen, M.; Guo, W.-L.; Li, Q.-Y.; Xu, J.-X.; Cao, Y.-J.; Liu, B.; Yu, X.-D.; Rao, P.-F.; Ni, L.; Lv, X.-C. The protective mechanism of *Lactobacillus plantarum* FZU3013 against non-alcoholic fatty liver associated with hyperlipidemia in mice fed a high-fat diet. *Food Funct.* **2020**, *11*, 3316–3331. [CrossRef]
31. Wang, G.; Jiao, T.; Xu, Y.; Li, D.; Si, Q.; Hao, J.; Zhao, J.; Zhang, H.; Chen, W. *Bifidobacterium adolescentis* and *Lactobacillus rhamnosus* alleviate non-alcoholic fatty liver disease induced by a high-fat, high-cholesterol diet through modulation of different gut microbiota-dependent pathways. *Food Funct.* **2020**, *11*, 6115–6127. [CrossRef] [PubMed]
32. Yin, H.; Huang, J.; Guo, X.; Xia, J.; Hu, M. Romboutsia lituseburensis JCM1404 supplementation ameliorated endothelial function via gut microbiota modulation and lipid metabolisms alterations in obese rats. *FEMS Microbiol. Lett.* **2023**, *370*, fnad016. [CrossRef] [PubMed]
33. Amiri, P.; Hosseini, S.A.; Ghaffari, S.; Tutunchi, H.; Ghaffari, S.; Mosharkesh, E.; Asghari, S.; Roshanravan, N. Role of butyrate, a gut microbiota derived metabolite, in cardiovascular diseases: A comprehensive narrative review. *Front. Pharmacol.* **2022**, *12*, 4178. [CrossRef] [PubMed]
34. Jia, B.; Kim, K.H.; Ruan, W.; Kim, H.M.; Jeon, C.O. Lantibiotic-encoding Streptococcus in the human microbiome are underlying risk factors for liver diseases. *J. Infect.* **2022**, *84*, e70–e72. [CrossRef] [PubMed]
35. Kim, Y.J.; Jeon, H.; Na, S.H.; Kwon, H.I.; Selasi, G.N.; Nicholas, A.; Park, T.I.; Lee, S.H.; Lee, J.C. *Stenotrophomonas maltophilia* outer membrane vesicles elicit a potent inflammatory response in vitro and in vivo. *FEMS Pathog. Dis.* **2016**, *74*, ftw104. [CrossRef] [PubMed]
36. Jin, M.; Zheng, L.; Wei, Y.; Cheng, J.; Zhang, D.; Yan, S.; Qin, H.; Wang, Q.; Ci, X.; Feng, H. *Enterobacter cloacae* aggravates metabolic disease by inducing inflammation and lipid accumulation. *Environ. Toxicol. Pharmacol.* **2022**, *90*, 103819. [CrossRef]
37. Keskitalo, A.; Munukka, E.; Toivonen, R.; Hollmén, M.; Kainulainen, H.; Huovinen, P.; Jalkanen, S.; Pekkala, S. *Enterobacter cloacae* administration induces hepatic damage and subcutaneous fat accumulation in high-fat diet fed mice. *PLoS ONE* **2018**, *13*, e0198262. [CrossRef]
38. Fei, N.; Bruneau, A.; Zhang, X.; Wang, R.; Wang, J.; Rabot, S.; Gérard, P.; Zhao, L. Endotoxin producers overgrowing in human gut microbiota as the causative agents for nonalcoholic fatty liver disease. *mBio* **2020**, *11*, e03263-19. [CrossRef]

nutrients

MDPI

Article

Effects of Celastrol-Enriched Peanuts on Metabolic Health and the Development of Atherosclerosis

Jiaxin Shi [1,†], Yitong Cheng [1,†], Chenxuan Wang [1,†], Min Liu [2], Mingxuan Qu [2], Shuaishuai Zhou [1], Leon Chen [2], Xiaohao Li [2], Junjie Luo [1], Yongting Luo [1,*], Chao Luo [2,*] and Peng An [1,*]

1 Department of Nutrition and Health, Key Laboratory of Precision Nutrition and Food Quality, China Agricultural University, Beijing 100193, China; s_jx0717@163.com (J.S.); ccc666678@126.com (Y.C.); wangchenxuan0609@163.com (C.W.); luojj@cau.edu.cn (J.L.)

2 Guangdong Agricultural Antibiotic Reduction and Replacement Technology Promotion Association, Shenzhen 518114, China

* Correspondence: luo.yongting@cau.edu.cn (Y.L.); jameslocke21@163.com (C.L.); anpeng@cau.edu.cn (P.A.)

† These authors contributed equally to this work.

Abstract: Background: Celastrol, a pentacyclic triterpenoid active component isolated from the root bark of the traditional medicinal plant Tripterygium wilfordii, displays significant anti-inflammatory, antioxidant, and immunomodulatory properties. However, its clinical application remains limited due to inadequate bioavailability. Methods: Regarding these issues, we innovatively developed a novel peanut cultivar (cel-peanut) enriched with celastrol through distant hybridization combined with metabolomics screening. Guided by the research concept of "natural anti-inflammatory diets for metabolic disease management", we established a high-fat diet-induced $ApoE^{-/-}$ atherosclerotic mouse model to systematically evaluate the anti-atherosclerosis effects and mechanisms of cel-peanut. Results: Our results revealed that cel-peanut significantly reduced serum levels of triglycerides (TGs) and increased high-density lipoprotein cholesterol (HDL-C). Concurrently, cel-peanut markedly decreased the atherosclerotic lesion area and enhanced collagen content within plaques. Mechanistic investigations demonstrated that cel-peanut reduced serum malondialdehyde (MDA) levels and suppressed the concentration of pro-inflammatory cytokine IL-6 in atherosclerotic lesions. Furthermore, cel-peanut promoted intestinal health by modulating the composition and functionality of gut microbiota, thereby attenuating atherosclerosis progression. Conclusions: Overall, these findings indicate that cel-peanut exerts therapeutic effects against atherosclerosis through its anti-inflammatory, antioxidant, and gut microbiota-modulating properties. This study proposes a novel nutritional intervention strategy for atherosclerosis and provides a promising adjuvant strategy for clinical atherosclerosis treatment.

Keywords: celastrol-enriched peanut; atherosclerosis; blood lipid; anti-inflammatory; intestinal flora

1. Introduction

Cardiovascular diseases are the leading cause of mortality, accounting for nearly 17.9 million lives each year [1]. Atherosclerosis (AS) is a chronic inflammatory disease that serves as the main pathological basis of most cardiovascular diseases [2]. Various risk factors, including obesity, genetic history, and age [3], have been considered as risk factors for atherosclerosis. In addition, there are additional non-traditional risk factors for atherosclerosis, such as poor diet quality, sedentary lifestyle, ambient air pollution, and psycho-social stress [4].

The pathogenesis of AS involves the following: increased endothelial permeability and initiating inflammation caused by minor damage, allowing for low-density lipoprotein infiltration and oxidative modification in the arterial wall; monocyte recruitment and transformation into macrophages and foam cells; platelet adhesion and growth factor release; migration and proliferation of medial smooth muscle cells into the intima, synthesizing the extracellular matrix (collagen and proteoglycans); and progressive lipid deposition in macrophages and smooth muscle cells. This chronic and complex process involves a continuous vicious cycle of lipid accumulation, inflammatory responses, and cellular proliferation, ultimately forming lipid-rich cores and fibrotic plaques [5]. Therefore, targeting inflammation could be an effective therapeutical strategy to prevent the development of atherosclerosis. Existing treatment strategies targeting inflammation include inhibiting cytokines, manipulating adaptive immunity, and promoting pro-resolution mechanisms [6]. Additionally, an increase in the intake of plant-based foods (whole grains, fruits, vegetables, legumes, and nuts) is associated with a reduced risk of atherosclerosis. Similarly, substituting butter and other animal/tropical fats with oils rich in unsaturated fats can benefit cardiovascular health. This type of diet affects the entire metabolism [7,8].

Natural products are an essential source for discovering and developing new compounds for the treatment of cardiovascular diseases [9–11]. Celastrol, a pentacyclic triterpenoid isolated from the roots of *Tripterygium wilfordii*, has shown great potential in the treatment of a wide variety of diseases and received considerable attention in recent years [12]. A large number of studies have shown that celastrol has a protective effect on obesity, diabetes, silicosis, and other diseases [13]. Importantly, growing evidence suggests celastrol could be a promising agent against atherosclerosis [14,15]. However, further clinical application of celastrol is still hampered by its limited hydrolysis, low oral bioavailability, and poor tolerance in vivo [16]. In addition, celastrol can have cytotoxic, hepatocyte, and even neurotic effects at high concentrations or in the case of prolonged exposure [17]. Thus, it may be useful to explore a more effective and safer strategy for the treatment of atherosclerosis through the proper utilization of celastrol.

Recently, advanced drug delivery systems based on nanotechnology were reported to deliver celastrol in the treatment of cancer [18] and inflammatory diseases [19]. However, shortcomings still exist in these studies, such as material instability, immunogenicity, and systemic toxicity [20,21]. Linoleic acid, lecithin, high-quality protein, minerals, vitamins, and fiber that exist within peanut are considered to be good carriers for fat-soluble natural compounds, which may effectively alleviate the toxicity produced by natural compounds via changing their pharmacokinetic properties [7,22–24].

This variety of peanut that rich in celastrol was screened and obtained through breeding techniques combining distant hybridization and metabolomics analysis. Considering the great potential of celastrol in the treatment of inflammation-associated diseases, the efficacy of celastrol-enriched peanut on atherosclerosis was investigated in a mouse model of atherosclerosis (*ApoE*$^{-/-}$ mice) fed a 10-week high-fat diet.

2. Materials and Methods

2.1. Celastrol-Enriched Peanut

The Paraguay Mountain Small Peanut is a small-fruited, black-skinned peanut variety characterized by thin shells, small yet plump seeds, and excellent flavor. However, this plant exhibits a relatively tall stature, long growth cycles, late maturation, limited branching, and low yields, making it unsuitable for large-scale cultivation in China. In contrast, the Yangjing variety, a local germplasm from Wuzhi Mountain in Hainan Province, is renowned for its early maturity, abundant branching, and relatively high yields. This hybrid cultivar was developed through distant hybridization combining the high-yield

Paraguay Mountain Small Peanut (maternal parent) with the Yangjing genotype (paternal parent). By integrating metabolomic analysis with distant hybridization, the secondary metabolic pathways of the plant were activated, achieving enrichment of celastrol while reducing its potential toxicity. This process preserved the superior flavor characteristics while maintaining stable high-yield traits. The combination of traditional hybrid breeding with modern metabolic pathway analysis has enabled synchronous optimization of phytochemical composition, sensory quality, and agronomic performance in this improved peanut variety.

Three types of animal feed were used in this experiment: (1) a high-fat purified diet (H10141, purchased from Beijing HFK Bio-Technology Co., Ltd., Beijing, China) with a fat–energy ratio of 41%, supplemented with 1.5% cholesterol, was used to induce high-fat and atherosclerosis models in mice; (2) a high-fat purified diet mixed with 20% regular peanuts per kilogram; and (3) a high-fat purified diet mixed with 20% celastrol-enriched peanuts per kilogram. The common peanuts (Luhua 11, celastrol content: 0.57 μg/kg) and celastrol-enriched peanuts (celastrol content: 1029.21 μg/kg) used in this study were provided by Hainan Misheng Biotechnology Co., Ltd. (Sanya, China).

2.2. Animals

Male apolipoprotein E-deficient mice (*ApoE*$^{-/-}$, C57BL/6J background), aged 6 weeks, were purchased from Beijing Vital River Laboratory Animal Technology Co., Ltd. (Beijing, China). The mice were housed under specific pathogen-free conditions, with a temperature range of 20 to 26 °C, humidity of 40–70%, pressure of 45 Pa, illumination of 15–20 Lux, and 12 h light/dark cycle. All the experimental animals were fed a high-fat diet (HFD) for 10 weeks to induce obesity and atherosclerosis. The mice were randomly divided into three groups (6 mice per group): the blank high-fat diet group (HFD group), the high-fat diet with regular peanut control group (HFD-peanut group), and the high-fat diet with celastrol-enriched peanut intervention group (HFD-Cel-peanut group). Each group was fed their corresponding diets accordingly. The intervention lasted for 8 weeks, during which the mice had ad libitum access to food and water. Weekly records of body weight and feed consumption were kept throughout the intervention period. All the mice were sacrificed following intraperitoneal administration of 1.25% tribromoethyl alcohol for anesthesia. Whole blood was obtained via cardiac puncture. Aortic tissues and other organs were harvested separately and stored in 4% formalin for histopathological analysis or at −80 °C for biochemical experiments. All the procedures were conducted in strict accordance with the Guiding Principles for the Care and Use of Laboratory Animals and were approved by the Ethics Committee on Animal Experiments of China Agricultural University (Beijing, China) (No. AW50804202-5-3).

2.3. Detection of Body Composition

After 8 weeks of intervention and just prior to euthanasia, the body fat and lean mass content of the mice were analyzed using the Awake Small Animal Body Composition Analysis and Imaging System (MesoQMR-060H-I, Shanghai Numai Electronic Technology Co., Ltd., Shanghai, China). For the measurement, a 40 g animal holder was selected, and the mice were placed into the holder. The holder was then inserted into the round opening beneath the instrument, ensuring the animal was positioned correctly for the test. The non-invasive nature of the MesoQMR system allowed for real-time monitoring, providing accurate and reliable data on the body composition of the mice without the need for anesthesia, thus minimizing potential stress and confounding factors during the assessment.

2.4. Analysis of Serum Lipid Profiles and Inflammatory Factors

After the whole blood samples were collected from the mice, they were allowed to stand at room temperature for 2 to 3 h. Subsequently, the samples were centrifuged at 3000 rpm for 15 min to separate the serum, which was then stored at −80 °C until further analysis. The levels of total cholesterol (TC), triglycerides (TG), low-density lipoprotein cholesterol (LDL-C), and high-density lipoprotein cholesterol (HDL-C) in the serum were quantified using commercially available assay kits (S03027, S0304, S03025, and S03029; Shenzhen Raydu Life Science Co., Ltd., Shenzhen, China). The processed samples were then analyzed automatically using a biochemical analyzer (Chemray 800, Shenzhen Raydu Life Science Co., Ltd., Shenzhen, China).

2.5. Hematoxylin–Eosin (HE) Staining for Aorta

The aortas of the mice were carefully immersed in 4% paraformaldehyde and fixed for over 48 h. Following fixation, the tissues were embedded in paraffin and sectioned into 5 μm thick slices using a microtome. These paraffin-embedded sections were then stained with a commercially available hematoxylin and eosin (HE) staining kit (G1120, Beijing Solarbio Science and Technology Co., Ltd., Beijing, China). The staining process began with dewaxing the sections, followed by rehydration in water. The tissues were then stained with hematoxylin solution for a duration of 5–20 min, after which they were thoroughly rinsed in running tap water. To differentiate the staining, the sections were treated with differentiation solution for 3 min, followed by two washes with tap water, each lasting 2 min. The next step involved re-staining the sections with Eosin Y Aqueous Solution for 10 s to 2 min and subsequently dehydrating the samples for 2–3 min each, followed by a 1 min rinse in 100% alcohol. After dehydration, the samples were placed in a series of alcohol solutions, 75%, 85%, 95%, and 100% alcohol, and the sections were cleared using xylene and mounted with neutral gum. The stained sections were then examined under an optical microscope, and the atherosclerotic plaques were analyzed and quantified using ImageJ software (version 1.8.0, National Institutes of Health, Bethesda, MD, USA).

2.6. Masson's Trichrome Stain

Weigert's iron hematoxylin solution, fuchsin ponceau acid solution, and aniline blue solution were utilized to stain the prepared paraffin sections, following the protocol provided in the Masson's trichrome stain kit (G1340, Beijing Solarbio Science and Technology Co., Ltd., Beijing, China). The staining process began with routine dewaxing of the paraffin sections in distilled water. Next, a 1:1 mixture of reagents A1 and A2 was applied to cover the sections, and the sections were left for 5–10 min. Afterward, the excess staining solution was washed away with distilled water, and the sections were differentiated with acid ethanol differentiation solution for 5–15 s, followed by another wash with distilled water for 30 s. The sections were then stained with Masson solution for 3–5 min, followed by a 30 s rinse in distilled water. Subsequently, a weak acid working solution was prepared by mixing distilled water and weak acid solution in a 2:1 ratio. This solution was applied to the sections for 30 s, after which the excess liquid was discarded. The sections were treated with phosphorolybdic acid solution for 1–2 min, followed by another 30 s wash with distilled water. The aniline blue stain was then applied for 1–2 min, and the sections were washed again with distilled water for 30 s. To complete the dehydration process, the sections were immersed in 95% ethanol for 2–3 s, followed by two washes in absolute ethanol for 5–10 s each. The sections were then cleared with xylene for 1–2 min, twice, and sealed with neutral gum. Finally, the stained sections were examined and photographed under an optical microscope (Leica CTR6, Leica, Wetzlar, Germany). The proportion of collagen in the stained tissue sections was analyzed and quantified using ImageJ software (version 1.8.0).

2.7. Analysis of MDA, IL-6, and TNF-α Levels in Serum

The levels of malondialdehyde (MDA) in serum were determined using a commercial assay kit (BC0020, Beijing Solarbio Science and Technology Co., Ltd., Beijing, China). Prior to measurement, the spectrophotometer was preheated for more than 30 min, and the distilled water was adjusted to zero. The measurement process involved preparing a measurement tube containing 600 μL of MDA working solution, 200 μL of the sample, and 200 μL of reagent 3, while a blank tube was prepared with 600 μL of MDA working solution, 200 μL of distilled water, and 200 μL of reagent 3. Both tubes were incubated in a 100 °C water bath for 60 min, followed by cooling in an ice bath. Afterward, the tubes were centrifuged at 10,000× *g* at room temperature for 10 min, and the supernatant was transferred to a 96-well plate to measure the absorbance at 532 nm and 600 nm. The differences in absorbance (ΔA_{532} and ΔA_{600}) were calculated by subtracting the blank readings from the measured values, and the final value for ΔA was obtained by subtracting ΔA_{600} from ΔA_{532}. For the high-fat blood blank tube, distilled water was diluted with a mixture of 33 μL distilled water and 67 μL ethanol. The MDA content (nmol/mL) was then calculated using the following formula: MDA content = 32.258 × ΔA, where ΔA represents the absorbance difference and other constants account for the total volume, sample volume, molar absorption coefficient of MDA, and dilution factor.

Additionally, for the quantitative detection of mouse interleukin-6 (IL-6) and tumor necrosis factor-α (TNF-α), an enzyme-linked immunosorbent assay (ELISA) was performed. The procedure involved coating a Corning™ Costar™ 9018 ELISA plate (Corning Incorporated-Life Sciences, Kennebunk ME, USA) with 100 μL of capture antibody in Coating Buffer and incubating the plate overnight at 4 °C. After washing the wells three times with Wash Buffer, the wells were blocked with 200 μL of ELISA/ELISPOT Diluent (1×) and incubated for 1 h at room temperature. The mouse IL-6 standard was reconstituted with distilled water, and the standard curve was prepared by performing 2-fold serial dilutions of the top standard across 8 points. Following this, 100 μL of each sample was added to the corresponding wells, and the plate was sealed and incubated for 2 h (or overnight at 4 °C for maximum sensitivity). After incubation, the detection antibody was added, followed by incubation for 1 h at room temperature. Subsequently, Avidin-HRP was added to the wells, and incubation continued for 30 min at room temperature. The plate was washed thoroughly after each step, with multiple wash cycles to ensure the effective removal of residual buffer. Finally, 100 μL of 1 × TMB Solution was added, and the plate was incubated for 15 min before adding 100 μL of Stop Solution. The absorbance was read at 450 nm, and if available, subtraction of the readings at 570 nm from those at 450 nm was performed to analyze the data.

2.8. Microbial Diversity Analysis

2.8.1. DNA Extraction of Sample

An E.Z.N.A. Soildnakit (Omega Bio-Tek, Norcross, GA, USA) was used to extract the total genomic DNA of the microbial community from the mouse feces samples, and the specific operation was carried out according to the instructions of the kit. The extracted DNA was detected by 1% agarose gel electrophoresis, and its concentration and purity were determined by Nano Drop 2000 (Thermoscientific, Waltham, MA, USA).

2.8.2. Construction of PCR Amplification and Sequencing Library

Using the extracted DNA as a template, the V3-V4 variable region of the 16SrRNA gene was amplified by PCR with primers 338 f (5′-ACTCCTACGGGAGGCCAGCAG-3′)

and 806 r (5′-GGACTACHVGGGTWTCTAAT-3′) [25]. The amplification procedure was as follows: pre-denaturing at 95 °C for 3 min; 27 cycles (denaturation at 95 °C for 30 s, annealing at 55 °C for 30 s, and extension at 72 °C for 30 s); 72 °C for 10 min; and store at 4 °C (PCR instrument: T100ThermalCycler, BIO-RAD, Hercules, CA, USA). The PCR reaction system was as follows: 5× TransStartFastPfu buffer 4 μL, 2.5 mM dNTPs 2 μL, upstream primer (5 μM) 0.8 μL, downstream primer (5 μM) 0.8 μL, TransStartFastPfuDNA polymerase 0.4 μL, template DNA 10 ng, and ddH2O make up to 20 μL. The PCR products were separated by 2% agarose gel electrophoresis, purified by using a DNA gel recovery and purification kit (PCR Clean-Up Kit C01-10000, Meiji Yuhua Biomedical Technology Co., Ltd, Shanghai, China), and the recovered products were quantitatively detected by Qubit 4.0 (Thermo Fisher Scientific, Waltham, MA, USA). The sequencing library was constructed by using the NEXTFLEXRapidDNA-SeqKit, and the steps were as follows: (1) connected the linker; (2) used magnetic beads to screen and remove the self-linking fragments of the linker; (3) amplified and enriched the library template by PCR; and (4) recovered the PCR products from the magnetic beads to obtain the final library. The library was sequenced on the Illumina PE300/PE250 platform (Shanghai Meiji Biomedical Technology Co., Ltd., Shanghai, China).

2.8.3. High-Throughput Sequencing Data Analysis

We used fastp [26] (v0.19.6) to control the quality of the original sequencing data: (1) The bases whose tail mass value was less than 20 were filtered, setting a 50 bp window; if the average mass value in the window was less than 20, we cut off the back-end bases and removed the reads whose length was less than 50 bp or contained N bases. (2) FLASH [27] (v1.2.11) was used to splice the pairs of PEreads into a sequence according to the overlap relationship between PEREADS, with the minimum overlap length of 10 bp and the maximum allowable mismatch ratio of 0.2, so as to screen and reject the unqualified sequences. (3) The samples were differentiated according to the barcodes and primers and the sequence direction was adjusted. The allowable mismatch number of barcodes was 0, and the maximum mismatch number of primers was two.

The amplicon sequence variant (ASV) was obtained by using DADA2 [28] plug-in in the Qiime2 process to denoise the sequence after quality control. Based on the Silva16SrRNA gene database (v138), the NaiveBayes classifier in Qiime2 was used to analyze the species taxonomy of the ASVs. At the same time, the function of the 16SrRNA gene data was predicted and analyzed by PICRUSt2 [29] (v2.2.0).

2.9. Statistical Analysis

The experimental results are expressed as the mean ± standard deviations (mean ± SDs). A statistical analysis was performed using GraphPad Prism software (version 8, San Diego, CA, USA). To assess the statistical differences among the three groups, one-way analysis of variance (ANOVA) followed by Tukey's multiple comparison test was conducted. A p-value of less than 0.05 was considered to indicate statistical significance.

A data analysis of the intestinal flora was completed on the Meggie Bio-cloud platform, and the specific methods were as follows: mothur [30] was used to calculate the Alpha diversity index (such as Sobs and Shannon index); principal component analysis (PCA) based on the Bray–Curtis distance algorithm and non-metric multidimensional scaling analysis (NMDS) were used to evaluate the similarity of and difference in the microbial community structure among the samples. A one-way ANOVA followed by Tukey's multiple comparison test was used to test the species abundance of the microbial communities in multiple groups of the samples, and the significance of the differences between the groups was evaluated. By LEfSe analysis [31] (LDA > 2, $p < 0.05$), the bacterial groups with significant differences between the groups from the phylum to genus level were identified. Based on the correlation coefficient of the top 10 dominant microorganisms and environmental factors, the heat map was drawn to reveal the potential relationship between the microorganisms and environmental factors.

3. Results

3.1. Determination of Feed Composition

The fat content of common peanuts and celastrol-enriched peanuts is 52.24% and 49.22%, protein content is 28.42% and 28.30%, and carbohydrate content is 16.68% and 16.26%, respectively (Table 1). The high-fat diet (H10141, Beijing HFK Bio-Technology Co., Ltd., Beijing, China) contains 21% fat, 20% protein, and 50% carbohydrates. Through calculation, the feed containing 20% regular peanuts (HFD-peanut) comprises 27.25% fat, 21.68% protein, and 43.34% carbohydrates. The feed containing 20% celastrol-enriched peanuts (HFD-Celastrol-peanut) comprises 26.64% fat, 21.66% protein, and 43.25% carbohydrates (Table 2).

Table 1. Nutrient composition of common peanut and celastrol-enriched peanut.

	Common Peanut	Celastrol-Enriched Peanut
Fat	52.24%	49.22%
Protein	28.42%	28.30%
Carbohydrate	16.68%	16.26%
Celastrol content	0.57 μg/kg	1029.21 μg/kg

Table 2. Nutrient composition of three feeds.

	HFD Group	HFD-Peanut Group	HFD-Cel-Peanut Group
Fat	21.00%	27.25%	26.64%
Protein	20.00%	21.68%	21.66%
Carbohydrate	50.00%	43.34%	43.25%

3.2. Improvements in Body Fat and Lean Mass Percentage

In order to establish an obesity model, 6-week-old mice were fed with HFD for 10 weeks. Then, the obesity mice were divided into the HFD group, HFD-peanut group, and HFD-Cel-peanut group and then fed for an additional 8 weeks (Figure 1A). In the first two weeks of the initial modeling period and the intervention period, we detected the food intake of mice by measuring the weight of the remaining feed. The results showed that the food intake of mice in both periods tended to be stable within two weeks. This indicates that a stable intake of intervention substances has no effect on the results. In the final weight plot, we observed that the body weight of the HFD-Cel-peanut group mice was lower than the HFD group and the control peanut group (Figure 1B). These results indicated that celastrol-enriched peanut could reduce body weight.

After 18 weeks, the body fat and lean content of mice were analyzed by the Awake Small Animal Body Composition Analysis and Imaging System. The results showed that compared with the HFD-peanut group, the body fat percentage of the HFD-Cel-peanut group was significantly decreased, while the lean meat percentage was significantly increased (Figure 1C,D).

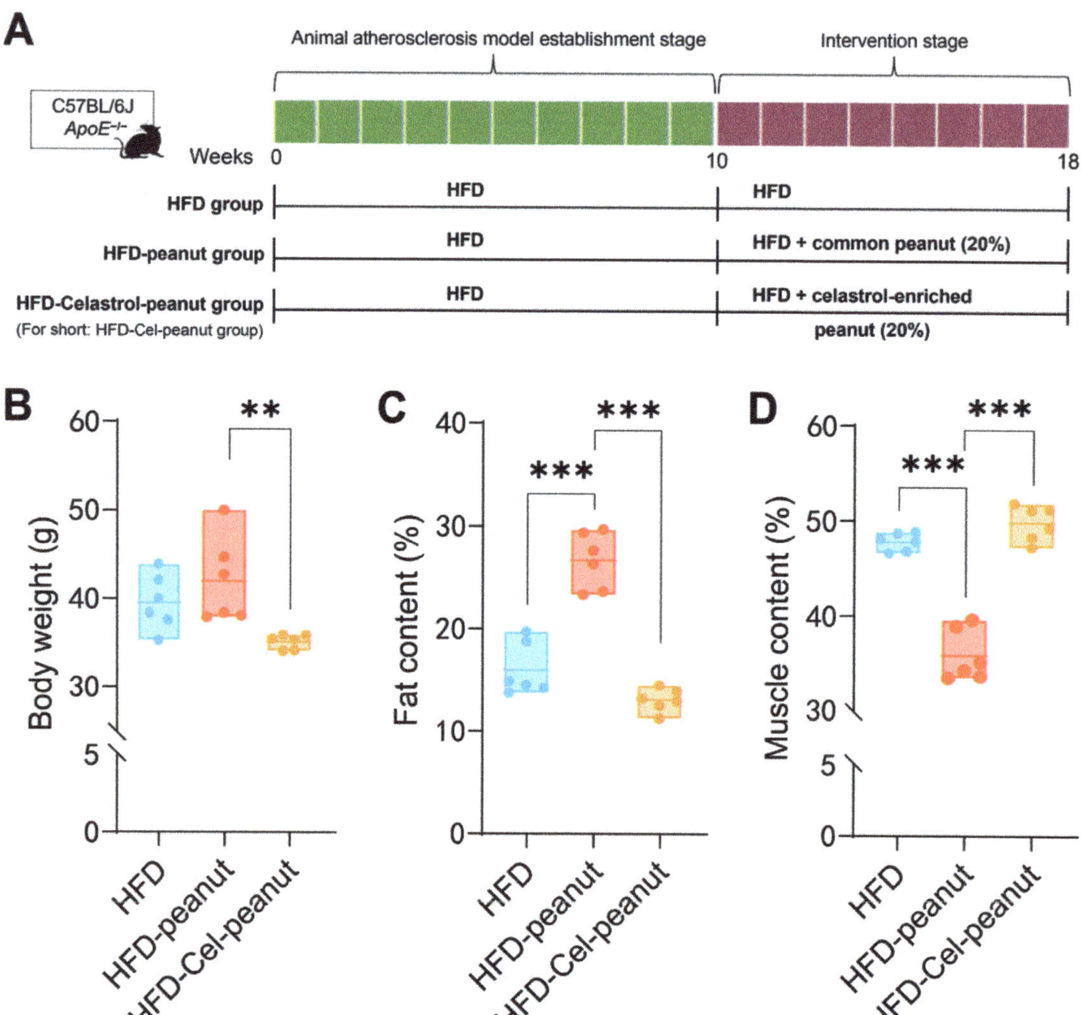

Figure 1. (**A**) Scheme of celastrol-enriched peanut intervention in HFD-induced atherosclerosis in *ApoE*$^{-/-}$ mice. (**B**) Effects of celastrol-enriched peanut on body weight in HFD-induced *ApoE*$^{-/-}$ mice. Body weight in HFD group, HFD-peanut group, and HFD-Cel-peanut group. Effects of celastrol-enriched peanuts on body composition in HFD-induced *ApoE*$^{-/-}$ mice. Fat content (**C**) and muscle content (**D**) percentage in HFD group, HFD-peanut group, and HFD-Cel-peanut group. Results are presented as means ± SDs, and n = 6 in each group. One-way ANOVA with Tukey's multiple comparison test; ** $p < 0.01$ and *** $p < 0.001$.

3.3. Celastrol-Enriched Peanut Improved the Blood Lipid Profiles

High blood lipids may cause atherosclerosis. Celastrol-enriched peanuts were shown to improve the blood lipid profiles (TG, TC, LDL-C, and HDL-C) in atherosclerotic mice. Reduced serum TG and increased HDL-cholesterol concentrations were observed in the HFD-Cel-peanut group when compared with the HFD-peanut group (Figure 2D–F). Additionally, the serum TC levels and LDL-C exhibited a reduction trend in the HFD-Cel-peanut group mice, but there is no significant difference (Figure 2E,G).

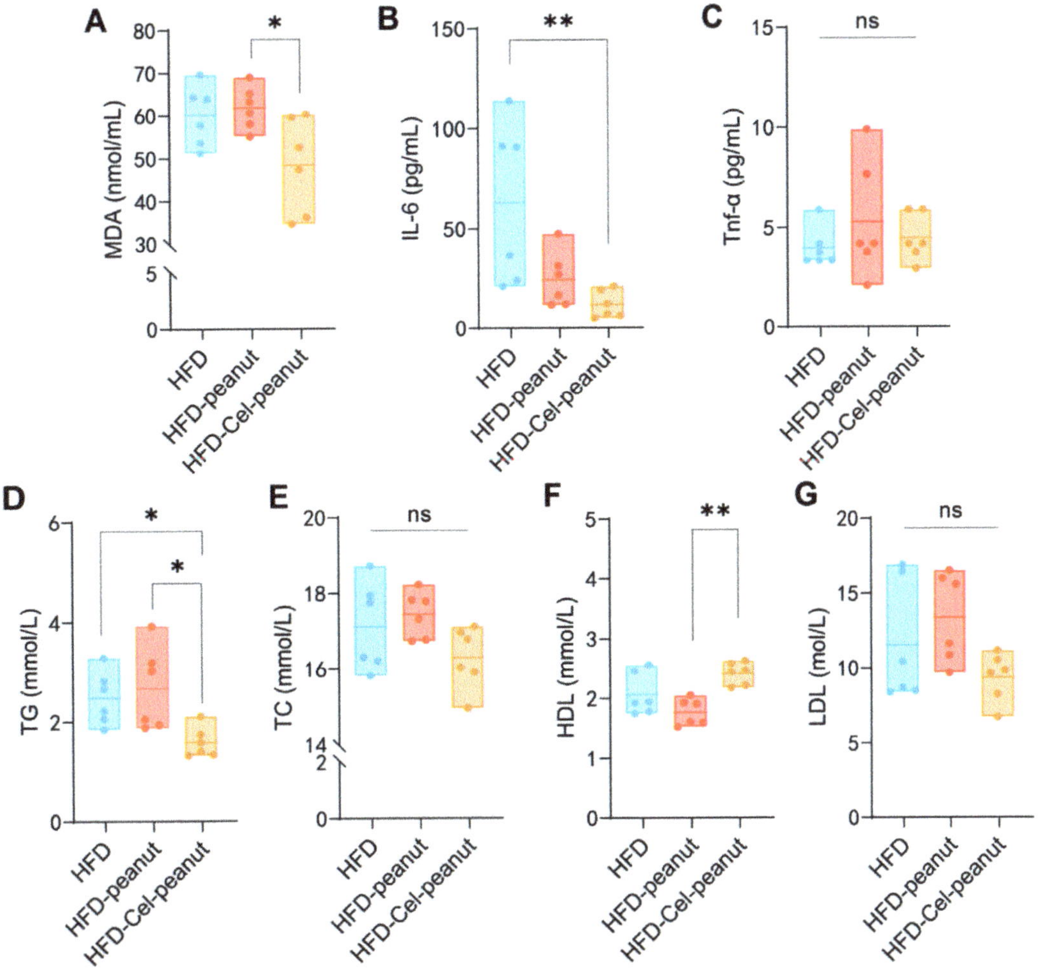

Figure 2. Effect of celastrol-enriched peanut on serum lipids in HFD-induced $ApoE^{-/-}$ mice. TG (**A**), TC (**B**), HDL-C (**C**), and LDL-C (**D**) levels of serum in dandelion polysaccharides and saline group. Effect of celastrol-enriched peanuts on antioxidant markers and inflammatory cytokines in HFD-induced $ApoE^{-/-}$ mice. MDA, TNF-α, and IL-6 concentrations (**E–G**) in serum. Results are presented as means ± SDs, and n = 6 in each group. One-way ANOVA with Tukey's multiple comparison test; * $p < 0.05$ and ** $p < 0.01$.

3.4. Celastrol-Enriched Peanut Reduces the Concentration of Oxidant-Related Markers and Inflammatory Cytokine

Malondialdehyde (MDA) is an oxidant-related marker. The celastrol-enriched peanuts reduced the MDA levels in the HFD-Cel-peanut group mice serum samples (Figure 2A), suggesting that celastrol-enriched peanut may attenuate high-fat diet-induced aortic damage. Inflammatory responses are involved in the pathophysiology of atherosclerosis. Subsequent studies confirmed the efficacy of celastrol-enriched peanut in reducing inflammation. The concentration of tumor necrosis factor-alpha (TNF-α) in the HFD-Cel-peanut group was significantly reduced compared with the HFD-peanut group (Figure 2C). Meanwhile, the serum IL-6 levels were found to be decreased in the HFD-Cel-peanut group relative to the mice in the HFD group (Figure 2B). These results suggests that the inhibition of AS by celastrol-enriched peanuts is partly due to its anti-inflammatory effect.

3.5. Celastrol-Enriched Peanut Reduced Atherosclerotic Plaques in the Aortic Root

A significant decrease in the atherosclerotic plaque's region was observed by HE staining of major tissues (Figure 3A). A cross-sectional analysis of the aortic roots further demonstrated a remarkable reduction in the plaque necrotic core area in the celastrol-peanut group mice (Figure 3B,C). The data suggest that celastrol-enriched peanut as a natural antioxidant agent could alleviate atherosclerosis lesions in the aortic root.

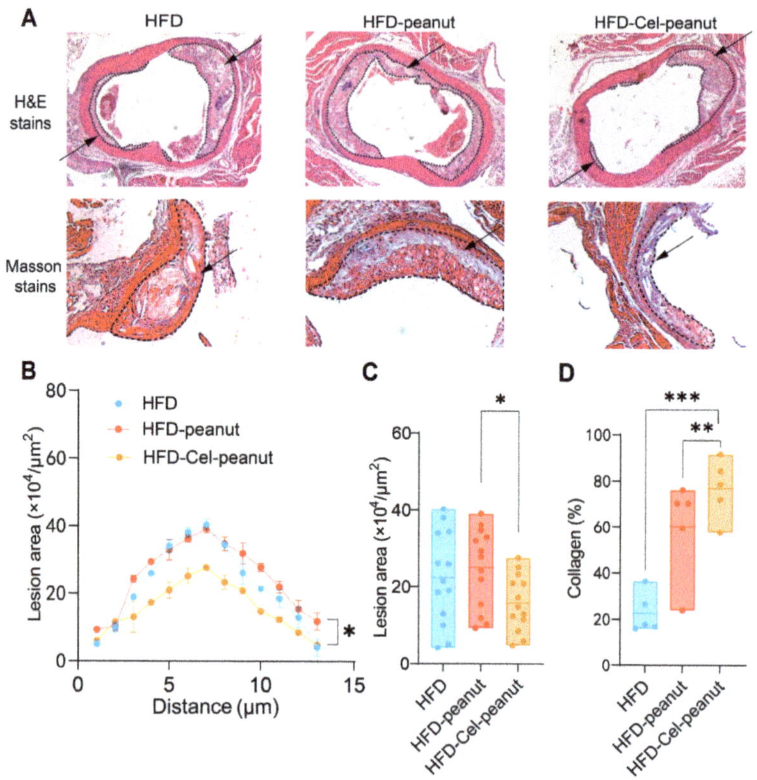

Figure 3. Effect of celastrol-enriched peanut on atherosclerotic lesion in HFD-induced *ApoE*$^{-/-}$ mice. Representative images for HE staining and Masson staining (**A**), curve chart (**B**), and quantitative chart of atherosclerotic lesion area by HE staining (**C**) and collagen area by Masson staining (**D**). For HE staining, results are presented as means ± SDs (n = 13 in each group). The arrows in the figure indicate the plaque area formed in the aorta. Each point represents the average plaque area of four mice, with two slices counted per mouse. For Masson staining, results are presented as means ± SDs (n = 5 in each group). * $p < 0.05$, ** $p < 0.01$, and *** $p < 0.001$; one-way ANOVA with Tukey's multiple comparison test.

3.6. Celastrol-Enriched Peanut Improved Stability in Aortic Roots

Masson staining, one of the most common methods for connective tissue staining, is used to differentiate muscle fibers (red) from collagen fibers (blue). It is generally accepted that higher collagen content in the aorta is associated with increased plaque stability and a reduced likelihood of rupture and thrombosis formation. Therefore, Masson staining results can serve as an indicator of AS plaque stability. Cel-peanut intervention displayed a marked increase in collagen fiber content (blue area; Figure 3A). A quantitative analysis further confirmed these findings, with collagen content after intervention being 54% higher than that of the HFD group and 16% higher than that of the HFD-peanut group (Figure 3D). These results suggest that HFD-Cel-peanut intervention significantly enhanced active collagen content, thereby improving plaque stability.

3.7. Biological Classification and Dilution Curve of Mouse Intestinal Flora

The intestinal flora of the HFD group, HFD-peanut group, and HFD-Cel-peanut group were sequenced and quality controlled. A total of 1,076,033 valid sequences were obtained, with a total base count of 450,620,837 bp and an average sequence length of 419 bp (Table S1). For the purpose of analysis, the sequences were classified by amplicon sequence variants (ASVs), and those ASVs accounting for less than 0.001% of the total sequence number were excluded. To assess whether the sample size was sufficient to represent the majority of microorganisms in the sample, a Pan/Core analysis and dilution curve analysis (using the Shannon and Sobs indices) were performed. The results indicate that as the number of samples increases, the total number of species gradually increases, while the number of common species decreases, leading to a gradual flattening of the curves (Figure S1A,B). Dilution curves (Figure S1C,D) were plotted based on the Shannon and Sobs diversity indices, and all three sets of curves tended to plateau as the number of reads increased. Additionally, the Coverage (coverage rate) for each sample library was calculated, with all the values exceeding 0.999. These findings indicate that the sample size is adequate, the sequencing depth is sufficient, and the experimental requirements are met. The data effectively represent the microbial composition within the samples and are suitable for further analysis.

3.8. Effect of Cel-Peanut Intervention on α-Diversity of Intestinal Flora in Mice

The α-diversity of intestinal flora is commonly used to assess the richness and diversity of microbial communities. Several widely used statistical indices, including the ACE index, Sobs index, Shannon index, and Simpson index, can be employed to evaluate these characteristics. The Sobs index reflects the number of amplicon sequence variants (ASVs) that are actually observed, while the ACE index estimates the total number of ASVs present in the sample. Both the ACE (Figure S2A) and Sobs (Figure S2B) indices together provide an indication of community richness. The results show no significant differences between the two indices after cel-peanut intervention, suggesting that this intervention does not affect the richness of the intestinal flora. The Shannon index (Figure S3A) and Simpson index (Figure S3B) are commonly used to represent regional biodiversity in ecology and to estimate microbial diversity within samples. Generally, higher Shannon values and lower Simpson values indicate greater α-diversity. The results show that the Shannon index did not change significantly following cel-peanut intervention, while the Simpson index increased significantly. These findings suggest that while the cel-peanut intervention did not alter community richness, it led to an enrichment of the dominant bacterial communities.

3.9. Effect of Cel-Peanut Intervention on β-Diversity

Principal component analysis (PCA) was performed to evaluate the community composition of the samples, providing insight into the differences between them. In the PCA plot (Figure 4A), the closer the distance between two samples, the more similar their species composition. The results indicated that samples within the same group were relatively close to each other, clustering together in the same region of the plot. In contrast, the distances between the HFD, HFD-peanut, and HFD-Cel-peanut groups were noticeably greater, with distinct separation along the PC1 axis. To further explore community differences, a non-metric multidimensional scaling (NMDS) analysis was conducted, using a two-dimensional scatter plot to visualize variations in the species composition between the samples or groups. The Bray–Curtis algorithm was employed to quantify the degree of aggregation or dispersion of the sample communities, based on the distances between them. Combined with the stress value (stress < 0.2, indicating a meaningful plot) and statistical analysis using the ANOSIM test, the results demonstrated significant differences in the community composition between the control and treatment groups. The closer two sample points were, the more similar their species composition. The findings revealed that several samples within the same group were evenly distributed along the PC1 axis, with a stress value of 0.107 and a p-value of less than 0.05, indicating a significant difference between the groups on the PC2 axis (Figure S4).

3.10. Effect of Cel-Peanut Intervention on the Composition of Intestinal Flora

The results above indicate that cel-peanut intervention affects the diversity of intestinal flora. As shown in the Venn diagram (Figure 4B), there are 101 common species shared among the HFD group, HFD-peanut group, and HFD-Cel-peanut group, with 8 species unique to the HFD group, 2 species unique to the HFD-peanut group, and 5 species unique to the HFD-Cel-peanut group.

Based on these findings, a further analysis of the flora composition of the three groups of mice was conducted. The composition of the intestinal flora was examined at the phylum level (Figure 4C). The dominant phyla across all three groups included *Bacillota*, *Bacteroidota*, *Thermodesulfobacteriota*, *Actinomycetota*, and *Patescibacteria*. A detailed comparison of the proportions of different bacterial phyla revealed that cel-peanut intervention primarily impacted *Bacillota*, *Bacteroidota*, and *Thermodesulfobacteriota*. Compared with the HFD group, *Bacillota* decreased from 63.33% to 45%, while *Bacteroidota* increased from 29.71% to 51.51%. When compared with the HFD-peanut group, *Bacillota* decreased from 53.42% to 45%, *Bacteroidota* increased from 25.66% to 51.51%, and *Thermodesulfobacteriota* decreased from 12.49% to 1.19%. The proportions of other bacterial phyla were relatively small, showing minimal differences from the HFD group after intervention. Additionally, compared with the HFD-peanut group, *Actinomycetota* and *Patescibacteria* decreased by approximately 1.5% and 3.5%, respectively.

The composition of the intestinal microbiota at the genus level was analyzed (Figure 4D). Compared with the HFD group, species that showed a significant decrease (greater than 1%) after cel-peanut intervention primarily included the following: *Allobaculum*, which decreased from 15.91% to 4.41%; *Dubosiella*, which decreased from 5.34% to 0%; and *Ileibacterium*, which decreased from 5.7% to 0%. Conversely, species that increased significantly (greater than 1%) included the following: *norank_f__Muribaculaceae*, which increased from 19.52% to 29.05%; *Bacteroides*, which increased from 3.41% to 9.53%; and *Ligilactobacillus*, which increased from 2.76% to 6.98%.

Compared with the HFD-peanut group, species showing a significant decrease (greater than 1%) after cel-peanut intervention primarily included the following: *Lachnospiraceae*, which decreased from 7.97% to 4.16%; *Desulfovibrio*, which decreased from 10.96% to 0.8%; *Dubosiella*, which decreased from 4.16% to 0%; *Candidatus_Saccharimonas*, which decreased from 4.35% to 0.9%; and *Clostridium*, which decreased from 3.1% to 0.6%. Species that increased significantly (greater than 1%) included the following: *norank_f__Muribaculaceae*, which increased from 16.13% to 29.05%; *Bacteroides*, which increased from 4.53% to 9.53%; *Ligilactobacillus*, which increased from 5.02% to 6.98%; and *Alistipes*, which increased from 1.3% to 2.6%.

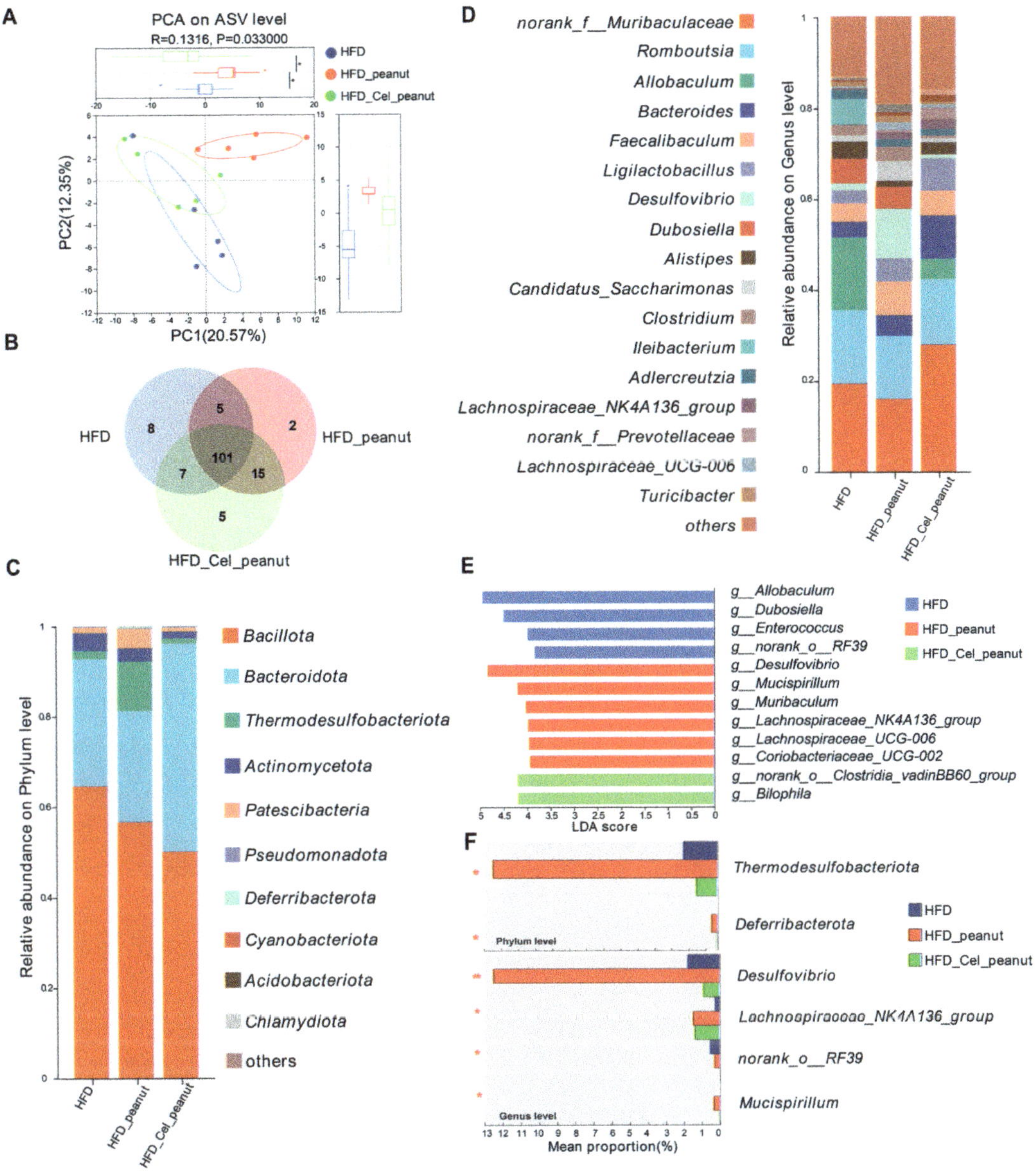

Figure 4. Effect of cel-peanut intervention on β-diversity of intestinal flora in *ApoE*$^{-/-}$ mice. (**A**) PCA analysis of intestinal microbiota and box plot based on PC1 and PC2 axis to evaluate sample community composition. (**B**) Intestinal flora species number Venn chart. (**C**) Intestinal bacterial community composition (phylum level). (**D**) Effect of cel-peanut intervention on intestinal flora composition (genus level). The horizontal coordinate represents grouping, and the vertical coordinate represents the relative abundance of the bacterial population (genus level). (**E**) Effect of cel-peanut intervention on characteristic bacterial genera in the intestinal flora of AS mice. (**F**) Effect of cel-peanut intervention on multi-group comparative analysis of species differences at the phylum level and genus level. In the figure, n = 5 means there are 5 mice; * $p < 0.05$ and ** $p < 0.01$, with significant differences.

3.11. Effect of Cel-Peanut Intervention on Characteristic Bacterial Genera

The LEfSe multi-level species difference analysis was performed at the genus level for the HFD group, HFD-peanut group, and HFD-Cel-peanut group. The Linear Discriminant Analysis (LDA) score was used to assess the impact of the species on the differences observed and to identify characteristic bacterial genera. The results (Figure 4E) revealed that the HFD group was significantly enriched in *g_Allobaculum*, *g_Dubosiella*, *g_Enterococcus*, and *g_norank_o_RF39*, among others. In contrast, *Desulfovibrio*, *g_Mucispirillum*, *g_Lachnospiraceae_UCG-006*, *g_Lachnospiraceae_NK4A136_group*, *g_Coriobacteriaceae_UCG-002*, and *g_Muribaculum* were significantly accumulated in the HFD-peanut group. The HFD-Cel-peanut group showed a significant enrichment in *g_Bilophila* and *g_norank_o_Clostridia_vadinBB60_group*.

3.12. Effect of Cel-Peanut Intervention on the Difference of Intestinal Flora

To evaluate the differences in the intestinal flora caused by cel-peanut, we conducted one-way ANOVA followed by Tukey's multiple comparison test on the intestinal flora of the three groups at both the phylum and genus levels to analyze significant differences in species abundance among the groups (Figure 4F).

At the phylum level, the HFD-peanut group was significantly enriched in *Thermodesulfobacteriota* and *Deferribacterota* ($p < 0.05$). However, after intervention with HFD-Cel-peanut, the relative abundance of these two phyla decreased significantly ($p = 0.004$; $p = 0.02$), even falling below the levels observed in the HFD group. At the genus level, the HFD-peanut group was significantly enriched in *Desulfovibrio*, *Lachnospiraceae_NK4A136_group*, and, to a lesser extent, *Mucispirillum* and *g_norank_o_RF39*. Following the HFD-Cel-peanut intervention, the relative abundance of *Desulfovibrio* and *Mucispirillum* decreased significantly ($p = 0.004$; $p = 0.02$), while the abundance of *Lachnospiraceae_NK4A136_group* remained comparable with that in the HFD-peanut group.

These results indicate that cel-peanut intervention can significantly reduce the relative abundance of harmful bacteria while maintaining or increasing the abundance of beneficial bacteria, thus improving the composition of the intestinal flora.

3.13. Correlation Analysis Between Intestinal Flora and Clinical Factors

3.13.1. Correlation Between Intestinal Flora and Blood Lipids

Changes in intestinal flora are strongly correlated with serum triglycerides (TGs), total cholesterol (TC), low-density lipoprotein cholesterol (LDL-C), and high-density lipoprotein cholesterol (HDL-C) concentrations (Figure 5A). TG levels are positively correlated with *Desulfovibrio*, *Candidatus_Saccharimonas*, *Clostridium*, and others while being negatively correlated with *Rikenellaceae_RC9_gut_group*, *Clostridium*, *Butyricimonas*, and others. TC levels exhibit a positive correlation with *Candidatus_Saccharimonas*, *Desulfovibrio*, *Dubosiella*, and others and a negative correlation with *norank_f_Prevotellaceae*, *Rikenellaceae_RC9_gut_group*, and others. LDL-C levels are positively correlated with *Desulfovibrio*, *Clostridium*, and others and negatively correlated with *norank_f_Prevotellaceae*, *Butyricimonas*, and others. HDL-C levels are positively correlated with *Rikenellaceae_RC9_gut_group*, *norank_f_Prevotellaceae*, *Butyricimonas*, and others while being negatively correlated with *Desulfovibrio*, *Candidatus_Saccharimonas*, *Clostridium*, and others.

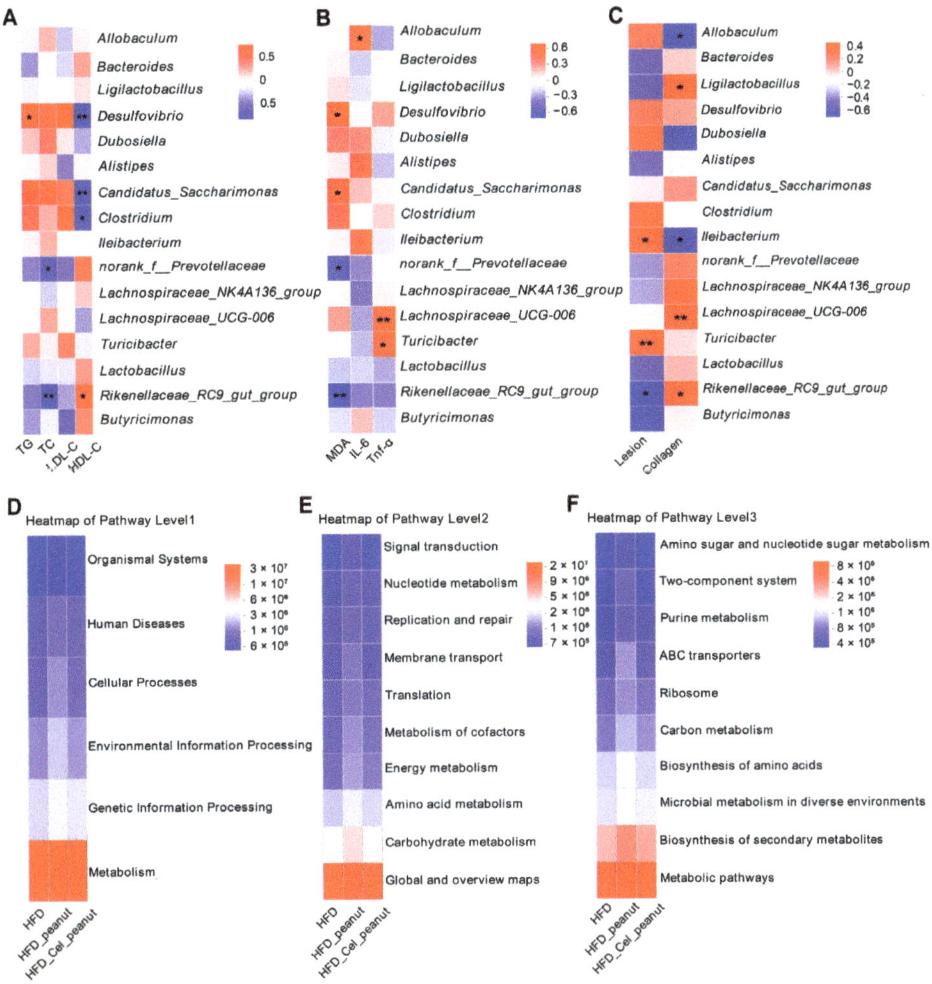

Figure 5. (**A**) Correlation analysis between intestinal flora and blood lipids. (**B**) Correlation analysis between intestinal flora and oxidative and inflammatory factors. (**C**) Correlation analysis between lesion area and collagen percentage. KEGG analysis of intestinal flora at pathway levels 1, 2, and 3. (**D**) KEGG results of intestinal flora at pathway level 1, (**E**) KEGG results of intestinal flora at pathway level 2, and (**F**) KEGG results of intestinal flora at pathway level 3. Red indicates positive correlation, blue indicates negative correlation, and the darker the color, the stronger the correlation, and the lighter the correlation is, the weaker the correlation. In the figure, * $p < 0.05$, and ** $p < 0.01$, with significant differences.

3.13.2. Correlation Between Intestinal Flora and Oxidative Factors, Inflammatory Factors

The correlation between the oxidative factors; inflammatory factors such as MDA, IL-6, and TNF-α; and the intestinal flora was investigated (Figure 5B). Among the antioxidant indicators, MDA was positively correlated with *Desulfovibrio*, *Candidatus_Saccharimonas*, and *Clostridium*, while it was negatively correlated with *norank_f_Prevotellaceae* and *Rikenellaceae_RC9_gut_group*. The inflammatory factor IL-6 was positively correlated with *Allobaculum*, *Alistipes*, and *Ileibacterium*, whereas TNF-α was strongly positively correlated with *Lachnospiraceae_UCG_006* and *Turicibacter*.

3.13.3. Correlation Between Intestinal Flora and AS Lesion Parameters

The correlation analysis of the intestinal flora and AS lesion parameters (including AS plaque area and collagen content) revealed (Figure 5C) that the plaque area was significantly positively correlated with *Turicibacter* and *Ileibacterium* and negatively correlated with *Rikenellaceae_RC9_gut_group*, *norank_f__Muribaculaceae*, and *Butyricimonas*. In contrast, thecollagen content was significantly positively correlated with *Lachnospiraceae_UCG-006*, *Rikenellaceae_RC9_gut_group*, *Ligilactobacillus*, and others, while it was negatively correlated with *Dubosiella*, *Ileibacterium*, and *Allobaculum*. Since collagen content is a key indicator of plaque stability, these findings suggest that plaque stability is closely related to alterations in the bacterial flora. Overall, the correlations reveal an inverse relationship between plaque area and collagen content in relation to bacterial flora composition. This inverse trend may be attributed to the progression of lesions into mid-to-late stages, during which plaque stability diminishes and collagen content declines, resulting in contrasting patterns between plaque area and bacterial composition.

3.14. Prediction of Intestinal Flora Function

To explore the significant role of intestinal flora in the HFD-Cel-peanut group, the KEGG pathway of PICRUSt (Phylogenetic Investigation of Communities by Reconstruction of Unobserved States) was used to predict the potential functions of the bacteria and to examine the correlation between differential flora and predicted functional pathways.

The results are presented for pathway levels 1, 2, and 3. At pathway levels 1 and 2, the most abundant pathways were related to metabolism and global overview maps, which were considerably more abundant than other pathways (Figure 5D,E). At pathway level 3, the metabolic pathway exhibited the highest abundance, followed by the biosynthesis of secondary metabolites (Figure 5F). These findings suggest that cel-peanut intervention holds promising potential for applications in metabolic pathways.

4. Discussion

With the popularity of the anti-inflammatory diet, the role of natural products in preventing and treating metabolic disorders has gained significant attention [32]. Celastrol, a triterpenoid extracted from the *Tripterygium wilfordii*, has emerged as a potent agent due to its anti-inflammatory and anti-obesity properties. Prior studies indicate that celastrol significantly reduces inflammation by inhibiting pro-inflammatory cytokines, such as IL-6, while also mitigating the harmful effects of oxidized low-density lipoprotein (oxLDL), both of which are crucial in the pathogenesis of atherosclerosis [33]. Furthermore, celastrol has been demonstrated to promote beneficial vascular remodeling, a process that is vital for maintaining cardiovascular health and mitigating diseases such as atherosclerosis [34]. Despite its promising benefits, several challenges hinder its clinical application. On one hand, celastrol is lipophilic, which limits its solubility in water and subsequently reduces its bioavailability. This poses restrictions for formulating effective delivery systems that maximize its absorption and utilization in the body. On the other hand, as an alkaloid, it still has some pharmacokinetic limitations and undesirable side effects that need to be overcome. The liver, kidney, cholangiocytes, heart, ear, and reproductive system may be affected by these toxic effects [35]. Recent evidence indicated that celastrol may be strictly limited due to the occurrence of severe side effects, which could be reduced by structural modification [36]. Delivery systems such as nanotechnology have been tried to diminish the potential toxicity of celastrol. An injectable thermosensitive micelle–hydrogel hybrid system loaded with celastrol was reported to be able to sustain and prolong the release of celastrol to inhibit posterior capsule opacification and had no apparent tissue toxicity [36,37]. However, in the context of food and pharmaceuticals, one of the significant challenges in utilizing bioactive compounds in nanoparticle form is the limited understanding of their cytotoxicity thresholds [38].

To tackle these problems, we designed a novel approach involving the selection and cultivation of celastrol-enriched peanuts. This method consists of distant hybridization and metabolomics analysis to enhance the natural content of celastrol in peanuts, offering a more effective delivery system while minimizing potential side effects. Meanwhile, it is essential to find out which combination of diet and medication is the most favorable and appropriate for each potential chronic disease [39]. To achieve a balance in our animal feed formulation, we monitored some key parameters, including the following: (1) to achieve the effect of making animals obese and ensure the effectiveness of their nutritional intervention; (2) to ensure that the macronutrient content of the new feed does not deviate too much from the original composition of the high-fat feed. Finally, replacing 20% of the high-fat feed with peanuts is an acceptable option.

Numerous studies have demonstrated that atherosclerosis is a chronic inflammatory disease, and high lipid levels can accelerate the development of atherosclerosis. These results suggested that celastrol-enriched peanut could affect the body fat and lean mass percentage and play a role in reducing fat and improving lean mass percentage. Our findings also clearly indicate that the inclusion of celastrol-enriched peanuts can significantly improve relevant biomarkers associated with this condition. Firstly, celastrol-enriched peanut improved the blood lipid levels of HFD-induced $ApoE^{-/-}$ mice. Specifically, it led to a significant decrease in the serum TG concentration and an increase in HDL-C. Since lipid dysregulation plays a pivotal role in the progression of atherosclerotic plaques [3], the improvement in atherosclerosis after the intervention with celastrol-enriched peanut may be partly attributed to its beneficial effect on blood lipids. Secondly, the intervention of celastrol-enriched peanut decreased the expression of oxidation-related markers and inflammatory factors in mice. Celastrol-enriched peanut reduced the levels of serum MDA, IL-6, and TNF-α. A convincing body of experimental and clinical data indicates that inflammation participates fundamentally in atherogenesis [40]. Our findings suggest that celastrol-enriched peanut can improve lipid peroxidation and prevent cell damage caused by inflammation.

As mentioned above, recent studies have highlighted the significant role of intestinal flora in the development of atherosclerotic diseases. Following cel-peanut intervention, the composition of the intestinal flora in mice changed significantly. At the phylum level, AS mice induced by a high-fat diet (HFD) were predominantly composed of *Bacillota* and *Bacteroidota*, whereas cel-peanut intervention significantly reduced the relative abundance of *Bacillota* and increased the relative abundance of *Bacteroidota*. Previous studies have indicated that downregulation of *Bacillota* and upregulation of *Bacteroidota* can help regulate lipid metabolism disorders [41]. At the genus level, Zheng et al. [42] observed a significant increase in the relative abundance of *Allobaculum* and the expression of ANGPTL4 in HFD mice. The increased ANGPTL4 expression inhibits lipid absorption. After cel-peanut intervention, the relative abundance of *Allobaculum* decreased, suggesting that cel-peanut may improve AS by promoting lipid absorption. Additionally, *Desulfovibrio* can absorb sulfate and produce hydrogen sulfide (H_2S), which is toxic to intestinal epithelial cells and may contribute to gastrointestinal diseases [43]; *Mucispirillum* is associated with intestinal inflammation, and its abundance can improve colitis symptoms through a fibrotic diet [44]. In the HFD-Cel-peanut group, the relative abundance of *norank_f_Muribaculaceae*, *Bacteroides*, *Ligilactobacillus*, and *Lachnospiraceae* was significantly increased. Previous studies have shown that *norank_f_Muribaculaceae* can alleviate intestinal inflammation [45]. *Bacteroides* plays a key role in intestinal metabolism, including the utilization of nitrogen-containing substances, fermentation of carbohydrates, and biotransformation of bile acids and other sterols. These changes may aid the digestion of food and nutrient production and support the growth of other bacteria to maintain intestinal homeostasis [46]. A high-fat diet reduces the relative abundance of *Ligilactobacillus*, but cel-peanut intervention significantly increases its abundance, thereby restoring the intestinal flora structure [47]. Furthermore, *Lachnospiraceae* is one of the primary bacteria that ferments dietary fiber to produce short-chain fatty acids (SCFAs) like butyrate, which serve as an important energy source for colon cells. *Butyrate* also has an anti-inflammatory property, which improves intestinal barrier integrity and promotes overall intestinal health [48].

To further investigate the relationship between intestinal flora and AS-related parameters, such as blood lipids, oxidative stress markers, inflammatory factors, lesion area, and collagen content, we analyzed the correlation between the abundance of intestinal flora and these clinical indicators. The results showed that after cel-peanut intervention, the relative abundance of *Desulfovibrio* and *Isobacteria* decreased significantly. Collagen content was negatively correlated with *Dubosiella* and *Ileibacterium* ($p < 0.05$), while the plaque area was positively correlated with *Rikenellaceae_RC9_gut_group*, *norank_f__Muribaculaceae*, and *Butyricimonas* ($p < 0.05$), suggesting a decrease in plaque area and an increase in collagen content.

5. Conclusions

Collectively, cel-peanut may increase the abundance of beneficial bacteria, decrease the abundance of harmful bacteria, regulate lipid metabolism, reduce inflammation, and improve the function of intestinal microflora, thereby promoting intestinal health, maintaining homeostasis, and ultimately slowing the progression of AS. These findings suggest that celastrol-enriched peanuts could serve as a beneficial component of an anti-inflammatory diet, potentially aiding in weight reduction and alleviating atherosclerosis. However, the specific mechanisms through which how celastrol influences atherosclerosis remain unclear, underscoring the need for further investigation in this area. Additionally, more clinical trials are necessary to assess the long-term effects and safety of celastrol in humans, particularly among diverse populations with varying levels of metabolic disorders.

In future research, we hope to utilize gradient dosing and varied durations of intervention to better determine the optimal dose and duration of action for celastrol. We will also compare the effects of celastrol-enriched peanuts with those of celastrol alone to highlight the advantages and disadvantages of the peanut carrier strategy. Moreover, we aim to explore the mechanisms by which celastrol and other bioactive compounds in peanuts work synergistically to achieve therapeutic effects. It may provide more reference for other researchers.

Supplementary Materials: The following supporting information can be downloaded at https://www.mdpi.com/article/10.3390/nu17091418/s1, Figure S1: Microbial species analysis and dilution curve; Figure S2: Effect of cel-peanut intervention on the richness of intestinal flora; Figure S3: Effect of cel-peanut intervention on intestinal flora diversity; Figure S4: NMDS analysis of intestinal microbiota and box plot based on PC1 and PC2 axes; Table S1: Sample name and information.

Author Contributions: Conceptualization, Y.L., C.L. and P.A.; investigation, J.S., Y.C., C.W., M.L., M.Q. and S.Z.; writing—original draft preparation, J.S., Y.C. and C.W.; writing—review and editing, J.S., L.C., X.L., J.L., Y.L., C.L. and P.A.; visualization, S.Z., J.S., Y.C., C.W., M.L. and M.Q.; supervision, L.C., X.L. and J.L.; project administration, Y.L., C.L. and P.A.; funding acquisition, P.A. All authors have read and agreed to the published version of the manuscript.

Funding: This work was supported by the Pinduoduo-China Agricultural University Research Fund (PC2023B01014); the State Key Laboratory of Cardiovascular Disease, Fuwai Hospital, Chinese

Academy of Medical Sciences (2024GZkf-05); the 111 projects from the Education Ministry of China (B18053); and the support of the 2115 Talent Development Program of China Agricultural University.

Institutional Review Board Statement: This study was approved by the Animal Experiment Ethics Committee of China Agricultural University AW50804202-5-3 (date of approval: 25 April 2023).

Informed Consent Statement: Informed consent was obtained from all the subjects involved in this study.

Data Availability Statement: The original contributions presented in this study are included in the article/Supplementary Materials; further inquiries can be directed to the corresponding authors.

Conflicts of Interest: The authors declare that the research was conducted in the absence of any commercial or financial relationships that could be construed as potential conflict of interests.

Abbreviations

$ApoE^{-/-}$	Apolipoprotein E knockout
AS	Atherosclerosis
CVD	Cardiovascular disease
HFD	High-fat diet
TG	Triglyceride
TC	Total cholesterol
HDL-C	High-density lipoprotein cholesterol
LDL-C	Low-density lipoprotein cholesterol
IL-6	Interleukin 6
MDA	Malondialdehyde
TNF-α	Tumor necrosis factor-α
HE	Hematoxylin–Eosin.
ASVs	Amplicon sequence variants
PCA	Principal component analysis
NMDS	Non-metric multidimensional scaling
LDA	Linear Discriminant Analysis
KEGG	Kyoto encyclopedia of genes and genomes
PICRUSt	Phylogenetic Investigation of Communities by Reconstruction of Unobserved States

References

1. GBD 2019 Diseases and Injuries Collaborators. Global burden of 369 diseases and injuries in 204 countries and territories, 1990–2019: A systematic analysis for the Global Burden of Disease Study 2019. *Lancet* **2020**, *396*, 1204–1222. [CrossRef]
2. Zhu, Y.; Xian, X.; Wang, Z.; Bi, Y.; Chen, Q.; Han, X.; Tang, D.; Chen, R. Research Progress on the Relationship between Atherosclerosis and Inflammation. *Biomolecules* **2018**, *8*, 80. [CrossRef]
3. Libby, P. The changing landscape of atherosclerosis. *Nature* **2021**, *592*, 524–533. [CrossRef] [PubMed]
4. Lechner, K.; von Schacky, C.; McKenzie, A.L.; Worm, N.; Nixdorff, U.; Lechner, B.; Krankel, N.; Halle, M.; Krauss, R.M.; Scherr, J. Lifestyle factors and high-risk atherosclerosis: Pathways and mechanisms beyond traditional risk factors. *Eur. J. Prev. Cardiol.* **2020**, *27*, 394–406. [CrossRef]
5. Kong, P.; Cui, Z.Y.; Huang, X.F.; Zhang, D.D.; Guo, R.J.; Han, M. Inflammation and atherosclerosis: Signaling pathways and therapeutic intervention. *Signal Transduct. Target. Ther.* **2022**, *7*, 131. [CrossRef]
6. Soehnlein, O.; Libby, P. Targeting inflammation in atherosclerosis-from experimental insights to the clinic. *Nat. Rev. Drug Discov.* **2021**, *20*, 589–610. [CrossRef]
7. An, P.; Wan, S.; Luo, Y.; Luo, J.; Zhang, X.; Zhou, S.; Xu, T.; He, J.; Mechanick, J.I.; Wu, W.C.; et al. Micronutrient Supplementation to Reduce Cardiovascular Risk. *J. Am. Coll. Cardiol.* **2022**, *80*, 2269–2285. [CrossRef]
8. Riccardi, G.; Giosue, A.; Calabrese, I.; Vaccaro, O. Dietary recommendations for prevention of atherosclerosis. *Cardiovasc. Res.* **2022**, *118*, 1188–1204. [CrossRef]
9. Chopra, B.; Dhingra, A.K. Natural products: A lead for drug discovery and development. *Phytother. Res.* **2021**, *35*, 4660–4702. [CrossRef]
10. Wu, X.; Wei, J.; Yi, Y.; Gong, Q.; Gao, J. Activation of Nrf2 signaling: A key molecular mechanism of protection against cardiovascular diseases by natural products. *Front. Pharmacol.* **2022**, *13*, 1057918. [CrossRef]

11. Zhong, L.; Tan, X.; Yang, W.; LI, P.; Ye, L.; Luo, Q.; Hou, H. Bioactive matters based on natural product for cardiovascular diseases. *Smart Mater. Med.* **2024**, *4*, 542–565. [CrossRef]
12. Zhao, Y.; Miettinen, K.; Kampranis, S.C. Celastrol: A century-long journey from the isolation to the biotechnological production and the development of an antiobesity drug. *Curr. Opin. Plant Biol.* **2024**, *81*, 102615. [CrossRef]
13. Liang, C.; Bai, Y.; Miao, R.; Yang, X.; Gao, L.; Liu, Y.; Zhou, J.; Guo, J.; Hu, D.; Wu, J. Celastrol as a candidate drug for silicosis: From bioinformatics and network pharmacology to experimental validation. *Int. Immunopharmacol.* **2023**, *125*, 111068. [CrossRef]
14. Xu, S.; Feng, Y.; He, W.; Xu, W.; Xu, W.; Yang, H.; Li, X. Celastrol in metabolic diseases: Progress and application prospects. *Pharmacol. Res.* **2021**, *167*, 105572. [CrossRef]
15. Gu, J.; Shi, Y.N.; Zhu, N.; Li, H.F.; Zhang, C.J.; Qin, L. Celastrol functions as an emerging manager of lipid metabolism: Mechanism and therapeutic potential. *Biomed. Pharmacother.* **2023**, *164*, 114981. [CrossRef] [PubMed]
16. Li, Z.; Zhang, J.; Duan, X.; Zhao, G.; Zhang, M. Celastrol: A Promising Agent Fighting against Cardiovascular Diseases. *Antioxidants* **2022**, *11*, 1597. [CrossRef]
17. Sun, Y.; Wang, C.; Li, X.; Lu, J.; Wang, M. Recent advances in drug delivery of celastrol for enhancing efficiency and reducing the toxicity. *Front. Pharmacol.* **2024**, *15*, 1137289. [CrossRef]
18. Zhou, M.; Liao, J.; Lai, W.; Xu, R.; Liu, W.; Xie, D.; Wang, F.; Zhang, Z.; Huang, J.; Zhang, R.; et al. A celastrol-based nanodrug with reduced hepatotoxicity for primary and metastatic cancer treatment. *EBioMedicine* **2023**, *94*, 104724. [CrossRef]
19. Fang, G.; Tang, B. Current advances in the nano-delivery of celastrol for treating inflammation-associated diseases. *J. Mater. Chem. B* **2020**, *8*, 10954–10965. [CrossRef]
20. Kedmi, R.; Ben-Arie, N.; Peer, D. The systemic toxicity of positively charged lipid nanoparticles and the role of Toll-like receptor 4 in immune activation. *Biomaterials* **2010**, *31*, 6867–6875. [CrossRef]
21. Lee, Y.; Jeong, M.; Park, J.; Jung, H.; Lee, H. Immunogenicity of lipid nanoparticles and its impact on the efficacy of mRNA vaccines and therapeutics. *Exp. Mol. Med.* **2023**, *55*, 2085–2096. [CrossRef] [PubMed]
22. Zhou, S.; Cheng, F.; He, J.; Xu, T.; Zhang, X.; Wan, S.; Qi, J.; He, J.; Chen, F.; Luo, J.; et al. Effects of high-quality protein supplementation on cardiovascular risk factors in individuals with metabolic diseases: A systematic review and meta-analysis of randomized controlled trials. *Clin. Nutr.* **2024**, *43*, 1740–1750. [CrossRef]
23. Zhao, Z.; Zhong, L.; Zhou, P.; Deng, Y.; Liu, G.; Li, P.; Zeng, J.; Zhang, Y.; Tang, X.; Zhang, M. Impact of Dietary Fatty Acid Composition on the Intestinal Microbiota and Fecal Metabolism of Rats Fed a High-Fructose/High-Fat Diet. *Nutrients* **2024**, *16*, 3774. [CrossRef]
24. Rahman, M.; Farooq, S. Role of peanut oleosomes in the delivery of curcumin embedded in interpenetrating emulsion-filled gels made with whey protein and chitosan. *Colloids Surf. A Physicochem. Eng. Asp.* **2025**, *707*, 135962. [CrossRef]
25. Liu, C.; Zhao, D.; Ma, W.; Guo, Y.; Wang, A.; Wang, Q.; Lee, D.J. Denitrifying sulfide removal process on high-salinity wastewaters in the presence of *Halomonas* sp. *Appl. Microbiol. Biotechnol.* **2016**, *100*, 1421–1426. [CrossRef]
26. Chen, S.; Zhou, Y.; Chen, Y.; Gu, J. fastp: An ultra-fast all-in-one FASTQ preprocessor. *Bioinformatics* **2018**, *34*, i884–i890. [CrossRef]
27. Magoc, T.; Salzberg, S.L. FLASH: Fast length adjustment of short reads to improve genome assemblies. *Bioinformatics* **2011**, *27*, 2957–2963. [CrossRef]
28. Callahan, B.J.; McMurdie, P.J.; Rosen, M.J.; Han, A.W.; Johnson, A.J.; Holmes, S.P. DADA2: High-resolution sample inference from Illumina amplicon data. *Nat. Methods* **2016**, *13*, 581–583. [CrossRef] [PubMed]
29. Douglas, G.M.; Maffei, V.J.; Zaneveld, J.R.; Yurgel, S.N.; Brown, J.R.; Taylor, C.M.; Huttenhower, C.; Langille, M. PICRUSt2 for prediction of metagenome functions. *Nat. Biotechnol.* **2020**, *38*, 685–688. [CrossRef] [PubMed]
30. Schloss, P.D.; Westcott, S.L.; Ryabin, T.; Hall, J.R.; Hartmann, M.; Hollister, E.B.; Lesniewski, R.A.; Oakley, B.B.; Parks, D.H.; Robinson, C.J.; et al. Introducing mothur: Open-source, platform-independent, community-supported software for describing and comparing microbial communities. *Appl. Environ. Microbiol.* **2009**, *75*, 7537–7541. [CrossRef]
31. Segata, N.; Izard, J.; Waldron, L.; Gevers, D.; Miropolsky, L.; Garrett, W.S.; Huttenhower, C. Metagenomic biomarker discovery and explanation. *Genome Biol.* **2011**, *12*, R60. [CrossRef] [PubMed]
32. Rahman, M.M.; Rahaman, M.S.; Islam, M.R.; Rahman, F.; Mithi, F.M.; Alqahtani, T.; Almikhlafi, M.A.; Alghamdi, S.Q.; Alruwaili, A.S.; Hossain, M.S.; et al. Role of Phenolic Compounds in Human Disease: Current Knowledge and Future Prospects. *Molecules* **2021**, *27*, 233. [CrossRef]
33. Gu, L.; Bai, W.; Li, S.; Zhang, Y.; Han, Y.; Gu, Y.; Meng, G.; Xie, L.; Wang, J.; Xiao, Y.; et al. Celastrol prevents atherosclerosis via inhibiting LOX-1 and oxidative stress. *PLoS ONE* **2013**, *8*, e65477. [CrossRef] [PubMed]
34. Tan, J.L.; Yi, J.; Cao, X.Y.; Wang, F.Y.; Xie, S.L.; Zhou, L.L.; Qin, L.; Dai, A.G. Celastrol: The new dawn in the treatment of vascular remodeling diseases. *Biomed. Pharmacother.* **2023**, *158*, 114177. [CrossRef]
35. Song, J.; He, G.N.; Dai, L. A comprehensive review on celastrol, triptolide and triptonide: Insights on their pharmacological activity, toxicity, combination therapy, new dosage form and novel drug delivery routes. *Biomed. Pharmacother.* **2023**, *162*, 114705. [CrossRef]

36. Xu, H.; Zhao, H.; Ding, C.; Jiang, D.; Zhao, Z.; Li, Y.; Ding, X.; Gao, J.; Zhou, H.; Luo, C.; et al. Celastrol suppresses colorectal cancer via covalent targeting peroxiredoxin 1. *Signal Transduct. Target. Ther.* **2023**, *8*, 51. [CrossRef]
37. Zhang, Y.; Liu, R.; Li, C.; Shi, L.; Guo, Z.; Zhu, L.; Li, W.; Li, J.; Li, Z. Celastrol-based nanomedicine hydrogels eliminate posterior capsule opacification. *Nanomedicine* **2022**, *17*, 1449–1461. [CrossRef]
38. Rezagholizade-Shirvan, A.; Soltani, M.; Shokri, S.; Radfar, R.; Arab, M.; Shamloo, E. Bioactive compound encapsulation: Characteristics, applications in food systems, and implications for human health. *Food Chem. X* **2024**, *24*, 101953. [CrossRef]
39. Dominguez, D.L.; Fernandez-Ruiz, V.; Camara, M. The frontier between nutrition and pharma: The international regulatory framework of functional foods, food supplements and nutraceuticals. *Crit. Rev. Food Sci. Nutr.* **2020**, *60*, 1738–1746. [CrossRef]
40. Libby, P.; Hansson, G.K. From Focal Lipid Storage to Systemic Inflammation: JACC Review Topic of the Week. *J. Am. Coll. Cardiol.* **2019**, *74*, 1594–1607. [CrossRef]
41. Xu, H.; Fang, F.; Wu, K.; Song, J.; Li, Y.; Lu, X.; Liu, J.; Zhou, L.; Yu, W.; Yu, F.; et al. Gut microbiota-bile acid crosstalk regulates murine lipid metabolism via the intestinal FXR-FGF19 axis in diet-induced humanized dyslipidemia. *Microbiome* **2023**, *11*, 262. [CrossRef] [PubMed]
42. Zheng, Z.; Lyu, W.; Ren, Y.; Li, X.; Zhao, S.; Yang, H.; Xiao, Y. Allobaculum Involves in the Modulation of Intestinal ANGPTLT4 Expression in Mice Treated by High-Fat Diet. *Front. Nutr.* **2021**, *8*, 690138. [CrossRef]
43. Kushkevych, I.; Dordevic, D.; Vitezova, M. Possible synergy effect of hydrogen sulfide and acetate produced by sulfate-reducing bacteria on inflammatory bowel disease development. *J. Adv. Res.* **2021**, *27*, 71–78. [CrossRef] [PubMed]
44. Kuffa, P.; Pickard, J.M.; Campbell, A.; Yamashita, M.; Schaus, S.R.; Martens, E.C.; Schmidt, T.M.; Inohara, N.; Nunez, G.; Caruso, R. Fiber-deficient diet inhibits colitis through the regulation of the niche and metabolism of a gut pathobiont. *Cell Host Microbe* **2023**, *31*, 2007–2022. [CrossRef]
45. Liu, Y.; Zhou, M.; Yang, M.; Jin, C.; Song, Y.; Chen, J.; Gao, M.; Ai, Z.; Su, D. Pulsatilla chinensis Saponins Ameliorate Inflammation and DSS-Induced Ulcerative Colitis in Rats by Regulating the Composition and Diversity of Intestinal Flora. *Front. Cell. Infect. Microbiol.* **2021**, *11*, 728929. [CrossRef]
46. McMillan, A.S.; Foley, M.H.; Perkins, C.E.; Theriot, C.M. Loss of Bacteroides thetaiotaomicron bile acid-altering enzymes impacts bacterial fitness and the global metabolic transcriptome. *Microbiol. Spectr.* **2024**, *12*, e03576-23. [CrossRef]
47. Zhu, J.; Liu, X.; Liu, N.; Zhao, R.; Wang, S. Lactobacillus plantarum alleviates high-fat diet-induced obesity by altering the structure of mice intestinal microbial communities and serum metabolic profiles. *Front. Microbiol.* **2024**, *15*, 1425764. [CrossRef]
48. Vacca, M.; Celano, G.; Calabrese, F.M.; Portincasa, P.; Gobbetti, M.; De Angelis, M. The Controversial Role of Human Gut Lachnospiraceae. *Microorganisms* **2020**, *8*, 573. [CrossRef]

nutrients MDPI

Article

Effects of Caprylic Acid and Eicosapentaenoic Acid on Lipids, Inflammatory Levels, and the JAK2/STAT3 Pathway in ABCA1-Deficient Mice and ABCA1 Knock-Down RAW264.7 Cells

Xinsheng Zhang [1], Peng Zhang [2], Yinghua Liu [1,*], Zhao Liu [1], Qing Xu [1], Yong Zhang [1], Lu Liu [1], Xueyan Yang [1], Liya Li [1] and Changyong Xue [1]

[1] Department of Nutrition, The First Medical Center, Chinese PLA General Hospital, Beijing 100853, China
[2] Guizhou Crops of Chinese People's Armed Police Force, Guiyang 550001, China
* Correspondence: liuyinghua77@163.com; Tel.: +86-10-66937619

Abstract: Our previous studies have found that caprylic acid (C8:0) can improve blood lipids and reduce inflammation levels and may be related to the upregulation of the p-JAK2/p-STAT3 pathway by ABCA1. This study aims to investigate the effects of C8:0 and eicosapentaenoic acid (EPA) on lipids, inflammatory levels, and the JAK2/STAT3 pathway in ABCA1-deficient mice ($ABCA1^{-/-}$) and ABCA1 knock-down (ABCA1-KD) RAW 264.7 cells. Twenty 6-week $ABCA1^{-/-}$ mice were randomly divided into four groups and fed a high-fat diet, or a diet of 2% C8:0, 2% palmitic acid (C16:0) or 2% EPA for 8 weeks, respectively. The RAW 264.7 cells were divided into the control or control + LPS group, and the ABCA1-KD RAW 264.7 cells were divided into ABCA1-KD with LPS (LPS group), ABCA1-KD with LPS + C8:0 (C8:0 group), and ABCA1-KD with LPS + EPA (EPA group). Serum lipid profiles and inflammatory levels were measured, and ABCA1 and JAK2/STAT3 mRNA and protein expressions were determined by RT-PCR and Western blot analyses, respectively. Our results showed that serum lipid and inflammatory levels increased in $ABCA1^{-/-}$ mice ($p < 0.05$). After the intervention of different fatty acids in $ABCA1^{-/-}$ mice, TG and TNF-α were significantly lower, while MCP-1 increased significantly in the C8:0 group ($p < 0.05$); however, LDL-C, TC, TNF-α, IL-6, and MCP-1 levels decreased significantly and IL-10 increased significantly in the EPA group ($p < 0.05$). In the aorta of $ABCA1^{-/-}$ mice, C8:0 significantly decreased p-STAT3 and p-JAK2 mRNA, while EPA significantly reduced TLR4 and NF-κBp65 mRNA. In the ABCA1-KD RAW 264.7 cells, TNF-α and MCP-1 were increased significantly and IL-10 and IL-1β were significantly decreased in the C8:0 group ($p < 0.05$). The protein expressions of ABCA1 and p-JAK2 were significantly higher, and the NF-κBp65 was significantly lower in the C8:0 and EPA groups ($p < 0.05$). Meanwhile, compared to the C8:0 group, the NF-κBp65 protein expression was significantly lower in the EPA group ($p < 0.05$). Our study showed that EPA had better effects than C8:0 on inhibiting inflammation and improving blood lipids in the absence of ABCA1. C8:0 may be involved mainly in inhibiting inflammation through upregulation of the ABCA1 and p-JAK2/p-STAT3 pathways, while EPA may be involved mainly in inhibiting inflammation through the TLR4/NF-κBp65 signaling pathway. The upregulation of the ABCA1 expression pathway by functional nutrients may provide research targets for the prevention and treatment of atherosclerosis.

Keywords: caprylic acid; EPA; inflammatory cytokine; ABCA1; JAK2; STAT3

1. Introduction

Atherosclerotic cardiovascular disease (ASCVD) is one of the leading causes of mortality worldwide [1]. In particular, in low- and middle-income countries, ASCVD accounts for about 80% of the disease burden [2]. Atherosclerosis (AS) is the pathological basis of

ASCVD, and is closely related to various risk factors, including hyperlipidemia, hypertension, chronic inflammation, immune factors, etc. Exploring the target of inhibiting AS has always been a hot topic in the treatment of ASCVD.

ATP-binding box transporter A1 (ABCA1) is a membrane protein that can promote intracellular cholesterol efflux and promote liver HDL production. Current studies have shown that ABCA1 not only promotes cholesterol reversal and reduces AS lipid deposition, but also participates in the inflammatory reaction process of AS. ABCA1 has been reported to inhibit the inflammatory response in the following ways [3–5]: first, ABCA1 directly activates Janus kinase 2 (JAK2) and the signal transducer and activator of transcription 3 (STAT3) downregulating downstream signaling molecules; the second is that ABCA1 indirectly inhibits the toll-like receptor-4 (TLR4) signaling pathway by promoting cholesterol efflux and reducing lipid raft in the cell membrane. These findings suggest that ABCA1 can play a direct role in cardioprotective effects by promoting cholesterol transport and inhibiting inflammation.

Dietary fatty acids are considered important factors affecting the progress of AS. Studies have reported that saturated fatty acids (SFAs) can increase the level of low-density lipoprotein cholesterol (LDL-C), thus promoting the occurrence of AS, while unsaturated fatty acids can improve blood lipids and play a protective role in cardiovascular diseases, especially omega-3 polyunsaturated fatty acids (ω-3 PUFAs), such as eicosapentaenoic acid (EPA) and docosahexaenoic acid (DHA) [6]. Fatty acids and inflammatory factors are closely related to the progress of AS [7]. Current studies suggest that PUFAs, such as linoleic acid (C18:2), omega-6 polyunsaturated fatty acids (ω-6 PUFAs), and ω-3 PUFAs from food sources, can reduce inflammation. Fish oil is rich in ω-3 PUFAs (DHA and EPA) and has anti-inflammatory effects. Its anti-inflammatory mechanism has been reported to be through inhibition of the TLR4 signaling pathway [8]. Medium-chain fatty acids (MCFAs), including caprylic acid (C8:0) and capric acid (C10:0), occur in milk fat, palm oil, and various feed materials [9]. MCFAs differ from long chain fatty acids (LCFAs) in digestion, absorption, and metabolism, and studies have found that MCFAs can reduce body weight and improve internal fat accumulation [10,11] and cholesterol metabolism [12,13]. Our previous experiments have confirmed that MCFAs can upregulate ABCA1 gene and protein expression in the apoE-deficient mouse liver, and C8:0 can promote cholesterol efflux in macrophages [14]. Further studies found that C8:0 could inhibit the levels of inflammatory cytokines in RAW 264.7 cells and in the serum of apoE-deficient mice, and confirmed that C8:0 could inhibit the inflammatory response based on the ABCA1-mediated JAK2/STAT3 pathway [15].

JAK2 is activated by ABCA1, undergoes autophosphorylation, and then phosphorylates its downstream target STAT3 [16], and then regulates the levels of nuclear factor kappa Bp65 (NF-κBp65), tumor necrosis factor α (TNF-α), interleukin-6 (IL-6), and monocyte chemoattractant protein-1 (MCP-1), which leads to the occurrence of AS [17]. This study aims to investigate the effects of C8:0 and EPA on lipid and inflammatory levels, and the JAK2/STAT3 pathway in ABCA1-deficient mice (ABCA1$^{-/-}$) and ABCA1 knock-down (ABCA1-KD) RAW 264.7 cells, and to confirm that C8:0 plays a regulatory role in improving blood lipid and inflammation mainly through ABCA1.

2. Materials and Methods

2.1. Materials

Fetal bovine serum (FBS), lipopolysaccharide (LPS), DMEM culture medium, and bovine serum albumin (BSA) were provided by Gibco (Grand Island, NE, USA). C8:0, palmitic acid (C16:0), and EPA were obtained from Sigma-Aldrich (St. Louis, MO, USA). Other reagents were available from Sigma-Aldrich.

2.2. Feed Configuration

For feed content, we applied the same method as our previous research [18]. Briefly, based on high-fat feed, 2% of the same amounts of different kinds of fatty acids were added.

Intervention feeds included a high-fat diet (HFD group), and high-fat diets of 2% C8:0 (C8:0 group), 2% eicosapentaenoic acid (EPA group), and 2% palmitic acid (C16:0 group). The feed was obtained from Beijing Huafukang Biotechnology Co., Ltd. (license No.: SCXK 2014-0008). The ingredient list and fatty acid compositions of the intervention diets are provided in Supplementary Materials (Tables S1 and S2).

2.3. Experimental Animals

To obtain ABCA1 knockout mice, we used DBA/1-ABCA1 tm1jdm/J female mice (ABCA1 heterozygous mice) purchased from Jackson Laboratory (stock#003897, Bar Harbor, ME). Because ABCA1 homozygotes cannot reproduce and have a 50% mortality rate, we used male C57BL/6J mice and heterozygous ABCA1 mice to reproduce more heterozygous mice and then obtained 20 homozygous female and male ABCA1 mice at 5 weeks of age. All animals were genetically identified prior to use to confirm that they were $ABCA1^{-/-}$ mice. Five animals per cage were housed in polycarbonate cages; temperature was maintained at 21–23 °C and humidity was maintained at 40–60%, with a 12 h light/dark cycle. Both the $ABCA1^{-/-}$ mice and the same week-old C57BL/6J mice were kept on a HFD prior to intervention, and the HFD was replaced with intervention diets for 8 weeks after random allocation based on fasting weight. Fasting weight was measured weekly during this period (fasting did not limit drinking water at night prior to measurement). The bedding and drinking water of the mice were replaced every 2–3 days and the feed intake of the mice was recorded. All experimental procedures were approved by the Animal Care and Use Committee of the Chinese PLA General Hospital.

2.4. Preparation of Fatty Acids

Fatty acids were prepared as in our previous research [15]. Briefly, the fatty acids were dissolved in a 95% ethanol solution and then diluted with serum-free medium containing 20 mg/mL of BSA, with 100 mmol/L added to the culture hole and 50 ng/mL of LPS added to the culture wells. Before the cell experiment, the obtained solution was incubated at 37 °C for 1 h.

2.5. ABCA1-KD in RAW 264.7 Cells

The RAW 264.7 cell line was obtained from the Peking Union Medical College, and the cells were cultured in DMEM with heat-inactivated FBS (10%) and penicillin–streptomycin solution (1%) in a humidified incubator with 95% air and 5% CO_2 at 37 °C. RAW 264.7 cells at the logarithmic growth stage were inoculated into 6-well cell culture plates (2×10^5 cells per well) and cultured overnight in an incubator. The ABCA1-KD RAW 264.7 cells were constructed with three types of siRNA of ABCA1-1530, ABCA1-1701, and ABCA1-4931 (Supplementary Materials, Table S3). The most effective plasmids that inhibited ABCA1 were screened by RT-PCR, as shown in Figure 1. ABCA1-1701 had the strongest inhibitory level and was selected to construct a siRNA plasmid to obtain ABCA1-KD RAW 264.7 cells. Two hours before transfection, the culture medium was changed to serum-free DMEM. According to the plasmid transfection instructions, cultured RAW 264.7 cells (2×10^5 cells/well) were transfected with the ABCA1-1701 plasmid using Lipofectamine 2000 reagent (Life Technologies, Carlsbad, CA, USA). The cells were then tested with the optimal concentration of G418 (500 µg/mL) for about 3 weeks. A limited dilution method was applied to isolate and obtain the maximum number of stably transfected cells. DMEM medium containing 10% fetal bovine serum was used during the experiment and then refilled with LPS medium (final concentration 100 ng/mL), and incubated for another 24 h after the addition of C8:0 or EPA to the culture medium. The ABCA1-KD RAW 264.7 cells were randomly divided into 5 groups (n = 5), including the control group (RAW 264.7 cells), ABCA1-KD group, ABCA1-KD + LPS group (LPS 100 ng/mL), ABCA1-KD + LPS + C8:0 (LPS 100 ng/mL, C8:0 100 µmol/L), and ABCA1-KD + LPS + EPA (LPS 100 ng/mL, EPA 100 µmol/L). Then the levels of interleukin-1β (IL-1β), IL-6, interleukin-10 (IL-10), TNF-α, and MCP-1 in the cell lysate were detected according to the instructions of the ELISA kit.

Cell assay was repeated, and the protein expressions of ABCA1, JAK2/STAT3, p-JAK2/p-ATAT3, and NF-κBp65 were determined by Western blot analyses.

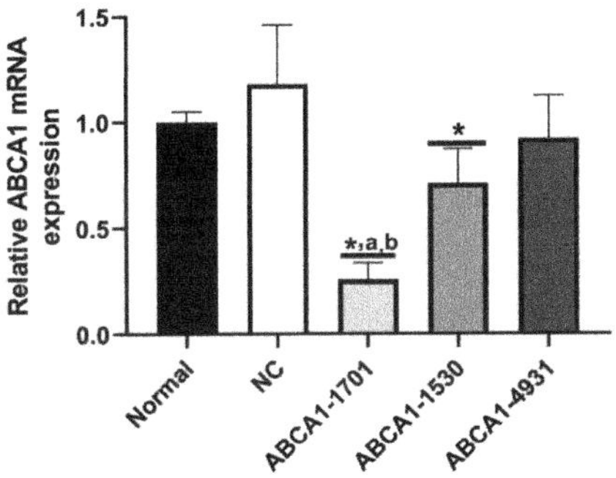

Figure 1. Effective plasmid screening of ABCA1 siRNA. Data in the figure are expressed as the mean ± SD with three samples in each group (n = 3). * $p < 0.05$, versus NC group; ^{a} $p < 0.05$, versus ABCA1-1530 group; ^{b} $p < 0.05$, versus ABCA1-4931 group.

2.6. Serum Lipid Profiles Measurement

Serum triglyceride (TG), total cholesterol (TC), high-density lipoprotein cholesterol (HDL-C), and LDL-C (Abcam, Cambridge, UK) were determined according to the commercial kit instructions, and HDL-C/LDL-C was calculated.

2.7. Inflammatory Level Measurement

After 8 weeks, the mice were sacrificed by intramuscular injection of 10 mg/kg of xylazine hydrochloride, blood was drawn from the abdominal aorta and then centrifuged at 4 °C and 3000 r/min for 10 min, and serum was collected for detection. After the cell experiment, the cell lysate from each group was collected and centrifuged at 3000 r/min at 4 °C for 10 min, and the supernatant was collected to be measured. The IL-1β, IL-6, IL-10, TNF-α, and MCP-1 were determined following the instructions of the ELISA kit (R&D Systems, Minneapolis, MN, USA).

2.8. Real-Time PCR Analysis

For RNA expression analysis, about 50 mg of aorta samples were taken, total RNA was isolated using TRIzol reagent (Omega Bio-Tek, Norcross, GA, USA), and then reverse transcription was performed using a reverse transcription kit (NEB, M MLV kit). The reaction mixtures were incubated at 95 °C for 2 min for the initial denaturation, followed by 45 cycles of 25 °C/5 min, 50 °C/15 min, 85 °C/5 min, and 4 °C/10 min for cDNA, and then 50 °C/2 min, 95 °C/10 min, 95 °C/30 s, and 60 °C/30 s. Relative expression levels were calculated with the ΔCt method. Primers were designed using Primer Express Software v3.0 (Applied Biosystems, SAN Jose, California, USA) (Table 1).

2.9. Western Blot Analysis

The 20 mg of mouse aorta tissue sample was extracted by protein lysis buffer and the cells were extracted with RIPA buffer (CST). Western blot analysis of mouse aorta tissue and cell samples referred to previous studies [18]. Immunoblotting for STAT3 (abcam, no.ab68153, 1:1000), JAK2 (abcam, no.ab108596, 1:1000), p-STAT3 (abcam, no.ab76315, 1:800), p-JAK2 (abcam, no.ab32101, 1:800), ABCA1 (abcam, no.Ab18180, 1:200), NF-κBp65 (abcam, no.ab32536, 1:1000), MYD88 (abcam, no.ab219413, 1:1000), TLR4 (Proteintech, no.19811-1-AP, 1:1000), and β-actin (Proteintech, no.66009-1-Ig, 1:5000) followed the procedures. The bands were visualized using a chemiluminescence detection system.

Table 1. Real-time PCR primer sequences.

Indicators	Primer	Sequence	Primer Bank ID
β-actin	Forward Reverse	5′-GGCTGTATTCCCCTCCATCG -3′ 5′-CCAGTTGGTAACAATGCCATGT -3′	6671509a1
JAK2	Forward Reverse	5′-TTGTGGTATTACGCCTGTGTATC-3′ 5′-ATGCCTGGTTGACTCGTCTAT-3′	6680508a1
STAT3	Forward Reverse	5′-CAATACCATTGACCTGCCGAT-3′ 5′-GAGCGACTCAAACTGCCCT-3′	13277852a1
MAPK	Forward Reverse	5′-GGCTCGGCACACTGATGAT-3′ 5′-TGGGGTTCCAACGAGTCTTAAA-3′	6754632a1
TLR4	Forward Reverse	5′-ATGGCATGGCTTACACCACC-3′ 5′-GAGGCCAATTTTGTCTCCACA-3′	10946594a1
MYD88	Forward Reverse	5′-TCATGTTCTCCATACCCTTGGT-3′ 5′-AAACTGCGAGTGGGGTCAG-3′	26354939a1
NF-κBp65	Forward Reverse	5′-CACCGGATTGAAGAGAAGCG-3′ 5′-AAGTTGATGGTGCTGAGGGA-3′	30047197a1

JAK2, Janus kinase 2; STAT3, signal transducer and activator of transcription 3; MAPK, mitogen-activated protein kinase; TLR4, toll-like receptor 4; MYD88, myeloid differentiation primary response 88; NF-κBp65, nuclear factor kappa Bp65.

2.10. Statistical Analysis

Based on our preliminary experiment [15], the sample size was estimated using G*Power software v3.1.9.3 (Heinrich-Heine University, Germany). With power = 80%, $\alpha = 0.05$, effect size = 0.85, the minimum sample size should be 5. In mouse experiments, the sample sizes for analysis of inflammatory levels, blood lipids, PCR, and Western blot were 5, 5, 5, and 4, respectively. The sample sizes for the analysis of inflammatory cytokines and Western blotting in cell experiments was 5 and 3, respectively. All data are expressed as mean ± standard deviation and for the detection of a significant difference ($p < 0.05$, two-tailed). The normality of the data was analyzed by Shapiro–Wilk test. The normal distribution data between the two groups were analyzed by Student's t test, and the non-normal distribution data between the two groups were analyzed by Mann–Whitney U and Wilcoxon signed-rank tests. One-way analysis of variance was used to analyze the multigroup data, and Tukey–Kramer multiple comparison analysis was used to analyze the differences between groups. SPSS 28.0 (SPSS, Inc., Chicago, IL, USA) was used to analyze the research data.

3. Results

3.1. Body Weight of ABCA1$^{-/-}$ Mice

After 2 weeks of intervention, the fasting body weight of the EPA, C8:0, and C16:0 groups decreased significantly compared to that of the HFD group ($p < 0.05$) (Figure 2A). There were no significant differences in the average feed intake among all groups during the intervention period ($p > 0.05$) (Figure 2B).

3.2. Serum Lipid Profiles in ABCA1$^{-/-}$ Mice

After 8 weeks of intervention, ABCA1$^{-/-}$-HFD mice showed a marked reduction in TC, TG, and non-HDL-C ($p < 0.05$) (Figure 3A,B,F). Next, we analyzed the serum lipids of ABCA1$^{-/-}$ mice with different fatty acid HFD. The EPA group had a significantly lower level of TC than that of the HFD, C8:0, and C16:0 groups ($p < 0.05$) (Figure 3A). The C8:0 and C16:0 groups had a significantly lower TG level than the HFD and EPA groups (Figure 3B) and had a significantly higher HDL-C level than the EPA group ($p < 0.05$) (Figure 3C). The EPA group exhibited a significant decrease in serum LDL-C and non-HDL-C levels compared to those of the C8:0 and C16:0 groups ($p < 0.05$) (Figure 3D,F).

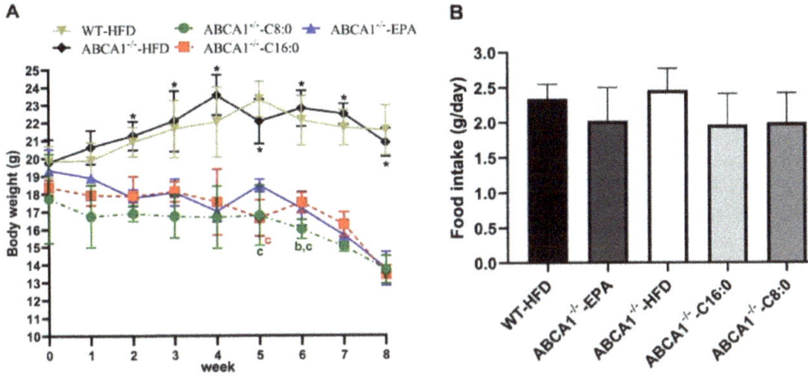

Figure 2. Fasting body weight and food intake of ABCA1$^{-/-}$ mice. (**A**) The fasting body weight was determined once per week; (**B**) Average daily food intake during the experiment. The data in the figure are expressed as mean ± SD with five samples in each group (n = 5). * $p < 0.05$ versus the ABCA1$^{-/-}$-C8:0, ABCA1$^{-/-}$-C16:0, and ABCA1$^{-/-}$-EPA groups; ^{b} $p < 0.05$ versus the ABCA1$^{-/-}$-C16:0 group; ^{c} $p < 0.05$ versus the ABCA1$^{-/-}$-EPA group.

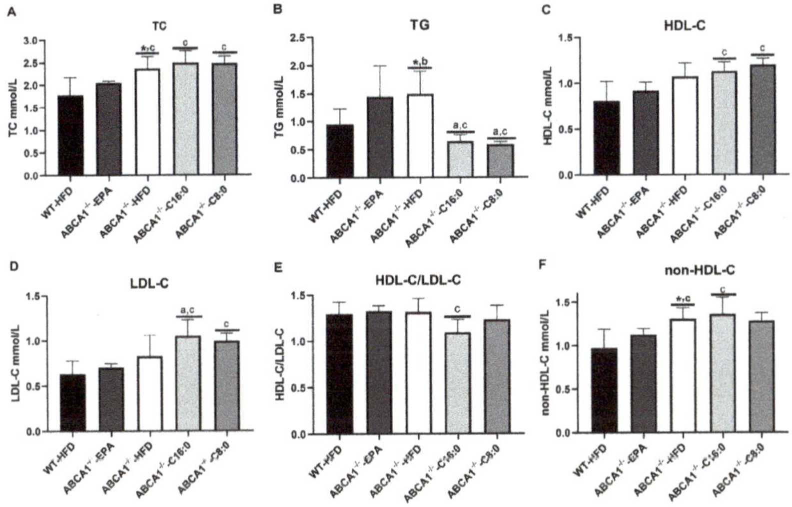

Figure 3. Serum lipid profiles in ABCA1$^{-/-}$ mice. (**A**) TC, (**B**) TG, (**C**) HDL-C, (**D**) LDL-C, (**E**) HDL-C/LDL-C, and (**F**) non-HLD-C. The data in the figure are expressed as mean ± SD with five samples in each group (n = 5). * $p < 0.05$ versus the WT-HFD group; ^{a} $p < 0.05$ versus the ABCA1$^{-/-}$ -HFD group; ^{b} $p < 0.05$ versus the ABCA1$^{-/-}$-C16:0 group; ^{c} $p < 0.05$ versus the ABCA1$^{-/-}$-EPA group.

3.3. Serum Inflammatory Factors in ABCA1$^{-/-}$ Mice

ABCA1 knockout can promote the release of different pro-inflammatory cytokines in mice. According to Figure 4, ABCA1$^{-/-}$-HFD mice had significantly higher levels of IL-1β, IL-6, TNF-α, and MCP-1, and had a significantly lower level of IL-10 than those of WT-HFD mice ($p < 0.05$). Then we analyzed the effects of different fatty acid HFDs on serum inflammation in ABCA1$^{-/-}$ mice. The EPA group exhibited a significant decrease in serum IL-1β, IL-6, TNF-α, and MCP-1 and a significant increase in serum IL-10 compared to that of the C8:0, C16:0, and HFD groups ($p < 0.05$) (Figure 4). Although the C8: 0 group had a significantly lower level of TNF-α than that of the HFD and C16: 0 groups, it had a significantly higher level of MCP-1 than that of the HFD group ($p < 0.05$) (Figure 4A,D).

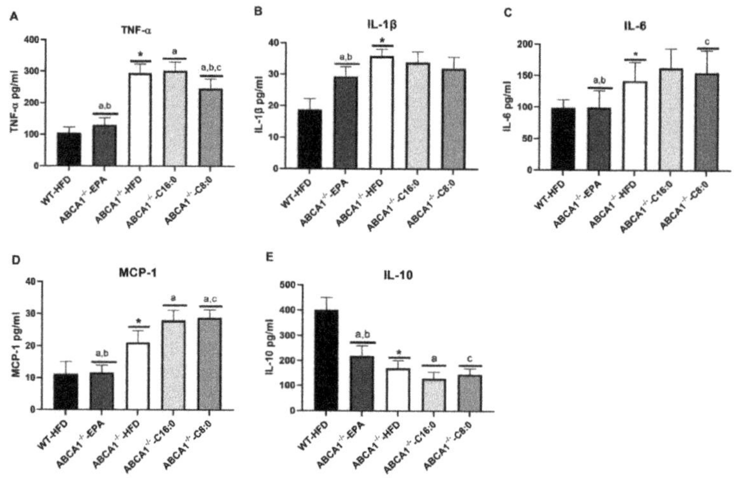

Figure 4. Serum levels of inflammatory cytokines in ABCA1$^{-/-}$ mice. (**A**) TNF-α, (**B**) IL-1β, (**C**) IL-6, (**D**) MCP-1, and (**E**) IL-10. The data in the figure are expressed as mean ± SD with five samples in each group (n = 5). * $p < 0.05$ versus the WT-HFD group; ^{a} $p < 0.05$ versus the ABCA1$^{-/-}$-HFD group; ^{b} $p < 0.05$ versus the ABCA1$^{-/-}$-C16:0 group; ^{c} $p < 0.05$ versus the ABCA1$^{-/-}$-EPA group.

3.4. The mRNA Expression Levels of TLR4 and JAK2/STAT3 in the ABCA1$^{-/-}$ Mouse Aorta

In ABCA1$^{-/-}$ mice, compared to the HFD group, the mRNA expression of TLR4 was significantly downregulated in the C8:0, EPA, and C16:0 groups ($p < 0.05$) (Figure 5D). EPA group mice had significantly lower TLR4 and NF-κBp65 mRNA expressions than those of the HFD and C16:0 groups, and had a significantly lower TLR4 mRNA expression than that of the C8:0 group ($p < 0.05$) (Figure 5D,F).

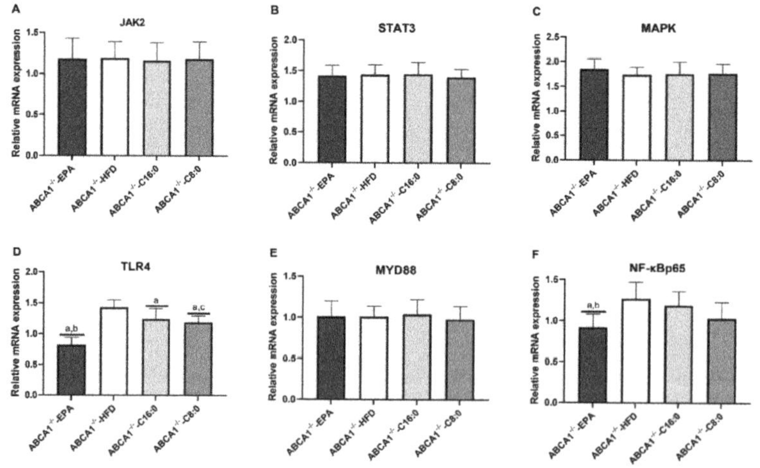

Figure 5. The mRNA expression levels of the signaling components TLR4 and JAK2/STAT3 in the ABCA1$^{-/-}$ mouse aorta. (**A**) JAK2, (**B**) STAT3, (**C**) MAPK, (**D**) TLR4, (**E**) MYD88, and (**F**) NF-κBp65. The data in the figure are expressed as mean ± SD with four samples in each group (n = 4). ^{a} $p < 0.05$ versus the ABCA1$^{-/-}$-HFD group; ^{b} $p < 0.05$ versus the ABCA1$^{-/-}$-C16:0 group; ^{c} $p < 0.05$ versus the ABCA1$^{-/-}$-EPA group.

3.5. The Relative Protein Expression Levels of TLR4 and JAK2/STAT3 in the ABCA1$^{-/-}$ Mouse Aorta

In ABCA1$^{-/-}$ mice, the C8:0 group had significantly lower expression levels of p-STAT3 and p-JAK2 than those of the HFD group ($p < 0.05$) (Figure 6B,C). The EPA group had a significantly lower expression level of NF-κBp65 than that of the HFD and C16:0 groups, and had a significantly lower expression level of TLR4 than that of the HFD, C16:0, and C8:0 groups ($p < 0.05$) (Figure 6D,F).

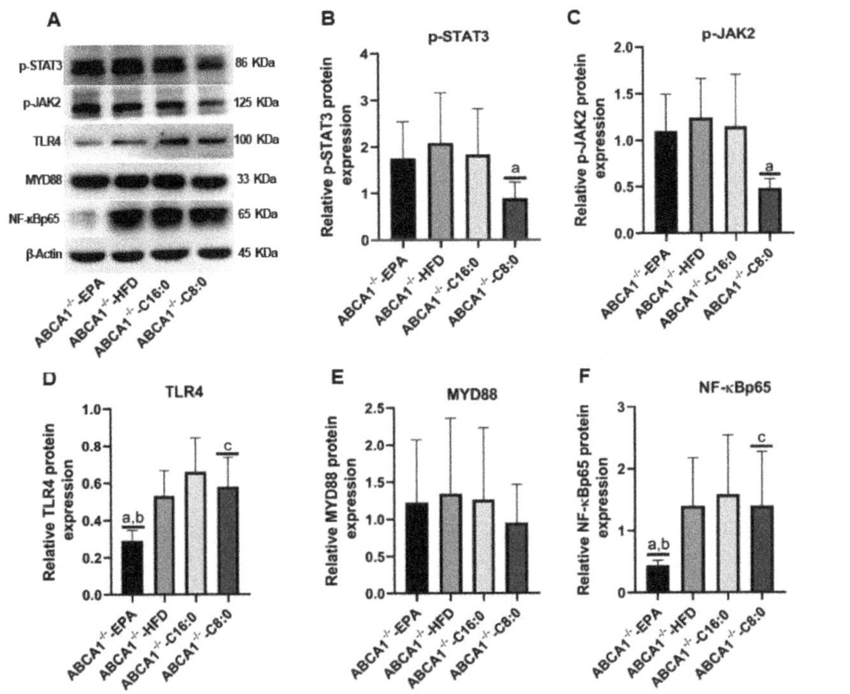

Figure 6. Relative protein expression of the TLR4 and JAK2/STAT3 signaling components in the ABCA1$^{-/-}$ mouse aorta. (**A**) bolt sections, (**B**) p-STAT3, (**C**) p-JAK2, (**D**) TLR4, (**E**) MYD88, and (**F**) NF-κBp65. The data in the figure are expressed as mean ± SD with four samples in each group (n = 4). ^{a} $p < 0.05$ versus the ABCA1 / -HFD group; ^{b} $p < 0.05$ versus the ABCA1 / -C16:0 group; ^{c} $p < 0.05$ versus the ABCA1$^{-/-}$-EPA group.

3.6. The Inflammatory Factors of ABCA1-KD RAW 264.7 Cells

After RAW 264.7 cells induced by LPS, the levels of TNF-α, MCP-1, IL-6, and IL-1β were significantly increased, while the levels of IL-10 decreased significantly ($p < 0.05$) (Figure 7A–E). Similarly, the levels of TNF-α, MCP-1, IL-6, and IL-1β inflammatory cytokines in the ABCA1-KD + LPS group decreased significantly compared to the control group + LPS group, while the level of IL-10 increased significantly ($p < 0.05$) (Figure 7A–E). In ABCA1-KD RAW 264.7 cells with LSP, the EPA group exhibited a significant decrease in TNF-α, MCP-1, IL-6, and IL-1β and a significant increase in IL-10 compared to that of the LPS groups ($p < 0.05$) (Figure 7). In addition, the EPA group had a significantly lower level of TNF-α and MCP-1 than that of the C8: 0 group (Figure 7A,B); however, it had significantly higher levels of IL-1β and IL-10 than those of the C8: 0 group ($p < 0.05$) (Figure 7D,E). The C8:0 group had a significantly higher level of TNF-α than that of the LPS group (Figure 7A), while it had significantly lower levels of MCP-1, IL-6, IL-1β, and IL-10 than those of the LPS group ($p < 0.05$) (Figure 7B–E).

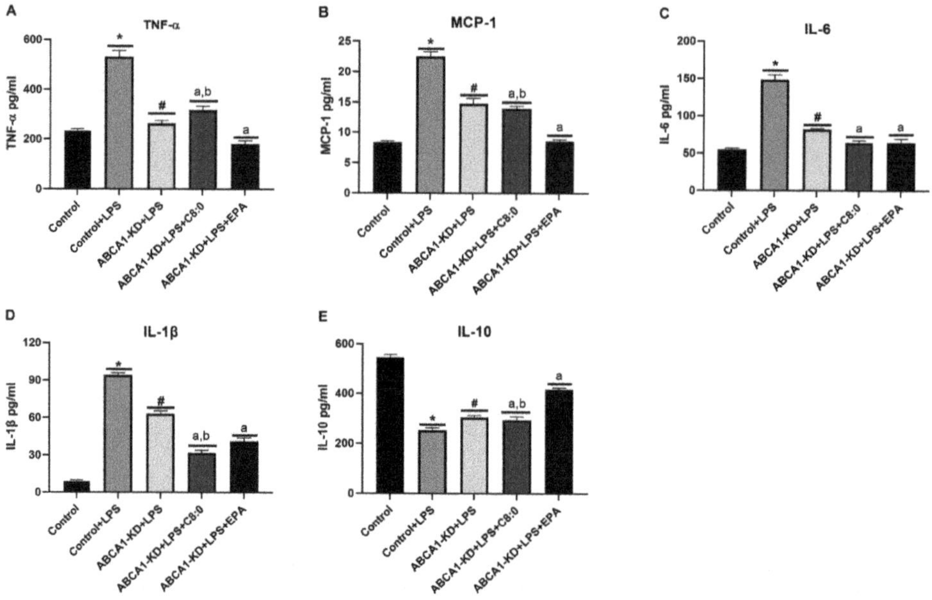

Figure 7. Inflammatory cytokine levels in LPS-stimulated ABCA1-KD RAW 264.7 cells. (**A**) TNF-α, (**B**) MCP-1, (**C**) IL-6, (**D**) IL-1β, and (**E**) IL-10. The data in the figure are expressed as mean ± SD with five samples in each group (n = 5). * $p < 0.05$ versus the control group; # $p < 0.05$ versus the control + LPS group; [a] $p < 0.05$ versus the ABCA1-KD + LPS group; [b] $p < 0.05$ versus the ABCA1 -KD + LPS + EPA group.

3.7. The Protein Expression of JAK2/STAT3 in ABCA1-KD RAW 264.7 Cells

After LPS-induced RAW 264.7 cells, the ABCA1 expression was significantly lower, whereas the NF-κBp65, p-JAK2, and p-STAT3 expressions were significantly higher ($p < 0.05$) (Figure 8D,F,H). Additionally, after LPS-induced ABCA1-KD RAW 264.7 cells, the ABCA1, p-STAT3, and p-JAK2 expressions were significantly lower than those of the Control + LPS group, whereas the NF-κBp65 expression was significantly higher than that of the control + LPS group ($p < 0.05$) (Figure 8B,D,F,H). The C8:0 group had significantly higher expressions of ABCA1 and p-JAK2 than those of the ABCA1-KD + LPS group, while they had significantly lower expression of NF-κBp65 than that of the ABCA1-KD + LPS group ($p < 0.05$) (Figure 8B,D,F). Similarly, the EPA group had significantly higher expressions of ABCA1 and p-JAK2 than those in the ABCA1-KD + LPS group ($p < 0.05$) (Figure 8B,D,F), but had a significantly lower expression of NF-κBp65 than that of the C8:0 group ($p < 0.05$) (Figure 8F).

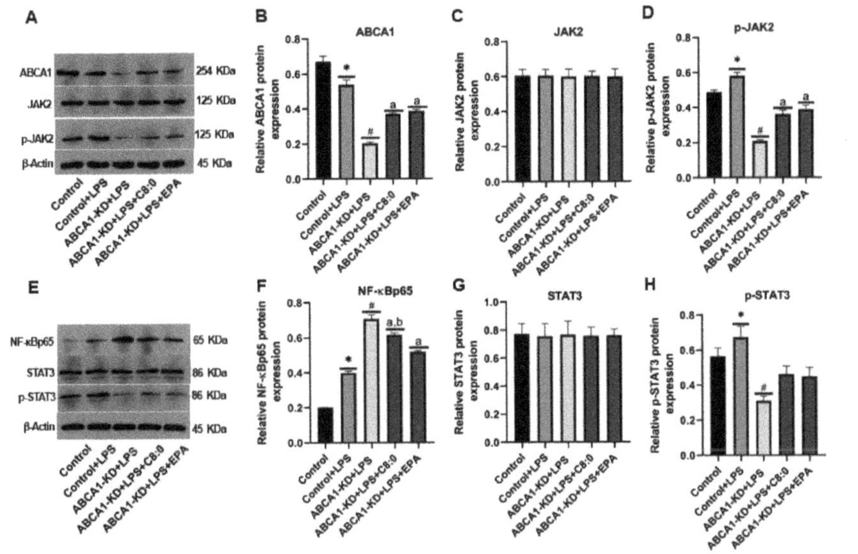

Figure 8. The relative protein expression of JAK2/STAT3 signaling components in LPS-stimulated ABCA1-KD RAW 264.7 cells. (**A**) and (**E**) bolt sections, (**B**) ABCA1, (**C**) JAK2, (**D**) p-JAK2, (**F**) NF-κBp65, (**G**) STAT3, and (**H**) p-STAT3. The data in the figure are expressed as mean ± SD with three samples in each group (n = 3). * $p < 0.05$ versus the control group; # $p < 0.05$ versus the control + LPS group; a $p < 0.05$ versus the ABCA1-KD + LPS group; b $p < 0.05$ versus the ABCA1-KD + LPS + EPA group.

4. Discussion

The present study showed that ABCA1 knockout resulted in dyslipidemia and increased inflammation in mice, which also resulted in significant fasting weight loss in the C8:0, C16:0, and EPA groups. Aiello et al. [19] reported that the survival rate and weight gain of ABCA1$^{-/-}$ mice after weaning were similar to those of wild-type mice, and the weight range of ABCA1$^{-/-}$ mice in this study was basically the same. In addition to ABCA1 defects, dietary differences have also been suggested as possible causes of weight loss. There was no significant difference in body weight between HFD-fed ABCA1$^{-/-}$ and wild-type mice in this study. On the contrary, Orso et al. [20] reported that ABCA1 knockout may cause insufficient vitamin absorption and platelet aggregation, as well as severe small intestinal lesions, resulting in decreased survival and body weight. In addition, homozygous female ABCA1-deficient mice are difficult to breed, probably due to altered hormone secretion and subsequent placental abnormalities caused by reduced estrogen and progesterone levels [21], which may also affect their metabolism and development. More recently, the important beneficial role that ABCA1 plays in modulating inflammation has been realized [22]. In ABCA1$^{-/-}$ mice, we found that C8:0 did not significantly improve LDL-C, TC, and HDL-C/LDL-C except for reducing TG, while EPA significantly improved LDL-C and TC, and a consistent effect was also observed on inflammation in ABCA1$^{-/-}$ mice and ABCA1-KD RAW 264.7 cells. Furthermore, C8:0 group mice had significantly decreased expression of p-STAT3 and p-JAK2 in the aorta, while EPA significantly decreased the expression of TLR4 and NF-κBp65 in the aorta of ABCA1$^{-/-}$ mice and ABCA1-KD RAW 264.7 cells. These results differ from our previous study of C57BL/6J mice [15]. These findings may help explore the different mechanisms of C8:0 and EPA in the regulation of blood lipids and inflammation.

ABCA1 belongs to the ABCA subfamily. ABCA1 was found to be highly expressed in hepatocytes, intestinal cells, macrophages, and endothelial cells [23]. Studies have shown that ABCA1 plays a crucial role in cholesterol reversal [22]. Fatty acids have been reported to regulate ABCA1 expression in mouse models by activating liver cyclic AMP-dependent protein kinase A and LXR/RXR pathways [4]. For example, linoleic acid suppressed the levels of ABCA1 transcripts and protein in human macrophages [24]. On the contrary, palmitic acid, ω-6 PUFAs and linolenic acid as a precursor to EPA, had the opposite effect [24,25]. In our previous studies, we found that MCT reduced LDL-C and TC levels and improved HDL-C levels in patients with high triglycerides [26,27]. We also observed that C8:0 could reduce TC and LDL-C levels, increase the HDL-C/LDL-C ratio, and improve atherosclerosis in apoE-deficient mice [18]. In recent years, in our mouse experiments, C8:0 was found to upregulate the expression of ABCA1 in the liver [14], in the mouse aorta [15], and in RAW 264.7 cells [15]. Tangier's disease is a high-risk ASCVD disease due to the lack of ABCA1, leading to high TG and TC and low HDL [28]. In this study, we found that ABCA1 knockout increased TG, TC, and non-HDL-C, but HDL-C did not decrease significantly, which may be related to the different intervention feeds and compensatory mechanisms. Drobnik et al. fed ABCA1$^{+/+}$ and ABCA1$^{-/-}$ mice with a cholesterol-free diet for 14 days and found a significant decrease in both serum HDL-C and TC in ABCA1$^{-/-}$ mice [29]. Haghpassand et al. reported that high fat feeding increased HDL cholesterol and apoA1 levels in wild-type mice or bone marrow-transplanted ABCA$^{-/-}$ mice [30]. A single deficiency of ABCA1 or ABCG1 in macrophages has been reported to not increase atherosclerosis, probably because ABCA1 deficiency leads to upregulation of ABCG1 expression [31]. Similarly, ABCG1-deficient mice were shown to have decreased plasma HDL cholesterol levels when fed a high-cholesterol diet. In addition to the significant reduction in TG in C8:0, there was no significant improvement in LDL-C, TC, and non-HDL-C levels. In contrast, EPA significantly reduced LDL-C, TC, and non-HDL-C levels compared to C8:0. It is suggested that the mechanism of C8:0 and EPA in reducing lipids is different, which is worthy of further study.

Research evidence has supported the role of ABCA1 in the regulation of cholesterol efflux [32] and its anti-inflammatory effects [33]. ABCA1 can regulate inflammation by participating in cellular cholesterol and phospholipid transport and the formation of lipid domains on the cell surface [3,33,34]. Dietary fatty acids not only affect blood lipids but also mediate inflammation levels, such as the way in which excessive intake of SFAs can increase the level of serum inflammatory cytokines in animals [35]. Furthermore, palmitic acid and stearic acid promoted the expression of TNF-α and IL-1β in macrophages [36]. Diets rich in fish oil can downregulate the expression of TLR4, TNF-α, IL-1, nucleotide-binding oligomerization domain protein1, and nucleotide-binding oligomerization domain protein2 in the liver of piglets [8]. Furthermore, supplementation with highly purified concentrated fish oil increased the levels of IL-10, IL-12, and IFN-γ while decreasing the levels of TNF-α and IL-6 [37]. In addition, EPA and DHA pretreatment may be beneficial for vascular inflammation in human saphenous veins undergoing a coronary bypass operation [38]. Although C8:0 belongs to SFA, both C8:0 and EPA can decrease the levels of MCP-1 and TNF-α and increase the level of IL-10 in mice and cells treated with LPS, in line with previous findings [15,18]. In mice, ABCA1 knockout increases inflammatory infiltration in vascular walls, peritoneal cavities, and blood circulation [19]. ABCA1/G1 deficiency improved LPS-induced inflammatory gene expression in mouse aortic endothelial cells [31]. In addition, THP-1 macrophage knockdown of ABCA1 inhibits downregulation of inflammatory cytokines by the apolipoprotein A-1 binding protein [39]. Patients with ABCA1 dysfunction tend to have chronic inflammation, suggesting that ABCA1 has a regulatory role in inflammation [40]. In this study, we found a significant decrease in inflammation levels by EPA after ABCA1 knockout; however, only TNF-α levels were significantly reduced by C8:0. In the ABCA1-KD RAW 264.7 cell assay, EPA was also found to significantly reduce inflammation levels compared to C8:0. The anti-inflammatory effects of C8:0 and EPA were different in ABCA1 deficiency. ABCA1 regulates both lipid metabolism and inflammation and may be the key protein in the mechanism of action of C8:0 and ω-3 PUFAs.

ABCA1 suppresses inflammation through multiple mechanisms. ABCA1 regulates the inflammatory response through NF-κBp65, TLR4/MYD88, JAK2/STAT3, cAMP/PKA, and apoptosis pathways [4,41]. SFAs, especially lauric acid, palmitic acid, and stearic acid, have been found to increase the level of IL-6 expression in macrophages through the TLR4 pathway, and stearic acid can promote the release of MCP-1 by activating TLR4 [42]. The mechanism of ω-6 PUFAs inhibiting the inflammatory response includes inhibition of the TLR-4/MYD88/NF-κBp65 pathway [43] and activation of GPR120 to inhibit the TAK1/NF-κBp65/JNK pathway [44]. Our previous results suggest that C8:0 can inhibit inflammation and improve atherosclerosis through the TLR4/NF-κBp65 signaling pathway in apoE$^{-/-}$ mice [18]. Further studies showed that C8:0 plays an important role in both lipid metabolism and inflammation, which may be related to the signaling pathways ABCA1 and JAK2/STAT3 [15]. Compared with EPA, the transcription levels of ABCA1, JAK2, and STAT3 in the mouse aorta increased significantly in C8:0, but there was no significant difference in the expressions of JAK2 and STAT3 in LPS-stimulated RAW 264.7 cells [15]. In this study, C8:0 significantly reduced the p-STAT3 and p-JAK2 in the aorta of ABCA1$^{-/-}$ mice. However, EPA significantly inhibited TLR4 and NF-κBp65 expression levels. C8:0 and EPA significantly increased ABCA1 and p-JAK2, while they decreased NF-κBp65. Meanwhile, EPA had a significantly lower NF-κBp65 protein expression than that of C8:0 in LPS-stimulated ABCA1-KD cells. However, the effects of C8:0 on inflammation levels and JAK2/STAT3 pathway protein expression were somewhat inconsistent in mice and cell lines. The reason may be that ABCA1 was knocked out and knocked down in mice and cells, respectively. In addition, different tissues analyzed in animal and cell experiments may have different results. Our study showed that C8:0 plays a regulatory role in improving blood lipids and inflammation primarily through ABCA1, while EPA mainly inhibits inflammation through the TLR4/NF-κBp65 pathway. The specific mechanism is worth further exploration.

However, there are some limitations to this study. (1) In the mouse experiment, the sample size was small because the ABCA1 homozygote mice could not reproduce. (2) The effects of ABCA1 knockout on different inflammatory pathways are unclear, and there are compensatory mechanisms, which will affect the results of the study. (3) In the future, we should observe the effects of C8:0 on inflammation and atherosclerosis in ABCA1- and apoE-gene-deficient mice. (4) The binding protein of C8:0 is still unknown and may be the key protein for its function; therefore, further study is necessary. (5) Dyslipidemia and inflammatory responses play a key role in the progression of atherosclerosis. In our study, no atherosclerotic lesions were found in ABCA1$^{-/-}$ mice fed a high-fat or palmitate diet for 8 weeks, which is consistent with previous findings [19,45]. Obviously, the mechanism of ABCA1 knockout in AS needs to be further studied, as well as the existing compensatory mechanism and the changing mechanism of the effects of C8:0 and EPA.

5. Conclusions

ABCA1 plays an important role in the regulation of lipid metabolism and inflammatory pathways. Our data showed that ABCA1 deficiency resulted in dyslipidemia and increased inflammation in mice, and that ABCA1 knockdown promoted increased inflammatory levels in RAW 264.7 cells. We found that EPA significantly improved cholesterol metabolism, while C8:0 showed only a significant decrease in TG. In addition, EPA inhibited inflammation levels significantly better than C8:0 in both ABCA1$^{-/-}$ mice and ABCA1-KD cells. These results differ from our previous studies of C57BL/6J mice and RAW 264.7 cells. The present study suggests that C8:0 can inhibit inflammation and improve blood lipids primarily through the upregulation of ABCA1 and p-JAK2/p-STAT3, while EPA can inhibit inflammation primarily through the TLR4/NF-κBp65 signaling pathway. The upregulation of the ABCA1 expression pathway by functional nutrients may provide research targets for the prevention and treatment of AS.

Supplementary Materials: The following supporting information can be downloaded at https://www.mdpi.com/article/10.3390/nu15051296/s1: Table S1, Compositions of experimental diets; Table S2, Fatty acid compositions of the experimental diets; Table S3, qRT-PCR Primer sequences in plasmid siRNA of ABCA1.

Author Contributions: X.Z. and P.Z. contributed to the collection and analysis of the data and writing of the manuscript. Z.L., L.L. (Liya Li), X.Y., and L.L. (Lu Liu) contributed to executing experiments and collecting data. Q.X. and Y.Z. contributed to the data collection. X.Z., P.Z., C.X., and Y.L. contributed to the design of the research and provided essential materials. Y.L. and C.X. contributed to the review of the manuscript. All authors have read and agreed to the published version of the manuscript.

Funding: This research was supported by the National Natural Science Fund of China (no. 81703204).

Institutional Review Board Statement: Not applicable.

Informed Consent Statement: Not applicable.

Data Availability Statement: Not applicable.

Conflicts of Interest: The authors declare no conflict of interest.

Abbreviations

ABCA1, ATP-binding box transporter A1; ABCA1$^{-/-}$, ABCA1-deficient; ABCA1-KD, ABCA1 knock-down; AS, atherosclerosis; ASCVD, atherosclerotic cardiovascular disease; BSA, bovine serum albumin; C10:0, capric acid; C16:0, palmitic acid; C18:2, linoleic acid; C8:0, caprylic acid; DHA, docosahexaenoic acid; EPA, eicosapentaenoic acid; EPA, eicosapentaenoic acid; FBS, fetal bovine serum; HDL-C, high-density lipoprotein cholesterol; IL-10, interleukin-10; IL-1β, interleukin-1β; IL-6, interleukin-6; JAK, Janus kinase 2; LCFAs, long-chain fatty acids; LDL-C, low-density lipoprotein cholesterol; LPS, lipopolysaccharide; MCFAs, medium-chain fatty acids; MCP-1, monocyte chemoattractant protein-1; NF-κBp65, nuclear factor kappa Bp65; non-HLD-C, non-high-density lipoprotein cholesterol; SFAs, saturated fatty acids; STAT3, signal transducer and activator of transcription 3; TC, total cholesterol; TG, triglyceride; TLR4, toll-like receptor-4; TNF-α, tumor necrosis factor α; ω-3 PUFAs, omega-3 polyunsaturated fatty acids; ω-6 PUFAs, omega-6 polyunsaturated fatty acids.

References

1. Yusuf, S.; Rangarajan, S.; Teo, K.; Islam, S.; Li, W.; Liu, L.; Bo, J.; Lou, Q.; Lu, F.; Liu, T.; et al. Cardiovascular risk and events in 17 low-, middle-, and high-income countries. *N. Engl. J. Med.* **2014**, *371*, 818–827. [CrossRef] [PubMed]
2. Yusuf, S.; Islam, S.; Chow, C.K.; Rangarajan, S.; Dagenais, G.; Diaz, R.; Gupta, R.; Kelishadi, R.; Iqbal, R.; Avezum, A.; et al. Use of secondary prevention drugs for cardiovascular disease in the community in high-income, middle-income, and low-income countries (the PURE Study): A prospective epidemiological survey. *Lancet* **2011**, *378*, 1231–1243. [CrossRef] [PubMed]
3. Westerterp, M.; Murphy, A.J.; Wang, M.; Pagler, T.A.; Vengrenyuk, Y.; Kappus, M.S.; Gorman, D.J.; Nagareddy, P.R.; Zhu, X.; Abramowicz, S.; et al. Deficiency of ATP-binding cassette transporters A1 and G1 in macrophages increases inflammation and accelerates atherosclerosis in mice. *Circ. Res.* **2013**, *112*, 1456–1465. [CrossRef] [PubMed]
4. Yin, K.; Liao, D.F.; Tang, C.K. ATP-binding membrane cassette transporter A1 (ABCA1): A possible link between inflammation and reverse cholesterol transport. *Mol. Med.* **2010**, *16*, 438–449. [CrossRef]
5. Fitzgerald, M.L.; Mujawar, Z.; Tamehiro, N. ABC transporters, atherosclerosis and inflammation. *Atherosclerosis* **2010**, *211*, 361–370. [CrossRef]
6. Yamagishi, K.; Hori, M.; Iso, H. Fish and omega-3 polyunsaturated fatty acids in relation to risk of cardiovascular disease. *Nihon Rinsho.* **2013**, *71*, 1552–1557.
7. Sacks, F.M.; Campos, H. Polyunsaturated fatty acids, inflammation, and cardiovascular disease: Time to widen our view of the mechanisms. *J. Clin. Endocrinol. Metab.* **2006**, *91*, 398–400. [CrossRef]
8. Chen, F.; Liu, Y.; Zhu, H.; Hong, Y.; Wu, Z.; Hou, Y.; Li, Q.; Ding, B.; Yi, D.; Chen, H. Fish oil attenuates liver injury caused by LPS in weaned pigs associated with inhibition of TLR4 and nucleotide-binding oligomerization domain protein signaling pathways. *Innate Immun.* **2013**, *19*, 504–515. [CrossRef]
9. Decuypere, J.A.; Dierick, N.A. The combined use of triacylglycerols containing medium-chain fatty acids and exogenous lipolytic enzymes as an alternative to in-feed antibiotics in piglets: Concept, possibilities and limitations. An overview. *Nutr. Res. Rev.* **2003**, *16*, 193–210. [CrossRef]

10. Nosaka, N.; Maki, H.; Suzuki, Y.; Haruna, H.; Ohara, A.; Kasai, M.; Tsuji, H.; Aoyama, T.; Okazaki, M.; Igarashi, O.; et al. Effects of margarine containing medium-chain triacylglycerols on body fat reduction in humans. *J. Atheroscler. Thromb.* **2003**, *10*, 290–298. [CrossRef]
11. Rego Costa, A.C.; Rosado, E.L.; Soares-Mota, M. Influence of the dietary intake of medium chain triglycerides on body composition, energy expenditure and satiety: A systematic review. *Nutr. Hosp.* **2012**, *27*, 103–108. [CrossRef]
12. Bourque, C.; St-Onge, M.P.; Papamandjaris, A.A.; Cohn, J.S.; Jones, P.J. Consumption of an oil composed of medium chain triacyglycerols, phytosterols, and N-3 fatty acids improves cardiovascular risk profile in overweight women. *Metabolism* **2003**, *52*, 771–777. [CrossRef]
13. St-Onge, M.P.; Lamarche, B.; Mauger, J.F.; Jones, P.J. Consumption of a functional oil rich in phytosterols and medium-chain triglyceride oil improves plasma lipid profiles in men. *J. Nutr.* **2003**, *133*, 1815–1820. [CrossRef]
14. Zhang, X.; Zhang, Y.; Liu, Y.; Wang, J.; Xu, Q.; Yu, X.; Yang, X.; Liu, Z.; Xue, C. Medium-chain triglycerides promote macrophage reverse cholesterol transport and improve atherosclerosis in ApoE-deficient mice fed a high-fat diet. *Nutr. Res.* **2016**, *36*, 964–973. [CrossRef]
15. Zhang, X.S.; Zhang, P.; Liu, Y.H.; Xu, Q.; Zhang, Y.; Li, H.Z.; Liu, L.; Liu, Y.M.; Yang, X.Y.; Xue, C.Y. Caprylic Acid Improves Lipid Metabolism, Suppresses the Inflammatory Response and Activates the ABCA1/p-JAK2/p-STAT3 Signaling Pathway in C57BL/6J Mice and RAW264.7 Cells. *Biomed. Environ. Sci.* **2022**, *35*, 95–106. [CrossRef]
16. Nofer, J.R. Signal transduction by HDL: Agonists, receptors, and signaling cascades. *Handb. Exp. Pharmacol.* **2015**, *224*, 229–256. [CrossRef]
17. Tang, C.; Houston, B.A.; Storey, C.; LeBoeuf, R.C. Both STAT3 activation and cholesterol efflux contribute to the anti-inflammatory effect of apoA-I/ABCA1 interaction in macrophages. *J. Lipid Res.* **2016**, *57*, 848–857. [CrossRef]
18. Zhang, X.; Xue, C.; Xu, Q.; Zhang, Y.; Li, H.; Li, F.; Liu, Y.; Guo, C. Caprylic acid suppresses inflammation via TLR4/NF-kappaB signaling and improves atherosclerosis in ApoE-deficient mice. *Nutr. Metab.* **2019**, *16*, 40. [CrossRef]
19. Aiello, R.J.; Brees, D.; Francone, O.L. ABCA1-deficient mice: Insights into the role of monocyte lipid efflux in HDL formation and inflammation. *Arterioscler. Thromb. Vasc. Biol.* **2003**, *23*, 972–980. [CrossRef]
20. Orso, E.; Broccardo, C.; Kaminski, W.E.; Bottcher, A.; Liebisch, G.; Drobnik, W.; Gotz, A.; Chambenoit, O.; Diederich, W.; Langmann, T.; et al. Transport of lipids from golgi to plasma membrane is defective in tangier disease patients and Abc1-deficient mice. *Nat. Genet.* **2000**, *24*, 192–196. [CrossRef]
21. Christiansen-Weber, T.A.; Voland, J.R.; Wu, Y.; Ngo, K.; Roland, B.L.; Nguyen, S.; Peterson, P.A.; Fung-Leung, W.P. Functional loss of ABCA1 in mice causes severe placental malformation, aberrant lipid distribution, and kidney glomerulonephritis as well as high-density lipoprotein cholesterol deficiency. *Am. J. Pathol.* **2000**, *157*, 1017–1029. [CrossRef] [PubMed]
22. Babashamsi, M.M.; Koukhaloo, S.Z.; Halalkhor, S.; Salimi, A.; Babashamsi, M. ABCA1 and metabolic syndrome; a review of the ABCA1 role in HDL-VLDL production, insulin-glucose homeostasis, inflammation and obesity. *Diabetes Metab. Syndr.* **2019**, *13*, 1529–1534. [CrossRef] [PubMed]
23. Langmann, T.; Klucken, J.; Reil, M.; Liebisch, G.; Luciani, M.F.; Chimini, G.; Kaminski, W.E.; Schmitz, G. Molecular cloning of the human ATP-binding cassette transporter 1 (hABC1): Evidence for sterol-dependent regulation in macrophages. *Biochem. Biophys. Res. Commun.* **1999**, *257*, 29–33. [CrossRef] [PubMed]
24. Mauerer, R.; Ebert, S.; Langmann, T. High glucose, unsaturated and saturated fatty acids differentially regulate expression of ATP-binding cassette transporters ABCA1 and ABCG1 in human macrophages. *Exp. Mol. Med.* **2009**, *41*, 126–132. [CrossRef]
25. Shen, J.; Hafeez, A.; Stevenson, J.; Yang, J.; Yin, C.; Li, F.; Wang, S.; Du, H.; Ji, X.; Rafols, J.A.; et al. Omega-3 fatty acid supplement prevents development of intracranial atherosclerosis. *Neuroscience* **2016**, *334*, 226–235. [CrossRef]
26. Liu, Y.; Wang, J.; Zhang, R.; Zhang, Y.; Xu, Q.; Zhang, J.; Zhang, Y.; Zheng, Z.; Yu, X.; Jing, H.; et al. A good response to oil with medium- and long-chain fatty acids in body fat and blood lipid profiles of male hypertriglyceridemic subjects. *Asia Pac. J. Clin. Nutr.* **2009**, *18*, 351–358.
27. Xue, C.; Liu, Y.; Wang, J.; Zhang, R.; Zhang, Y.; Zhang, J.; Zhang, Y.; Zheng, Z.; Yu, X.; Jing, H.; et al. Consumption of medium- and long-chain triacylglycerols decreases body fat and blood triglyceride in Chinese hypertriglyceridemic subjects. *Eur. J. Clin. Nutr.* **2009**, *63*, 879–886. [CrossRef]
28. Parks, J.S.; Chung, S.; Shelness, G.S. Hepatic ABC transporters and triglyceride metabolism. *Curr. Opin. Lipidol.* **2012**, *23*, 196–200. [CrossRef]
29. Drobnik, W.; Lindenthal, B.; Lieser, B.; Ritter, M.; Christiansen Weber, T.; Liebisch, G.; Giesa, U.; Igel, M.; Borsukova, H.; Büchler, C.; et al. ATP-binding cassette transporter A1 (ABCA1) affects total body sterol metabolism. *Gastroenterology* **2001**, *120*, 1203–1211. [CrossRef]
30. Haghpassand, M.; Bourassa, P.A.; Francone, O.L.; Aiello, R.J. Monocyte/macrophage expression of ABCA1 has minimal contribution to plasma HDL levels. *J. Clin. Investig.* **2001**, *108*, 1315–1320. [CrossRef]
31. Westerterp, M.; Tsuchiya, K.; Tattersall, I.W.; Fotakis, P.; Bochem, A.E.; Molusky, M.M.; Ntonga, V.; Abramowicz, S.; Parks, J.S.; Welch, C.L.; et al. Deficiency of ATP-Binding Cassette Transporters A1 and G1 in Endothelial Cells Accelerates Atherosclerosis in Mice. *Arterioscler. Thromb. Vasc. Biol.* **2016**, *36*, 1328–1337. [CrossRef]
32. Wang, N.; Lan, D.; Chen, W.; Matsuura, F.; Tall, A.R. ATP-binding cassette transporters G1 and G4 mediate cellular cholesterol efflux to high-density lipoproteins. *Proc. Natl. Acad. Sci. USA* **2004**, *101*, 9774–9779. [CrossRef]

33. Westerterp, M.; Bochem, A.E.; Yvan-Charvet, L.; Murphy, A.J.; Wang, N.; Tall, A.R. ATP-binding cassette transporters, atherosclerosis, and inflammation. *Circ. Res.* **2014**, *114*, 157–170. [CrossRef]
34. Chai, A.B.; Ammit, A.J.; Gelissen, I.C. Examining the role of ABC lipid transporters in pulmonary lipid homeostasis and inflammation. *Respir. Res.* **2017**, *18*, 41. [CrossRef]
35. Nguyen, M.T.; Favelyukis, S.; Nguyen, A.K.; Reichart, D.; Scott, P.A.; Jenn, A.; Liu-Bryan, R.; Glass, C.K.; Neels, J.G.; Olefsky, J.M. A subpopulation of macrophages infiltrates hypertrophic adipose tissue and is activated by free fatty acids via Toll-like receptors 2 and 4 and JNK-dependent pathways. *J. Biol. Chem.* **2007**, *282*, 35279–35292. [CrossRef]
36. Haversen, L.; Danielsson, K.N.; Fogelstrand, L.; Wiklund, O. Induction of proinflammatory cytokines by long-chain saturated fatty acids in human macrophages. *Atherosclerosis* **2009**, *202*, 382–393. [CrossRef]
37. Abou-Saleh, H.; Ouhtit, A.; Halade, G.V.; Rahman, M.M. Bone Benefits of Fish Oil Supplementation Depend on its EPA and DHA Content. *Nutrients* **2019**, *11*, 2701. [CrossRef]
38. Daci, A.; Ozen, G.; Uyar, I.; Civelek, E.; Yildirim, F.I.A.; Durman, D.K.; Teskin, O.; Norel, X.; Uydes-Dogan, B.S.; Topal, G. Omega-3 polyunsaturated fatty acids reduce vascular tone and inflammation in human saphenous vein. *Prostaglandins Other Lipid Mediat.* **2017**, *133*, 29–34. [CrossRef]
39. Zhang, M.; Zhao, G.J.; Yin, K.; Xia, X.D.; Gong, D.; Zhao, Z.W.; Chen, L.Y.; Zheng, X.L.; Tang, X.E.; Tang, C.K. Apolipoprotein A-1 Binding Protein Inhibits Inflammatory Signaling Pathways by Binding to Apolipoprotein A-1 in THP-1 Macrophages. *Circ. J.* **2018**, *82*, 1396–1404. [CrossRef]
40. Soro-Paavonen, A.; Westerbacka, J.; Ehnholm, C.; Taskinen, M.R. Metabolic syndrome aggravates the increased endothelial activation and low-grade inflammation in subjects with familial low HDL. *Ann. Med.* **2006**, *38*, 229–238. [CrossRef]
41. He, P.; Gelissen, I.C.; Ammit, A.J. Regulation of ATP binding cassette transporter A1 (ABCA1) expression: Cholesterol-dependent and–independent signaling pathways with relevance to inflammatory lung disease. *Respir. Res.* **2020**, *21*, 250. [CrossRef] [PubMed]
42. Lee, J.Y.; Sohn, K.H.; Rhee, S.H.; Hwang, D. Saturated fatty acids, but not unsaturated fatty acids, induce the expression of cyclooxygenase-2 mediated through Toll-like receptor 4. *J. Biol. Chem.* **2001**, *276*, 16683–16689. [CrossRef] [PubMed]
43. Calder, P.C. Long-chain fatty acids and inflammation. *Proc. Nutr. Soc.* **2012**, *71*, 284–289. [CrossRef] [PubMed]
44. Talukdar, S.; Olefsky, J.M.; Osborn, O. Targeting GPR120 and other fatty acid-sensing GPCRs ameliorates insulin resistance and inflammatory diseases. *Trends Pharmacol. Sci.* **2011**, *32*, 543–550. [CrossRef]
45. Aiello, R.J.; Brees, D.; Bourassa, P.A.; Royer, L.; Lindsey, S.; Coskran, T.; Haghpassand, M.; Francone, O.L. Increased atherosclerosis in hyperlipidemic mice with inactivation of ABCA1 in macrophages. *Arterioscler. Thromb. Vasc. Biol.* **2002**, *22*, 630–637. [CrossRef]

nutrients

MDPI

Brief Report

The Interplay Between Depression, Probiotics, Diet, Immunometabolic Health, the Gut, and the Liver—A Secondary Analysis of the Pro-Demet Randomized Clinical Trial

Oliwia Gawlik-Kotelnicka [1,*], Jakub Rogalski [2], Karolina H. Czarnecka-Chrebelska [3], Jacek Burzyński [4], Paulina Jakubowska [1], Anna Skowrońska [1] and Dominik Strzelecki [1]

1 Department of Affective and Psychotic Disorders, Medical University of Lodz, 92-216 Lodz, Poland; paulina.jakubowska1@stud.umed.lodz.pl (P.J.); anna.zabka@gmail.com (A.S.); dominik.strzelecki@umed.lodz.pl (D.S.)
2 University Clinical Hospital No. 2, Medical University of Lodz, 90-549 Lodz, Poland; jakub.rogalski1@stud.umed.lodz.pl
3 Department of Biomedicine and Genetics, Medical University of Lodz, 92-213 Lodz, Poland; karolina.czarnecka@umed.lodz.pl
4 Department of Biostatistics and Translational Medicine, Medical University of Lodz, 92-215 Lodz, Poland; jacek.burzynski@umed.lodz.pl
* Correspondence: oliwia.gawlik@umed.lodz.pl

Abstract: (1) Background: Depression, metabolic alternations, and liver diseases are highly comorbid. Studies have shown that probiotics might be helpful in the treatment of the above-mentioned states. The aim of this secondary analysis was to search for possible predictors of probiotics' efficacy on liver-related outcome measures. (2) Methods: Data from 92 subjects from a randomized clinical trial on the effect of probiotics on depression were analyzed. The shift in liver steatosis and fibrosis indices was assessed in the context of baseline immunometabolic, psychometric, dietary, and intestinal permeability factors. Correlation analysis and linear regression models were used. (3) Results: A total of 30% of the variance of the improvement in the score of the aspartate transferase to platelet ratio index was explained by probiotic use, higher pre-intervention triglycerides, cholesterol, C-reactive protein levels, increased cereal intake, and a lower consumption of sweets. Then, the model of the change in alanine transferase indicated that probiotics were efficient when used by subjects with higher basal levels of intestinal permeability markers. (4) Conclusions: Probiotics being used along with a healthy diet may provide additional benefits, such as decreased cardiovascular risk, for patients with measures consistent with the immunometabolic form of depression. Probiotic augmentation may be useful for liver protection among subjects with a suspected "leaky gut" syndrome. ClinicalTrials.gov: NCT04756544.

Keywords: probiotics; liver dysfunction; cardiovascular risk; depression; intestinal permeability; diet

1. Introduction

Depression, metabolic disorders, and numerous liver pathologies, including steatotic liver disease and drug- or alcohol-induced liver injury, often co-occur [1–6]. It is suggested that gut microbiota dysbiosis, as well as the issue of intestinal permeability (also known as "leaky gut syndrome", a weakened gut barrier state resulting in various inflammatory agents, toxic substances, and bacterial components crossing the gut lining into systemic circulation [7]) and improper dietary habits, may mediate the clinical relationship between these disorders [8–13]. Interestingly, previous studies revealed the possible beneficial role of probiotic use and dietary interventions in treating the above-mentioned states [14–18]. However, there are numerous inconsistencies regarding the role of baseline metabolic and microbiota-related parameters, as well as dietary patterns, in predicting the influence of probiotics on liver-derived indices. The parental Pro-Demet randomized controlled trial

(RCT), which assessed probiotics' efficacy in depression, showed their minimal impact on depressive outcome measures as an add-on treatment dependent on the patient's pre-treatment metabolic status, including their hepatic steatosis index (HSI) [19]. At the same time, a secondary analysis of the same RCT revealed a statistically significantly better improvement in alanine aminotransferase (ALT)-based liver biomarkers after the probiotic intervention in antidepressant-treated subjects in comparison to those not treated with antidepressive drugs. Moreover, a similar relationship was found regarding the main mental disorder diagnosis—a better improvement in fatty liver means after probiotics supplementation was observed among subjects diagnosed with depressive episodes vs. those with mixed depressive and anxiety disorder diagnoses [20].

All in all, the target subpopulation for probiotic supplementation among patients with depression is not fully understood. Specifically, it is not known whether immunometabolic features comorbid with depression, microbiota and gut permeability proxy biomarkers, or lifestyle factors are predictive of the efficacy of probiotics for liver-related non-invasive biomarkers in a clinical population with depressive disorders.

Therefore, this analysis aimed to search for possible predictors of probiotics' influence on non-invasive biomarkers of liver steatosis and fibrosis among inflammation and metabolic parameters; intestinal permeability biomarkers—such as intestinal fatty acid-binding protein (I-FABP/FABP-2); microbiota metabolites—such as blood short-chain fatty acids (bSCFAs); or dietary habits.

We hypothesized that pre-treatment abnormalities in microbiota-intestine markers, as well as immunometabolic abnormalities comorbid with depression, would serve as possible predictors of probiotics' efficacy for liver function based on non-invasive blood indices. Dietary habits were hypothesized to be additional explanatory factors.

2. Materials and Methods

2.1. Study Participants

A total of 116 patients with depressive disorders, according to the 11th International Classification of Diseases, were randomized and assigned to the probiotic (PRO) or placebo (PLC) groups. The PRO group received a mixture of *Lactobacillus helveticus* Rosell®-52 and *Bifidobacterium longum* Rosell®-175 for 60 days. During the trial, anthropometric, psychometric, and metabolic parameters, as well as inflammatory and microbiota proxy biomarkers, both circulating and fecal, were assessed in both groups according to the study protocol [21]. Moreover, detailed dietary habits, physical activity levels, and medication and dietary supplement intake were assessed pre-intervention.

The eligibility criteria and study timeline may be found elsewhere [21,22].

Finally, data from 92 subjects (74 women and 14 men, aged (Mdn (IQR)) 32.0 (22.5–42.1) years) were analyzed in this study. In total, 63 (68.5%) subjects were using antidepressants; the median ALT value was 16.2 (IQR: 12.9–23.3) U/L. A participant flow diagram and detailed sample characteristics of this population have been published previously [20]. A shortened form of the sample's characteristics is shown in the Appendix A. Importantly, there were no baseline differences in their pre-intervention circulating I-FABP; bSCFAs; psychometric, metabolic, or inflammatory parameters; or dietary habits.

2.2. Primary Outcome Measures

Non-invasive liver-related biomarkers were analyzed (Table 1) [23–25].

The change in values of liver-derived blood-based biomarkers (pre-intervention vs. post-intervention) was assessed as a potential improvement/worsening in liver function in general without indicating a histopathological change in the level of steatosis/liver fibrosis [26,27].

Table 1. Non-invasive blood-based liver function biomarkers.

The Name of the Non-Invasive Liver-Related Biomarker	Abbreviation	Liver Abnormality Detection	Formula	Cut-Off Point for Detecting/Ruling Out Liver Abnormalities
Alanine Transaminase	ALT	(acute/chronic) hepatic cytotoxic injury	-	the upper limit of normal
Aspartate Aminotransferase	AST		-	the upper limit of normal
Alanine Aminotransferase to Aspartate Aminotransferase Ratio	ALT/AST ratio	fatty liver disease	[ALT value]/[AST value]	1.33
Hepatic Steatosis Index	HSI		$8 \times$ [ALT value]/[AST value] + [BMI in kg/m^2] + 2 * + 2 **	36
Framingham Steatosis Index	FSI		$7.981 + 0.011 \times$ [age] $-$ $0.146 \times$ [se×] *** + $0.173 \times$ [BMI in kg/m^2] + $0.007 \times$ [TG in mg/dL] + $0.593 \times$ [HTN] **** + $0.789 \times$ [DM] ***** + $1.1 \times$ [ALT/AST ratio] ******	−1.2
AST to Platelet Ratio Index	APRI	liver fibrosis	[AST value]/[AST value upper limit of normal]/[PLT value] $\times$ 100	0.5
Fibrosis-4 Index	FIB-4		[age] $\times$ [AST value]/[PLT value] $\times$ $\sqrt{[\text{ALT value}]}$	1.3

Abbreviations: ALT = alanine transaminase; APRI = AST-to-platelet ratio index; AST = aspartate aminotransferase; BMI = body mass index; DM = diabetes mellitus, FIB-4 = fibrosis-4 index; FSI = Framingham Steatosis Index; HSI = hepatic steatosis index; HTN = hypertension; PLT = platelets count; TG = triglycerides. * if DM diagnosis; ** if female; *** if female = 1, if male = 0; **** if HTN = 1, if no HTN = 0; ***** if DM = 1, if no DM = 0; ****** if ALT/AST ratio $\geq$ 1.33 = yes, if no = 0.

Importantly, the aspartate aminotransferase (AST)-to-platelets ratio index (APRI) and fibrosis-4 index (FIB-4), when used in the general population, are effective in the cardiovascular risk (CVR) assessment [28,29].

The rest of the outcome measures are shown in Appendix A.

2.3. Statistical Analysis

Correlations between non-invasive hepatic steatosis indices and clinical parameters were assessed using Spearman's rank correlation. We selected variables for further analysis based on Spearman's rank correlation coefficients. To explore multivariate associations between non-invasive hepatic-related indices and other clinical parameters, we developed linear regression models with a backward feature elimination method. All independent variables were checked for collinearity and possible interactions. For each model, adjusted R^2 was used as a measurement of explained variability. The significance threshold was set at $p < 0.05$. The significance threshold for linear regression models (six models of changes in liver-derived parameters) was set at $p = 0.008$ using Bonferroni correction.

3. Results

First, it was shown that variables such as age, baseline ALT, circulating lipid profile, dietary habits, physical activity, or I-FABP correlated with changes in liver steatosis and fibrosis markers values ($|r| \geq 0.20$) (Table 2). Interestingly, there were noticeable differences in sets of those factors between the PRO and PLC groups.

Table 2. Spearman's correlation between changes in liver-derived markers and baseline factors; * $p < 0.05$, ** $p < 0.01$, *** $p < 0.001$; red—the higher value of a baseline parameter is a possible positive predictor of the decrease in liver-related marker level; green—the higher value of the parameter is a possible negative predictor of the decrease in liver-related marker level. $n = 92$.

R	≥0.40	0.30 to 0.39	0.20 to 0.29	0.10 to 0.19	−0.09 to 0.09	−0.10 to −0.19	−0.20 to −0.29	−0.30 to −0.39	≤−0.40

	% ΔHSI	% ΔALT	% ΔALT/AST	% ΔFSI	% ΔAPRI	% ΔFIB-4
PRO						
HSI	−0.04	−0.06	−0.06	0.04	−0.06	0.02
ALT	−0.33 *	−0.33 *	−0.34 *	0.06	−0.17	0.12
ALT/AST	−0.25	−0.22	−0.26	0.01	−0.03	0.16
FSI	0.07	−0.03	0.04	0.18	−0.12	−0.09
APRI	−0.38 **	−0.45 **	−0.45 **	−0.07	−0.26	0.17
FIB-4	−0.35 *	−0.25	−0.35 *	0.13	0.05	0.27
AST	−0.41 **	−0.56 ***	−0.46 ***	0.05	−0.35 *	0.1
age	−0.37 **	−0.15	−0.28	0.21	0.14	0.30 *
sBP	0.16	0.13	0.15	0.09	0.01	−0.2
dBP	0.27	0.21	0.23	0.01	0.1	−0.21
weight	0.22	0.06	0.2	0.04	−0.16	−0.19
VAI	0.2	0.1	0.22	0.25	−0.17	−0.33 *
fGlc	−0.22	−0.15	−0.17	−0.02	0.03	0.27
TG	0.15	0.05	0.15	0.35 *	−0.19	−0.33 *
HDL-c	−0.2	−0.1	−0.22	0.11	0.04	0.17
LDL-c	0.05	0.08	0.1	0.17	0.21	0.07
Non-HDL-c	0.06	0.06	0.11	0.16	0.14	−0.04
CHOL	−0.01	0	0.03	0.19	0.13	0.01
TG/HDL-c	0.17	0.08	0.2	0.32 *	−0.17	−0.34 *
TyG	0.05	−0.01	0.06	0.30 *	−0.2	−0.22
CRP	−0.09	−0.14	−0.11	−0.09	−0.17	−0.04
I-FABP	−0.28 *	−0.43 **	−0.39 **	0.09	−0.32 *	0.01
bSCFAs	−0.05	−0.1	−0.11	0.04	0.16	0.18
fruits	0.07	0.08	−0.01	0.02	0.25	0.13
vegetables and seeds	0.09	−0.03	0.01	0.03	−0.04	0.05
oils	0.04	−0.01	0.06	0.05	−0.05	−0.04
sweets	0.08	0.14	0.02	−0.04	0.27	0.18
meat	−0.04	−0.15	−0.06	−0.02	−0.05	−0.01
diary and eggs	−0.08	0.08	−0.05	−0.02	0.11	0.14
cereal	0.19	0.14	0.23	−0.14	−0.1	−0.22
drinks	0.2	0.09	0.11	−0.18	0.04	−0.05
processed food products	0.17	0.09	0.11	−0.16	0.07	−0.02
physical activity	0.02	0.05	−0.03	−0.32	−0.14	0.07
MADRS	0.06	0.12	0.03	0.14	0.22	0.1
D-DASS	0.17	0.22	0.06	−0.1	0.27	0.11
S-DASS	−0.03	−0.07	−0.11	0.08	0.05	0.22
PLC						
	% ΔHSI	% ΔALT	% ΔALT/AST	% ΔFSI	% ΔAPRI	% ΔFIB-4
HSI	−0.19	−0.22	−0.23	−0.15	−0.18	0.01
ALT	−0.14	−0.31 *	−0.24	−0.1	−0.3	−0.09
ALT/AST	−0.23	−0.36 *	−0.33 *	−0.04	−0.1	0.11
FSI	−0.07	−0.19	−0.09	−0.05	−0.29	−0.13
APRI	−0.12	−0.18	−0.19	−0.25	−0.33*	−0.19
FIB-4	0.06	0.02	−0.05	−0.11	−0.16	−0.13
AST	−0.07	−0.26	−0.13	−0.12	−0.42 **	−0.24
age	−0.04	−0.08	−0.12	0.1	−0.09	−0.01

Table 2. *Cont.*

sBP	0.12	−0.1	0.02	−0.17	−0.25	−0.2
dBP	0.05	−0.11	0.1	−0.01	−0.23	−0.17
weight	−0.08	−0.13	−0.1	−0.16	−0.26	−0.1
VAI	0.13	0.01	0.15	0.02	−0.26	−0.22
fGlc	−0.02	0.07	−0.01	−0.35 *	−0.06	−0.12
TG	0.11	−0.06	0.18	0.16	−0.33 *	−0.28
HDL-c	−0.09	−0.14	−0.13	0.18	−0.1	0.01
LDL-c	0.2	−0.18	0.13	0.14	−0.45 **	−0.3
non-HDL-c	0.2	−0.15	0.17	0.12	−0.46 **	−0.35 *
CHOL	0.17	−0.2	0.11	0.15	−0.49 **	−0.32 *
TG/HDL-c	0.17	0.03	0.23	0.09	−0.2	−0.21
TyG	0.14	−0.01	0.2	0.1	−0.26	−0.25
CRP	0.05	−0.13	−0.01	0.03	−0.33 *	−0.26
I-FABP	−0.16	−0.15	−0.23	0.07	0.07	0.21
bSCFAs	0.23	0.37 *	0.27	0.21	0.08	0
fruits	0.09	0.2	0.05	−0.17	0.46 **	0.39 *
oils	−0.01	0.19	−0.03	0.07	0.34 *	0.2
vegetables and seeds	0.3	0.34 *	0.26	−0.2	0.33 *	0.15
sweets	−0.08	−0.12	−0.09	0.27	0.09	−0.06
meat	0.17	0.25	0.21	0.09	0.01	−0.19
diary and eggs	0.13	0.08	−0.01	0.04	−0.12	−0.28
cereal	0.34 *	0.35 *	0.32 *	−0.1	0.1	−0.08
drinks	0.04	0.28	0.23	0.01	0.02	−0.15
processed food products	0.11	0.16	0.18	0.19	−0.01	−0.25
physical activity ($n = 41$)	−0.38	−0.28	−0.47	0.3	0	0.51 *
MADRS	0.02	0.16	0.06	−0.12	0.11	0.03
D-DASS	−0.06	−0.03	0.03	−0.02	−0.34 *	−0.3
S-DASS	−0.1	0.02	−0.14	0.12	−0.05	0.1

Abbreviations: ALT—alanine aminotransferase; APRI—AST-to-platelet ratio; AST—aspartate aminotransferase; bSCFAs—blood short-chain fatty acids; CHOL—cholesterol; CRP—C-reactive protein; dBP—diastolic blood pressure; D-DASS—Depression subscale of the Depression, Anxiety, and Stress Scale; fGlc—fasting serum glucose; FIB-4—Fibrosis-4 Index; FSI—Framingham Steatosis Index; HDL-c—high-density lipoprotein cholesterol; HSI—Hepatic Steatosis Index; I-FABP—intestinal fatty acid-binding protein; LDL-c—low-density lipoprotein cholesterol; MADRS—Montgomery Asberg Depression Rating Scale; PLC—placebo group; PRO—probiotic group; sBP—systolic blood pressure; S-DASS—Stress subscale of the Depression, Anxiety, and Stress Scale; TG—triglycerides; TyG—triglyceride-glucose index; VAI—visceral adiposity index.

Based on the correlation heatmap, the following factors were chosen for regression models: age, weight, diastolic blood pressure (dBP), triglycerides (TG), cholesterol, C-reactive protein (CRP), I-FABP, bSCFAs, depression subscale of Depression, Anxiety, and Stress Scale (D-DASS), fruits, oils, vegetable and seeds, sweets, meat, or cereal intake, and physical activity level.

Second, the multiple linear regression (MLR) models, including PRO or PLC allocation and its interactions with other independent variables, were valid for the changes in ALT and APRI values ($p < 0.008$) (Table 3). The forest plots of MLR results are shown in Figure 1.

Table 3. The summary of the multiple linear regression models with interactions for the change in liver steatosis or cardiovascular risk-related indices, including the type of intervention (probiotic vs. placebo).

Dependent Variable	R^2adj	F	*p*	Independent Variable	Coefficient (β [95% CI])	*p*-Value
Δ ALT	0.186	3.74	0.001	PRO vs. PLC	0.76 (0.15–1.36)	0.014
				I-FABP	−0.31 (−0.54–−0.08)	0.008
				PRO vs. PLC * I-FABP	−0.39 (−0.81–0.02)	0.061
				bSCFAs	0.09 (−0.12–0.30)	0.378
				PRO vs. PLC * bSCFAs	−0.62 (−1.15–−0.09)	0.023
				cholesterol	−0.31 (−0.53–−0.08)	0.009
				weight	−0.30 (−0.53–−0.07)	0.010
Δ APRI	0.304	4.88	<0.001	PRO vs. PLC	−0.85 (−1.33–−0.38)	<0.001
				D-DASS	−0.26 (−0.82–0.29)	0.349
				PRO vs. PLC * D-DASS	0.77 (0.30–1.25)	0.002
				cholesterol	−0.26 (−0.48–−0.05)	0.018
				TG	−16.36 (−24.91–−7.81)	<0.001
				CRP	−1.72 (−4.11–0.67)	0.157
				cereals	−10.95 (−20.06–−1.85)	0.019
				sweets and snacks	0.28 (0.07–0.50)	0.010

Symbols: Δ—the change between the post- and pre-intervention values. Abbreviations: bSCFAs—blood short-chain fatty acids; CRP—C-reactive protein; D-DASS—Depression subscale of the Depression, Anxiety, and Stress Scale; HDL-c—high-density lipoprotein cholesterol; I-FABP—intestinal fatty acid-binding protein; PLC—placebo group; PRO—probiotic group; R^2adj—adjusted squared coefficient of determination; TG—triglycerides; VAI—visceral adiposity index. * means interaction.

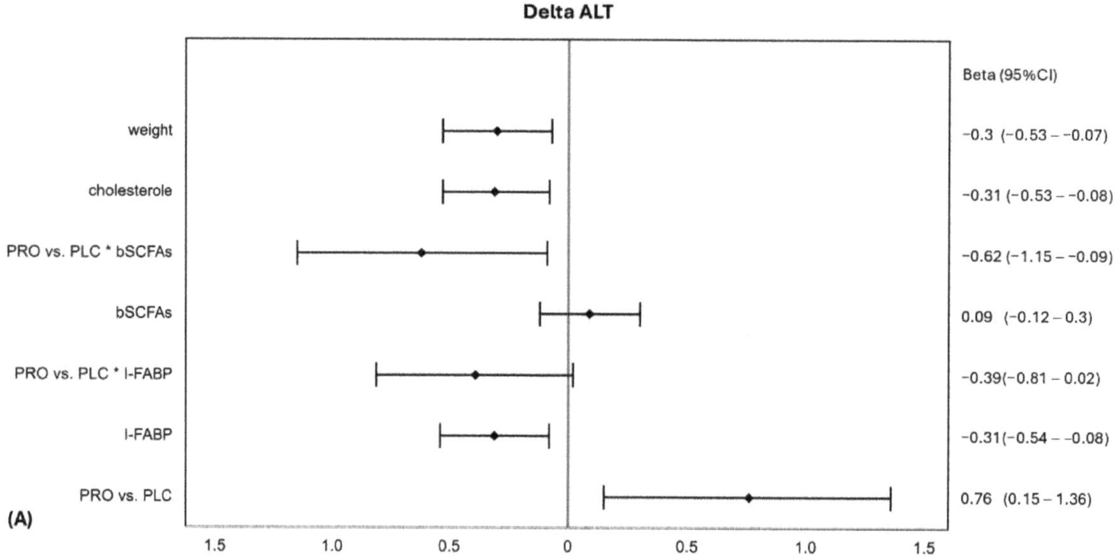

Figure 1. *Cont.*

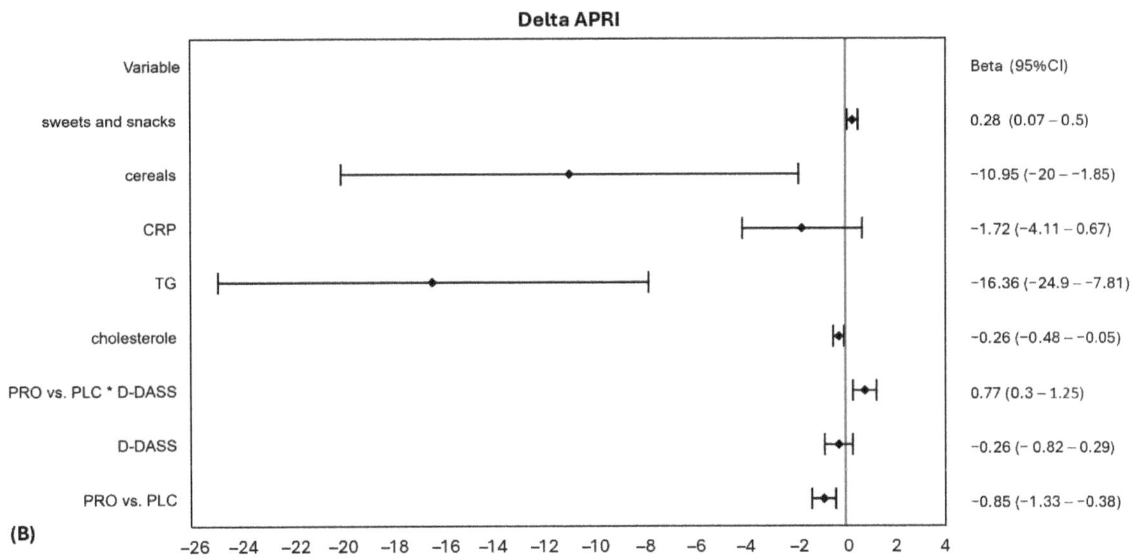

Figure 1. Forest plots of the multiple linear regression models with interactions, including the type of intervention (probiotic vs. placebo). (**A**) For the changes in alanine aminotransferase (ALT); (**B**) for the changes in aspartate aminotransferase (AST)-to-platelets ratio index (APRI). * means interaction. Abbreviations: bSCFAS = blood short-chain fatty acids; CRP = C-reactive protein; D-DASS = Depression subscale of Depression, Anxiety, and Stress Scale; I-FABP = intestinal fatty-acid binding protein; TG = triglycerides.

4. Discussion

4.1. Correlation Analyses Results

Based on the correlation analysis, as expected, pre-treatment liver steatosis and fibrosis parameters were associated with more improvement in steatosis indices values only in the PRO group.

Interestingly, the pre-intervention diet, especially fruits, vegetables, seeds, and cereal products intake, was connected with the change in liver-derived markers only in the PLC group. We hypothesize that all study participants had improved their dietary habits during the Pro-Demet intervention, as stated earlier [20]. The healthier the pre-intervention diet, the less possible any further improvement in dietary habits. Thus, participants in the PLC group gained no additional benefits from the intervention.

The higher the basal level of I-FABP, the better improvement in hepatic indices was shown in the PRO group. As FABP2 is a validated marker of enterocyte microdamage and higher intestinal permeability [30], an underlying "leaky gut" syndrome may be a proposed explanatory factor of the probiotic's influence on liver function.

The lipid profile and CRP level were consistently shown to be connected with changes in CVR indices in the PLC, but not PRO, group, possibly making immunometabolic status not the only and not the most robust determinant of the PRO efficacy.

Finally, it is crucial to bear in mind that the above findings are only preliminary, and causal effects cannot be determined based on the results of correlation analysis. Thus, these analyses were performed to select parameters for regression models.

4.2. Predictors of Probiotics Possible Efficacy for Liver Dysfunction Improvement

As shown earlier, PRO intervention alone did not change ALT levels compared with PLC in the population with depressive disorders. However, significant differences in probiotics efficacy for this parameter were found when stratified subjects by the antidepressant use [20]. Here, our MLR model for the change in ALT values indicated that PRO acted differently when used by subjects with higher basal levels of I-FABP or bSCFAs, and these compounds were proposed to be indicators of the microbiota–gut wall homeostasis. I-FABP is utilized as a marker of the enterocyte lesion and the "leaky gut" syndrome [30,31]. On the other hand, circulating SCFAs, intestinal microbiota metabolites, may provide information on the gut ecosystem status—their levels and ratios are proposed to be biomarkers of the chronic inflammatory diseases state or treatment efficacy [32–34]. Thus, our study's probiotic intervention effect may depend on the basal microbiota–intestinal function. Indeed, it has been demonstrated repeatedly that probiotics improve the pre-intervention gut microbiota composition and intestinal barrier status, especially following disruptive events [35,36]. Moreover, it was shown that restoring the gut microbiota balance with rifaximin helped to reduce the rate of increased intestinal permeability and decrease liver-derived inflammation and liver-related outcomes in animal models [37]. Therefore, we conclude that probiotics may act similarly on the microbiota–gut–liver axis in humans. Moreover, excessive inflammatory cytokines release, mediated by the hepato-cytotoxic injury [38], might constitute a target for probiotics' anti-inflammatory properties, as probiotics were shown to decrease not only ALT values but also CRP levels in non-alcoholic fatty liver disease (NAFLD) subjects [39]. A recent systematic review has pointed to the curative action of probiotics for endocrine disorders through modulating inflammation [40]. Further, our previous analysis had shown that in the PRO group, subjects treated with antidepressants had greater improvement in ALT values than those who did not receive antidepressants [20]. Moreover, we have previously found increased I-FABP values under the antidepressant treatment in the Pro-Demet entry population [41]. Indeed, antidepressants were shown to lower microbiota richness and diversity as well as increase intestinal permeability in pre-clinical models [42–44]. All of the above-mentioned findings make the current analysis results complementary to previous ones.

To sum up, probiotics might be beneficial for liver tests in patients with depression comorbid with microbiota–gut dysfunction. Nevertheless, the adjusted R^2 in the MLR model was found to be relatively small, indicating that other factors, not included in our study, may also have a significant impact on ALT changes.

4.3. The Assessment of Probiotics Efficacy and Diet in the Cardiovascular Risk Reduction

As for CVR indices, 30% of the variance of the improvement in APRI score may be explained by higher pre-intervention TG, cholesterol and CRP levels, high cereals intake and low sweets consumption, and probiotics use. Higher levels of depressive symptoms, however, counteracted the curative action of probiotics. These findings have confirmed some of the previous studies results that among people with immunometabolic alternations, probiotics in combination with other nutrients or the improvement of specific lifestyle changes, especially dietary habits, may result in better outcomes [45–47]. For instance, the consumption of a whole-grain pasta lowered plasma CRP, or the low-to-high-density lipoprotein cholesterol ratio (LDL/HDL) in obese volunteers, compared to pasta without a synbiotic [46]. Indeed, whole-grain cereal products contain dietary fiber, which acts as a prebiotic, and dietary fiber was found to be associated with a decreased risk of all-cause mortality [48,49]. Thus, the supplementation of probiotics along with a diet rich in fiber may act similarly to the intake of synbiotics. Regarding sweets intake, a diet low in added fructose was shown to have favorable effects on NAFLD patients [18]. Sweets are usually fortified not only with different sugars but also with artificial sweeteners, colors or preservatives. Both added sugars and artificial additives are well recognized as some of the factors increasing cardiovascular risk [50,51]. So, they may counteract the benefits of probiotics. As regards lifestyle modification in a broad sense, nutraceutical supplementation including probiotics decreased a 10-year CVR score by 40% compared to lifestyle changes alone [47]. Concerning whole dietary approaches, a dietary weight loss program, combined with probiotics supplementation, had favorable effects on total cholesterol levels in patients with coronary artery disease [52]. Moreover, our analysis results revealed that the probiotic intervention might be effective when used by participants with low baseline depressiveness. This may be because more severe depression was previously shown to be connected with poor dietary habits, e.g., a higher intake of sweets and fast food, as well as low compliance with the Mediterranean diet [53] or higher consumption of sugar-sweetened beverages in adolescents [54]. Specifically, anhedonia or anxiety was found to drive the high consumption of fried or sugar-enriched food products [55]. Thus, dietary and possibly other lifestyle improvements combined with probiotics may be necessary to affect clinical outcomes, especially in people with immunometabolic abnormalities. This may be due to fiber-derived microbiota metabolites, mainly SCFAs, which have been shown to possess anti-inflammatory properties, regulating metabolic health and even protecting the liver [56–58].

So, healthy dietary habits in patients with depression and immunometabolic disturbances may condition the improvement of CVR after probiotics.

4.4. The Generalizability of the Results

The generalizability of the findings to other populations may be, however, limited. First, the study population consisted of individuals with mild to moderate depressive disorders, the majority of whom used antidepressants. Many studies have shown that both depression and its pharmacological treatment are associated with distinct gut microbial profiles and altered gut wall permeability [42,59,60]. Similarly, metabolic abnormalities, low-grade inflammation, and unhealthy diet are more common among patients with depression than in the general population [55,61]. Second, the study population was primarily female, and chronic liver dysfunction is more prevalent in males than females due to several potential factors, including sex hormones or alcohol abuse [62].

Moreover, the long-term effects of probiotic intervention for liver function remain uncertain. In the systematic review, half of the patients with dysbiosis at enrollment were shown to have improved gut microbiota composition after the probiotic supplementation. Still, the follow-up period lasted only up to 30 days [36]. This would resemble the situation of those patients in our study with higher levels of FABP2 or bSCFAs that showed some improvement in ALT values. As this improvement is hypothesized to be associated with the decreased severity of dysbiosis and 'leaky gut', as discussed earlier, an ALT improvement might last as long as the gut microbiota balance. Longer-term studies in adult populations are lacking [63]. However, a probiotic effect may last long when administered very early in life; e.g., perinatal probiotic supplementation resulted in a very long-term (up to several years) decreased prevalence of allergy in children [64]. But the results of different studies are conflicting [65].

4.5. Limitations

The main limitation of our study is its modest sample size; thus, some analyses, especially when examining subgroups or interactions, might be underpowered. This fact limits making firm conclusions or assessing causal effects. Additionally, the explanatory nature of this secondary analysis of the primary trial data makes conclusions about the cause-and-effect relationship even more constricted. Furthermore, we used only non-invasive blood tests to assess liver function, hepatic steatosis, or any other specific liver dysfunction. Moreover, probiotic effects are strain-specific; psychobiotic strains were used due to the design of the parent study [66]. However, a meta-analysis focusing on the pro- or synbiotics influence on liver enzymes revealed that there was a massive diversity of probiotic strains used among NAFLD patients, the most common genera were *Lactobacillus*, *Bifidobacterium*, and *Streptococcus*; thus, the overlap with psychobiotics seems to be significant [65]. Nonetheless, the results of our study may enable the design of better future trial protocols to elucidate predictors of probiotics efficacy for liver-related markers in clinical populations with depression.

Despite the above-listed limitations, the strength of the present study lies in its novelty in terms of analyzed biomarkers and preliminary assessment of the complex net of interaction between clinical depression, liver, gut wall, microbiota, and diet. To the best of our knowledge, this is the first study that assessed possible conditions for probiotics action toward proxy liver abnormalities markers in patients with depressive disorders.

5. Conclusions

As regards patients with depression, PRO augmentation may be useful for liver protection among subjects with the suspected "leaky gut" syndrome. Further, the PRO intervention combined with the fiber-rich diet may provide additional benefits, such as a decrease in CVR, among patients with immunometabolic alterations.

The interplay between probiotics, diet, microbiota, gut, depression, and liver function may constitute the direction of future research.

Author Contributions: Conceptualization, O.G.-K.; methodology, O.G.-K., J.R., J.B. and A.S.; software, O.G.-K.; formal analysis, J.B. and K.H.C.-C.; investigation, O.G.-K., A.S., K.H.C.-C. and P.J.; resources, O.G.-K. and A.S.; writing—original draft preparation, O.G.-K. and J.R.; writing—review and editing, J.R., K.H.C.-C. and D.S.; visualization, O.G.-K. and P.J.; supervision, D.S.; project administration, O.G.-K. and A.S.; funding acquisition, D.S., A.S. and P.J. All authors have read and agreed to the published version of the manuscript.

Funding: Medical University of Lodz, grant numbers: 503/1-155-02/503-11-003-20, 502-03/1-155-02/502-14-386-18, and 564/1-000-00/564-20-070.

Institutional Review Board Statement: The study was conducted according to the Declaration of Helsinki and approved by the Ethics Committee of the Medical University of Lodz (15 December 2020; reference number RNN/228/20/KE).

Informed Consent Statement: Informed consent was collected from all the trial participants.

Data Availability Statement: The dataset is available from the corresponding author upon request.

Conflicts of Interest: The authors declare no conflicts of interest.

Appendix A

Appendix A.1

1. Sample Characteristics (n = 92) Parameter	Number (%) or Mdn (IQR)
MetS according to IDF	20 (21.74%)
Antidepressants	63 (68.47%)
Antipsychotics	4 (4.35%)
Other pharmacological treatment	33 (35.87%)
Comorbidities	48 (52.17%)
Smoking status	13 (4.13%)
Dietary supplements	48 (52.17%)
Physical activity (MET-min/week)	1783.50 (1026.50–2892.00)
ALT (U/L)	16.20 (12.90–23.30)
ALT/AST	0.75 (0.63–0.89)
HSI	32.13 (28.49–35.14)
FSI	−2.64 (−3.50–−1.61)
APRI	0.24 (0.19–0.30)
FIB-4	0.61 (0.46–0.80)
Weight (kg)	68.30 (56.50–79.60)
BMI (kg/m^2)	24.31 (21.21–27.15)
WC (cm)	83.25 (72.00–93.50)
fGlc (mmol/L)	5.07 (4.86–5.38)
HDL-c (mmol/L)	1.61 (1.43–1.90)
non-HDL-c (mmol/L)	3.60 (2.88–4.36)
TG (mmol/L)	0.95 (0.80–1.39)
Sweets and snacks	2.57 (2.14–3.14)

1. Sample Characteristics (n = 92) Parameter	Number (%) or Mdn (IQR)
Diary and eggs	3.17 (2.67–3.67)
Cereal products	3.20 (2.60–3.40)
Oils	2.67 (2.33–3.00)
Fruits	2.70 (2.40–3.20)
Vegetables and seeds	3.36 (2.91–3.82)
Meat (including fish)	2.25 (1.86–2.75)
Drinks (excluding water)	2.00 (1.71–2.43)
Processed food products	2.36 (2.10–2.71)
MADRS score	19.00 (16.00–24.00)
DASS score	64.50 (47.00–80.00)
Depression	21.00 (14.00–27.00)
Anxiety	16.00 (10.00–23.00)
Stress	24.00 (20.00–34.00)
CRP (mg/L)	1.20 (0.50–2.85)
TNF-α (pg/mL)	6.00 (1.84–7.57)
I-FABP (ng/mL)	1843.38 (1169.14–2485.55)
bSCFAs (pg/mL)	4341.41 (3376.19–5820.68)

Dietary habits: 1—never or almost never; 2—once a month; 3—several times a month; 4—several times a week; 5—every day; 6—several times a day. Abbreviations: ALT = alanine aminotransferase; APRI = aspartate aminotransferase-to-platelets ratio index; BMI = body mass index; bSCFAs = blood short-chain fatty acids; CRP = C-reactive protein; DASS = Depression, Anxiety, and Stress Scale; fGlc = fasting glucose; FSI = Framingham Steatosis Index; HDL-c = HDL cholesterol; HSI = hepatic steatosis index; IDF = International Diabetes Federation; I-FABP = intestinal fatty acid-binding protein; IQR = interquartile range; MADRS = Montgomery–Asberg Depression Rating Scale; Mdn = median; MET = metabolic equivalent of task; MetS = metabolic syndrome; TG = triglycerides; TNF-α = tumor necrosis factor alpha; WC = waist circumference.

Appendix A.2. Secondary Outcomes

Delta (Δ) was defined as a post-(V2) minus pre-intervention (V1) value.

%delta (%Δ) was defined as (Δ/V1) * 100%.

The Depression, Anxiety, and Stress Scale (DASS) was used to measure three negative emotional states. This analysis used data measured by the Depression subscale of DASS (D-DASS) [67].

The triglycerides to high-density lipoprotein cholesterol (TG/HDL-c) ratio has been proposed as a marker of insulin resistance and MetS occurrence [68].

The visceral adiposity index (VAI) is a sex-specific index including WC, BMI, TG and HDL-c to estimate visceral adiposity. It is calculated by using the following formulas: for males: VAI = WC [cm]/(39.68 + (1.88 × BMI) × (TG [mmol/L]/1.03) × (1.31/HDL-c [mmol/L]); for females: VAI = WC [cm]/(36.58 + (1.89 × BMI)) × (TG [mmol/L]/0.81) × (1.52/HDL-c [mmol/L]) [69].

TyG index is a proxy marker for identifying insulin resistance. It is calculated as Ln(fasting TG [mg/dL] × fasting blood glucose [mg/dL]/2 [70].

Intestinal fatty acid-binding protein (FABP2/I-FABP) increased levels occur when an intestinal epithelial cell lesion is found; it is used as a marker of "leaky gut" [71].

Short-chain fatty acids (SCFAs) include butyrate, propionate, and acetate, and are metabolites of gut microbiota produced from fibers. They play a role in supporting the intestinal barrier, preventing neuroinflammation and metabolic dysfunctions [72].

References

1. Sahoo, S.; Mishra, E.; Premkumar, M. Antidepressants in People with Chronic Liver Disease and Depression: When Are They Warranted and How to Choose the Suitable One? *J. Clin. Exp. Hepatol.* **2024**, *14*, 101390. [CrossRef] [PubMed]
2. Ueberberg, B.; Frommberger, U.; Messer, T.; Zwanzger, P.; Kuhn, J.; Anghelescu, I.; Ackermann, K.; Assion, H.J. Drug-Induced Liver Injury (DILI) in Patients with Depression Treated with Antidepressants: A Retrospective Multicenter Study. *Pharmacopsychiatry* **2020**, *53*, 60–64. [CrossRef] [PubMed]
3. Hsu, J.H.; Chien, I.C.; Lin, C.H. Increased Risk of Chronic Liver Disease in Patients with Major Depressive Disorder: A Population-Based Study. *J. Affect. Disord.* **2019**, *251*, 180–185. [CrossRef] [PubMed]

4. Gu, Y.; Zhang, W.; Hu, Y.; Chen, Y.; Shi, J. Association between Nonalcoholic Fatty Liver Disease and Depression: A Systematic Review and Meta-Analysis of Observational Studies. *J. Affect. Disord.* **2022**, *301*, 8–13. [CrossRef] [PubMed]
5. Huang, X.; Liu, X.; Yu, Y. Depression and Chronic Liver Diseases: Are There Shared Underlying Mechanisms? *Front. Mol. Neurosci.* **2017**, *10*, 134. [CrossRef]
6. Manikat, R.; Nguyen, M.H. Nonalcoholic Fatty Liver Disease and Non-Liver Comorbidities. *Clin. Mol. Hepatol.* **2023**, *29*, S86–S102. [CrossRef]
7. Dmytriv, T.R.; Storey, K.B.; Lushchak, V.I. Intestinal Barrier Permeability: The Influence of Gut Microbiota, Nutrition, and Exercise. *Front. Physiol.* **2024**, *15*, 1380713. [CrossRef]
8. Kronsten, V.T.; Tranah, T.H.; Pariante, C.; Shawcross, D.L. Gut-Derived Systemic Inflammation as a Driver of Depression in Chronic Liver Disease. *J. Hepatol.* **2022**, *76*, 665–680. [CrossRef]
9. Liu, L.; Wang, H.; Chen, X.; Zhang, Y.; Zhang, H.; Xie, P. Gut Microbiota and Its Metabolites in Depression: From Pathogenesis to Treatment. *eBioMedicine* **2023**, *90*, 104527. [CrossRef]
10. Schwenger, K.J.; Clermont-Dejean, N.; Allard, J.P. The Role of the Gut Microbiome in Chronic Liver Disease: The Clinical Evidence Revised. *JHEP Rep.* **2019**, *1*, 214. [CrossRef]
11. Fang, J.; Yu, C.H.; Li, X.J.; Yao, J.M.; Fang, Z.Y.; Yoon, S.H.; Yu, W.Y. Gut Dysbiosis in Nonalcoholic Fatty Liver Disease: Pathogenesis, Diagnosis, and Therapeutic Implications. *Front. Cell Infect. Microbiol.* **2022**, *12*, 997018. [CrossRef] [PubMed]
12. Mega, A.; Marzi, L.; Kob, M.; Piccin, A.; Floreani, A. Food and Nutrition in the Pathogenesis of Liver Damage. *Nutrients* **2021**, *13*, 1326. [CrossRef] [PubMed]
13. Mrozek, W.; Socha, J.; Sidorowicz, K.; Skrok, A.; Syrytczyk, A.; Piątkowska-Chmiel, I.; Herbet, M. Pathogenesis and Treatment of Depression: Role of Diet in Prevention and Therapy. *Nutrition* **2023**, *115*, 112143. [CrossRef] [PubMed]
14. Bischoff, S.C.; Bernal, W.; Dasarathy, S.; Merli, M.; Plank, L.D.; Schütz, T.; Plauth, M. ESPEN Practical Guideline: Clinical Nutrition in Liver Disease. *Clin. Nutr.* **2020**, *39*, 3533–3562. [CrossRef] [PubMed]
15. Firth, J.; Marx, W.; Dash, S.; Carney, R.; Teasdale, S.B.; Solmi, M.; Stubbs, B.; Schuch, F.B.; Carvalho, A.F.; Jacka, F.; et al. The Effects of Dietary Improvement on Symptoms of Depression and Anxiety: A Meta-Analysis of Randomized Controlled Trials. *Psychosom. Med.* **2019**, *81*, 265. [CrossRef]
16. Merkouris, E.; Mavroudi, T.; Miliotas, D.; Tsiptsios, D.; Serdari, A.; Christidi, F.; Doskas, T.K.; Mueller, C.; Tsamakis, K. Probiotics' Effects in the Treatment of Anxiety and Depression: A Comprehensive Review of 2014–2023 Clinical Trials. *Microorganisms* **2024**, *12*, 411. [CrossRef]
17. Maslennikov, R.; Ivashkin, V.; Efremova, I.; Poluektova, E.; Shirokova, E. Probiotics in Hepatology: An Update. *World J. Hepatol.* **2021**, *13*, 1154. [CrossRef]
18. Semmler, G.; Datz, C.; Trauner, M. Eating, Diet, and Nutrition for the Treatment of Non-Alcoholic Fatty Liver Disease. *Clin. Mol. Hepatol.* **2023**, *29*, S244–S260. [CrossRef]
19. Gawlik-Kotelnicka, O.; Margulska, A.; Płeska, K.; Skowró Nska, A.; Strzelecki, D. Metabolic Status Influences Probiotic Efficacy for Depression—PRO-DEMET Randomized Clinical Trial Results. *Nutrients* **2024**, *16*, 1389. [CrossRef]
20. Gawlik-Kotelnicka, O.; Burzyński, J.; Rogalski, J.; Skowrońska, A.; Strzelecki, D. Probiotics May Be Useful for Drug-Induced Liver Dysfunction in Patients with Depression–A Secondary Analysis of a Randomized Clinical Trial. *Clin. Nutr. ESPEN* **2024**, *63*, 604–614. [CrossRef]
21. Gawlik-Kotelnicka, O.; Skowrońska, A.; Margulska, A.; Czarnecka-Chrebelska, K.H.; Łoniewski, I.; Skonieczna-Żydecka, K.; Strzelecki, D. The Influence of Probiotic Supplementation on Depressive Symptoms, Inflammation, and Oxidative Stress Parameters and Fecal Microbiota in Patients with Depression Depending on Metabolic Syndrome Comorbidity—PRO-DEMET Randomized Study Protocol. *J. Clin. Med.* **2021**, *10*, 1342. [CrossRef] [PubMed]
22. Gawlik-Kotelnicka, O.; Margulska, A.; Skowrońska, A.; Strzelecki, D. PRO-DEMET Randomized Controlled Trial on Probiotics in Depression—Pilot Study Results. *Nutrients* **2023**, *15*, 1400. [CrossRef] [PubMed]
23. Long, M.T.; Pedley, A.; Colantonio, L.D.; Massaro, J.M.; Hoffmann, U.; Muntner, P.; Fox, C.S. Development and Validation of the Framingham Steatosis Index to Identify Persons with Hepatic Steatosis. *Clin. Gastroenterol. Hepatol.* **2016**, *14*, 1172–1180.e2. [CrossRef] [PubMed]
24. Lee, J.H.; Kim, D.; Kim, H.J.; Lee, C.H.; Yang, J.I.; Kim, W.; Kim, Y.J.; Yoon, J.H.; Cho, S.H.; Sung, M.W.; et al. Hepatic Steatosis Index: A Simple Screening Tool Reflecting Nonalcoholic Fatty Liver Disease. *Dig. Liver Dis.* **2010**, *42*, 503–508. [CrossRef] [PubMed]
25. Park, J.H.; Choi, J.; Jun, D.W.; Han, S.W.; Yeo, Y.H.; Nguyen, M.H. Low Alanine Aminotransferase Cut-Off for Predicting Liver Outcomes; A Nationwide Population-Based Longitudinal Cohort Study. *J. Clin. Med.* **2019**, *8*, 1445. [CrossRef]
26. Basheer, M.; Naffaa, M.; Assy, N. Non-Invasive Biomarkers of Liver Fibrosis in Nonalcoholic Fatty Liver Disease. *Clin. Mol. Hepatol.* **2023**, *29*, 398–400. [CrossRef]
27. Jang, H.; Kim, Y.; Lee, D.H.; Joo, S.K.; Koo, B.K.; Lim, S.; Lee, W.; Kim, W. Outcomes of Various Classes of Oral Antidiabetic Drugs on Nonalcoholic Fatty Liver Disease. *JAMA Intern. Med.* **2024**, *184*, 375–383. [CrossRef]
28. Schreiner, A.D.; Zhang, J.; Moran, W.P.; Koch, D.G.; Marsden, J.; Livingston, S.; Mauldin, P.D.; Gebregziabher, M. FIB-4 and Incident Severe Liver Outcomes in Patients with Undiagnosed Chronic Liver Disease: A Fine-Gray Competing Risk Analysis. *Liver Int.* **2023**, *43*, 170–179. [CrossRef]

29. De Matteis, C.; Cariello, M.; Graziano, G.; Battaglia, S.; Suppressa, P.; Piazzolla, G.; Sabbà, C.; Moschetta, A. AST to Platelet Ratio Index (APRI) Is an Easy-to-Use Predictor Score for Cardiovascular Risk in Metabolic Subjects. *Sci. Rep.* **2021**, *11*, 14834. [CrossRef]
30. Arnone, D. Increased Levels of Intestinal-Type Fatty Acid-Binding Protein (I-FABP) in Mood Disorders. *Psychol. Med.* **2023**, *53*, 4827–4828. [CrossRef]
31. Lau, E.; Marques, C.; Pestana, D.; Santoalha, M.; Carvalho, D.; Freitas, P.; Calhau, C. The Role of I-FABP as a Biomarker of Intestinal Barrier Dysfunction Driven by Gut Microbiota Changes in Obesity. *Nutr. Metab.* **2016**, *13*, 31. [CrossRef] [PubMed]
32. Saresella, M.; Marventano, I.; Barone, M.; La Rosa, F.; Piancone, F.; Mendozzi, L.; d'Arma, A.; Rossi, V.; Pugnetti, L.; Roda, G.; et al. Alterations in Circulating Fatty Acid Are Associated with Gut Microbiota Dysbiosis and Inflammation in Multiple Sclerosis. *Front. Immunol.* **2020**, *11*, 543824. [CrossRef]
33. Deleu, S.; Machiels, K.; Raes, J.; Verbeke, K.; Vermeire, S. Short Chain Fatty Acids and Its Producing Organisms: An Overlooked Therapy for IBD? *eBioMedicine* **2021**, *66*, 103293. [CrossRef] [PubMed]
34. Gandhi, P.; Gandhi, I.; Hoeschen, A.; Mosher, W.; MacMillan, M.L.; Rashidi, A.; El Jurdi, N.H.; Khoruts, A.; Weisdorf, D.J.; Blazar, B.R.; et al. Plasma Short Chain Fatty Acids as a Predictor of Response to Therapy for Life-Threatening Acute Graft-Versus-Host Disease. *Blood* **2020**, *136*, 14. [CrossRef]
35. Zheng, Y.; Zhang, Z.; Tang, P.; Wu, Y.; Zhang, A.; Li, D.; Wang, C.Z.; Wan, J.Y.; Yao, H.; Yuan, C.S. Probiotics Fortify Intestinal Barrier Function: A Systematic Review and Meta-Analysis of Randomized Trials. *Front. Immunol.* **2023**, *14*, 1143548. [CrossRef] [PubMed]
36. McFarland, L.V. Use of Probiotics to Correct Dysbiosis of Normal Microbiota Following Disease or Disruptive Events: A Systematic Review. *BMJ Open* **2014**, *4*, e005047. [CrossRef]
37. Han, J.W.; Kim, D.I.; Nam, H.C.; Chang, U.I.; Yang, J.M.; Song, D.S. Association between Serum Tumor Necrosis Factor-α and Sarcopenia in Liver Cirrhosis. *Clin. Mol. Hepatol.* **2021**, *28*, 219–231. [CrossRef]
38. Yan, M.; Man, S.; Ma, L.; Guo, L.; Huang, L.; Gao, W. Immunological Mechanisms in Steatotic Liver Diseases: An Overview and Clinical Perspectives. *Clin. Mol. Hepatol.* **2024**, *30*, 620–648. [CrossRef]
39. Huang, Y.; Wang, X.; Zhang, L.; Zheng, K.; Xiong, J.; Li, J.; Cong, C.; Gong, Z.; Mao, J. Effect of Probiotics Therapy on Nonalcoholic Fatty Liver Disease. *Comput. Math. Methods Med.* **2022**, *2022*, 7888076. [CrossRef]
40. Nemati, M.; Ebrahimi, B.; Montazeri-Najafabady, N. Probiotics Ameliorate Endocrine Disorders via Modulating Inflammatory Pathways: A Systematic Review. *Genes. Nutr.* **2024**, *19*, 7. [CrossRef]
41. Gawlik-Kotelnicka, O.; Czarnecka-Chrebelska, K.; Margulska, A.; Pikus, E.; Wasiak, J.; Skowrońska, A.; Brzeziańska-Lasota, E.; Strzelecki, D. Associations between Intestinal Fatty-Acid Binding Protein and Clinical and Metabolic Characteristics of Depression. *Prog. Neuropsychopharmacol. Biol. Psychiatry* **2025**, *136*, 111170. [CrossRef] [PubMed]
42. Cussotto, S.; Strain, C.R.; Fouhy, F.; Strain, R.G.; Peterson, V.L.; Clarke, G.; Stanton, C.; Dinan, T.G.; Cryan, J.F. Differential Effects of Psychotropic Drugs on Microbiome Composition and Gastrointestinal Function. *Psychopharmacology* **2019**, *236*, 1671–1685. [CrossRef] [PubMed]
43. Hatamnejad, M.R.; Baradaran Ghavami, S.; Shirvani, M.; Asghari Ahmadabad, M.; Shahrokh, S.; Farmani, M.; Sherkat, G.; Asadzadeh Aghdaei, H.; Zali, M.R. Selective Serotonin Reuptake Inhibitors and Inflammatory Bowel Disease; Beneficial or Malpractice. *Front. Immunol.* **2022**, *13*, 980189. [CrossRef] [PubMed]
44. Sjöstedt, P.; Enander, J.; Isung, J. Serotonin Reuptake Inhibitors and the Gut Microbiome: Significance of the Gut Microbiome in Relation to Mechanism of Action, Treatment Response, Side Effects, and Tachyphylaxis. *Front. Psychiatry* **2021**, *12*, 682868. [CrossRef] [PubMed]
45. Dang, L.; Li, D.; Mu, Q.; Zhang, N.; Li, C.; Wang, M.; Tian, H.; Jha, R.; Li, C. Youth-Derived Lactobacillus Rhamnosus with Prebiotic Xylo-Oligosaccharide Exhibits Anti-Hyperlipidemic Effects as a Novel Synbiotic. *Food Res. Int.* **2024**, *195*, 114976. [CrossRef]
46. Angelino, D.; Martina, A.; Rosi, A.; Veronesi, L.; Antonini, M.; Mennella, I.; Vitaglione, P.; Grioni, S.; Brighenti, F.; Zavaroni, I.; et al. Glucose- and Lipid-Related Biomarkers Are Affected in Healthy Obese or Hyperglycemic Adults Consuming a Whole-Grain Pasta Enriched in Prebiotics and Probiotics: A 12-Week Randomized Controlled Trial. *J. Nutr.* **2019**, *149*, 1714–1723. [CrossRef]
47. Dahlberg, C.J.; Ou, J.J.; Babish, J.G.; Lamb, J.J.; Eliason, S.; Brabazon, H.; Gao, W.; Kaadige, M.R.; Tripp, M.L. A 13-Week Low Glycemic Load Diet and Lifestyle Modification Program Combining Low Glycemic Load Protein Shakes and Targeted Nutraceuticals Improved Weight Loss and Cardio-Metabolic Risk Factors. *Can. J. Physiol. Pharmacol.* **2017**, *95*, 1414–1425. [CrossRef]
48. Garzón, A.G.; Veras, F.F.; Brandelli, A.; Drago, S.R. Bio-Functional and Prebiotics Properties of Products Based on Whole Grain Sorghum Fermented with Lactic Acid Bacteria. *J. Sci. Food Agric.* **2024**, *104*, 2971–2979. [CrossRef]
49. Ramezani, F.; Pourghazi, F.; Eslami, M.; Gholami, M.; Mohammadian Khonsari, N.; Ejtahed, H.S.; Larijani, B.; Qorbani, M. Dietary Fiber Intake and All-Cause and Cause-Specific Mortality: An Updated Systematic Review and Meta-Analysis of Prospective Cohort Studies. *Clin. Nutr.* **2024**, *43*, 65–83. [CrossRef]
50. Girigosavi, K.B.; Etta, I.; Kambham, S.; Panjiyar, B.K. Sweet Surprises: An In-Depth Systematic Review of Artificial Sweeteners and Their Association with Cerebrovascular Accidents. *Curr. Nutr. Rep.* **2024**, *13*, 97–105. [CrossRef]
51. Yeterian, M.; Parikh, M.A.; Frishman, W.H.; Peterson, S.J. The Bittersweet Reality: The Cardiovascular Risk of Artificial Sweeteners. *Cardiol. Rev.* 2024, *online ahead of print*. [CrossRef]

52. Moludi, J.; Alizadeh, M.; Behrooz, M.; Maleki, V.; Seyed Mohammadzad, M.H.; Golmohammadi, A. Interactive Effect of Probiotics Supplementation and Weight Loss Diet on Metabolic Syndrome Features in Patients with Coronary Artery Diseases: A Double-Blind, Placebo-Controlled, Randomized Clinical Trial. *Am. J. Lifestyle Med.* **2021**, *15*, 653. [CrossRef] [PubMed]
53. Paans, N.P.G.; Gibson-Smith, D.; Bot, M.; van Strien, T.; Brouwer, I.A.; Visser, M.; Penninx, B.W.J.H. Depression and Eating Styles Are Independently Associated with Dietary Intake. *Appetite* **2019**, *134*, 103–110. [CrossRef] [PubMed]
54. Dabravolskaj, J.; Patte, K.A.; Yamamoto, S.; Leatherdale, S.T.; Veugelers, P.J.; Maximova, K. Association Between Diet and Mental Health Outcomes in a Sample of 13,887 Adolescents in Canada. *Prev. Chronic Dis.* **2024**, *21*, 240187. [CrossRef] [PubMed]
55. Alrehaili, S.; Afifi, A.A.; Algheshairy, R.M.; Bushnaq, T.; Alharbi, T.A.F.; Alharbi, H.F. Prevalence of Anhedonia, Anxiety, and Their Impact on Food Consumption among Postgraduate Qassim University Students. *Front. Nutr.* **2024**, *11*, 1445125. [CrossRef] [PubMed]
56. Olaniyi, K.S.; Areloegbe, S.E.; Badejogbin, O.C.; Ajadi, I.O.; Ajadi, M.B. Butyrate-Mediated Modulation of Paraoxonase-1 Alleviates Cardiorenometabolic Abnormalities in a Rat Model of Polycystic Ovarian Syndrome. *Cardiovasc. Drugs Ther.* 2024, *online ahead of print*. [CrossRef]
57. Ziętek, M.; Celewicz, Z.; Kikut, J.; Szczuko, M. Implications of Scfas on the Parameters of the Lipid and Hepatic Profile in Pregnant Women. *Nutrients* **2021**, *13*, 1749. [CrossRef]
58. Tan, J.K.; Macia, L.; Mackay, C.R. Dietary Fiber and SCFAs in the Regulation of Mucosal Immunity. *J. Allergy Clin. Immunol.* **2023**, *151*, 361–370. [CrossRef]
59. Wasiak, J.; Gawlik-Kotelnicka, O. Intestinal Permeability and Its Significance in Psychiatric Disorders–A Narrative Review and Future Perspectives. *Behav. Brain Res.* **2023**, *448*, 114459. [CrossRef]
60. Gamboa, J.; Le, G.H.; Wong, S.; Alteza, E.A.; Zachos, K.A.; Teopiz, K.M.; McIntyre, R.S. Impact of Antidepressants on the Composition of the Gut Microbiome: A Systematic Review and Meta-Analysis of in Vivo Studies. *J. Affect. Disord.* **2024**, *369*, 819–833. [CrossRef]
61. Teixeira, A.L.; Scholl, J.N.; Bauer, M.E. Psychoneuroimmunology of Mood Disorders. *Methods Mol. Biol.* **2024**, *2868*, 49–72. [CrossRef]
62. Cooper, K.M.; Delk, M.; Devuni, D.; Sarkar, M. Sex Differences in Chronic Liver Disease and Benign Liver Lesions. *JHEP Rep.* **2023**, *5*, 100870. [CrossRef]
63. Merenstein, D.; Pot, B.; Leyer, G.; Ouwehand, A.C.; Preidis, G.A.; Elkins, C.A.; Hill, C.; Lewis, Z.T.; Shane, A.L.; Zmora, N.; et al. Emerging Issues in Probiotic Safety: 2023 Perspectives. *Gut Microbes* **2023**, *15*, 2185034. [CrossRef] [PubMed]
64. Lundelin, K.; Poussa, T.; Salminen, S.; Isolauri, E. Long-Term Safety and Efficacy of Perinatal Probiotic Intervention: Evidence from a Follow-up Study of Four Randomized, Double-Blind, Placebo-Controlled Trials. *Pediatr. Allergy Immunol.* **2017**, *28*, 170–175. [CrossRef] [PubMed]
65. Davies, G.; Jordan, S.; Brooks, C.J.; Thayer, D.; Storey, M.; Morgan, G.; Allen, S.; Garaiova, I.; Plummer, S.; Gravenor, M. Long Term Extension of a Randomised Controlled Trial of Probiotics Using Electronic Health Records. *Sci. Rep.* **2018**, *8*, 7668. [CrossRef] [PubMed]
66. Darwesh, M.A.K.; Bakr, W.; Omar, T.E.I.; El-Kholy, M.A.; Azzam, N.F. Unraveling the Relative Abundance of Psychobiotic Bacteria in Children with Autism Spectrum Disorder. *Sci. Rep.* **2024**, *14*, 24321. [CrossRef] [PubMed]
67. Makara-Studzińska, M.; Załuski, M.; Amczyk, K.A.D.; Tyburski, E. Polish Version of the Depression Anxiety Stress Scale (DASS-42)-Adaptation and Normalization. *Psychiatr. Pol.* **2024**, *58*, 63–78. [CrossRef] [PubMed]
68. Kosmas, C.E.; Rodriguez Polanco, S.; Bousvarou, M.D.; Papakonstantinou, E.J.; Peña Genao, E.; Guzman, E.; Kostara, C.E. The Triglyceride/High-Density Lipoprotein Cholesterol (TG/HDL-C) Ratio as a Risk Marker for Metabolic Syndrome and Cardiovascular Disease. *Diagnostics* **2023**, *13*, 929. [CrossRef]
69. Amato, M.C.; Giordano, C.; Galia, M.; Criscimanna, A.; Vitabile, S.; Midiri, M.; Galluzzo, A. Visceral Adiposity Index: A Reliable Indicator of Visceral Fat Function Associated with Cardiometabolic Risk. *Diabetes Care* **2010**, *33*, 920–922. [CrossRef]
70. Simental-Mendía, L.E.; Rodríguez-Morán, M.; Guerrero-Romero, F. The Product of Fasting Glucose and Triglycerides as Surrogate for Identifying Insulin Resistance in Apparently Healthy Subjects. *Metab. Syndr. Relat. Disord.* **2008**, *6*, 299–304. [CrossRef]
71. Stevens, B.R.; Goel, R.; Seungbum, K.; Richards, E.M.; Holbert, R.C.; Pepine, C.J.; Raizada, M.K. Increased Human Intestinal Barrier Permeability Plasma Biomarkers Zonulin and FABP2 Correlated with Plasma LPS and Altered Gut Microbiome in Anxiety or Depression. *Gut* **2018**, *67*, 1555. [CrossRef]
72. Yu, S.; Wang, L.; Jing, X.; Wang, Y.; An, C. Features of Gut Microbiota and Short-Chain Fatty Acids in Patients with First-Episode Depression and Their Relationship with the Clinical Symptoms. *Front. Psychol.* **2023**, *14*, 1088268. [CrossRef]

nutrients

MDPI

Article

Preoperative Multistrain Probiotic Supplementation Does Not Affect Body Weight Changes or Cardiometabolic Risk Factors in Bariatrics: Randomized, Double-Blind, Placebo-Controlled Clinical Trial

Marta Potrykus [1], Sylwia Czaja-Stolc [2,*], Marta Stankiewicz [2], Michał Szymański [1], Igor Łoniewski [3,4], Łukasz Kaska [5] and Monika Proczko-Stepaniak [1]

1 Department of Oncological, Transplant, and General Surgery, Medical University of Gdansk, 80-211 Gdańsk, Poland; martapotrykus@gumed.edu.pl (M.P.); szymanski@gumed.edu.pl (M.S.); monika.proczko-stepaniak@gumed.edu.pl (M.P.-S.)

2 Department of Clinical Nutrition and Dietetics, Medical University of Gdansk, 80-211 Gdańsk, Poland; marta.stankiewicz@gumed.edu.pl

3 Sanprobi sp. z o.o. sp. k., 70-535 Szczecin, Poland; sanprobi@sanprobi.pl

4 Department of Biochemical Science, Pomeranian Medical University in Szczecin, 71-460 Szczecin, Poland

5 Independent Public Health Care Center of the Ministry of Internal Affairs and Administration, 80-210 Gdańsk, Poland; lukasz.kaska@wp.pl

* Correspondence: sylwia.czaja-stolc@gumed.edu.pl; Tel.: +48-(58)-349-27-24

Abstract: Emerging evidence suggests that microbiota plays a crucial role in the development, progression, and therapeutic options in obesity and its comorbidities. This study assessed preoperative probiotic therapy's impact on bariatric treatment outcomes. A 12-week randomized, double-blind, placebo-controlled trial with 48 patients undergoing bariatric surgery was conducted. Participants received probiotics—Sanprobi Barrier—which contained nine strains of bacteria: *Bifidobacterium bifidum* W23, *Bifidobacterium lactis* W51 and W52, *Lactobacillus acidophilus* W37, *Levilactobacillus brevis* W63, *Lacticaseibacillus casei* W56, *Ligilactobacillus salivarius* W24, *Lactococcus lactis* W19, and *Lactococcus lactis* W58. Primary outcomes included excess body weight loss, body weight loss, and excess body mass index loss, with secondary objectives focusing on metabolic profiles. Surgical treatment of obesity significantly improved anthropometric and metabolic parameters. No significant differences were observed in primary outcomes or in secondary outcomes between groups at any time point post-surgery. Preoperative probiotics administration did not affect clinical outcomes 1, 3, or 6 months following bariatric surgery.

Keywords: probiotics; intestinal microbiota; bariatric surgery; obesity; metabolic disorders; weight loss

1. Introduction

Obesity is a disorder characterized by the accumulation of an excessive amount of body fat, leading to detrimental health consequences [1]. According to the latest data from the World Health Organization (WHO), in 2022, every eighth person worldwide suffered from obesity [2]. With the consistent rise in mortality and morbidity rates in individuals with excess body weight, gaining a comprehensive understanding of the mechanisms underlying prolonged and excessive overeating is of paramount importance [2] In 2019, an elevated body mass index (BMI) caused approximately 5 million deaths attributed to noncommunicable diseases (NCDs), including cardiovascular diseases, diabetes, cancer, neurological disorders, chronic respiratory diseases, neurological disorders, and digestive disorders [3].

Although bariatric surgery (BS) has shown remarkable efficacy in treating obesity and its comorbidities, there remains a subset of patients who fail to achieve the desired outcomes [4]. Obesity is a serious healthcare challenge due to its multifactorial nature.

Genetic predisposition, lifestyle factors, and dietary habits are recognized as leading causes of obesity, yet an emerging focus has been placed on the gut microbiota's influence [5]. The gut microbiota in individuals with obesity significantly differs from that observed in individuals with normal body weight. People with excess body weight tend to show reduced bacterial diversity within the gut microbiome, often with an increased ratio of Bacillota (Firmicutes) to Bacteroidota (Bacteroidetes) [6]. Studies suggest that a 20% increase in Firmicutes and a proportional decrease in Bacteroidetes may result in an additional intake of approximately 150 kilocalories per day [7]. The intestinal microbiota contributes to increasing energy harvest by producing short-chain fatty acids (SCFA) and simple sugars through the breakdown of polysaccharides. Microorganisms stimulate higher nutrient absorption by enhancing blood vessel density in the intestine [8]. Notably, the dominance of specific bacteria associated with obesity inhibits fasting-induced adipose tissue factor (FIAF). This inhibition increases fat accumulation by diminishing fat oxidation in the liver and muscles [9]. Moreover, intestinal microbiota has been shown to reduce the secretion of intestinal hormones such as peptide YY (PYY) and glucagon-like peptide-1 (GLP-1). These hormones play a pivotal role in regulating satiety, and their decreased secretion may lead to heightened food consumption [10]. Probiotic supplementation before BS may influence postoperative outcomes through various mechanisms. Probiotic supplementation helps maintain a healthy balance of gut bacteria by promoting the growth of beneficial strains that compete with pathogenic bacteria for nutrients and colonization niches, producing substances called bacteriocins that inhibit the growth of detrimental microorganisms [11]. Probiotics regulate cytokine levels by enhancing anti-inflammatory cytokines while diminishing pro-inflammatory ones [12]. Additionally, probiotics strengthen the integrity and functionality of the intestinal barrier, thereby preventing the translocation of harmful substances from the gut epithelium into the bloodstream, which may alleviate adipose tissue inflammation associated with obesity [13]. Overall, preoperative probiotics may create a healthier gut environment, modulate the immune response, help alleviate the inflammatory response caused by surgery, and enhance the effect of bariatric treatment.

Conclusions drawn from studies investigating the impact of probiotic therapy post-bariatric surgery are inconsistent. Some suggest potential benefits, such as improvements in weight loss and metabolic state, while others indicate inconspicuous clinical effects. The variability in findings provoked thoughts on alternative approaches to supporting the intestinal microbiome to enhance the effectiveness of bariatric treatment. To the best of our current knowledge, there is a lack of scientific literature concerning probiotic therapy before surgical obesity treatment. Therefore, we have decided to examine whether implementing probiotic therapy preoperatively could enhance the outcomes of bariatric treatment. The primary aim of this study was to assess the impact of probiotic therapy on weight loss, with secondary objectives focused on evaluating metabolic profiles.

2. Materials and Methods

2.1. Study Design

The study was designed as a randomized, double-blind, placebo-controlled clinical trial with a 12-week probiotics intervention period. Participants were randomly divided into two research arms—the probiotic group receiving multistrain probiotics and the placebo group. Allocation to groups was performed at a 1:1 ratio using an Microsoft Excel version 2019 random number generator. The study was unblinded after the statistical analysis. The project was conducted between August 2021 and April 2023 at the University Clinical Center (UCC) in Gdańsk (Poland). The protocol was approved by the Independent Bioethics Committee for Scientific Research at the Medical University of Gdańsk (No. NKNNB/447/2021) in accordance with the Declaration of Helsinki. The study was registered with clinical trials under the identifier NCT05407090.

This study is the first to evaluate the effect of preoperative probiotic supplementation; hence there are no previous studies on which we could base our sample size calculation. Based on data from Sanchez et al. [14] (weight reduction due to probiotics in patients with obesity), assuming $\alpha = 0.05$ and power = 80%, the initial calculation resulted in 20 patients per group. However, considering protocols variations and potential patient dropouts to ensure the study's validity and reliability, we decided to include 40 patients per group, which gives a total of 80 participants. However, during the study, it was noted that the attrition rate among patients exceeded the anticipated rate of 10–15%, reaching levels of 20–30%. Consequently, the study's recruited patient cohort was increased to 110 individuals.

2.2. Participants

One hundred and ten patients qualified for BS were enrolled in the study after screening interviews. The patients were qualified for Laparoscopic Sleeve Gastrectomy (LSG) or One Anastomosis Gastric Bypass (OAGB). The inclusion criteria included eligibility for BS based on International Federation for the Study of Obesity (IFSO) guidelines [15], Caucasian race, and age over 18. Patients were excluded from the study if they met any of the exclusion criteria: allergy/intolerance to any of the ingredients of the preparations; inflammatory bowel diseases; current antibiotic therapy; immunosuppression; biological treatment; long-term antibiotic therapy; probiotic therapy in the 1 month before study enrollment; neurodegenerative diseases, and antipsychotic drugs. Operational treatments were performed in accordance with the Enhanced Recovery After Bariatric Surgery (ERABS) protocol [16].

2.3. Study Protocol

Baseline and follow-up evaluations were performed in the University Clinical Center (UCC) in Gdańsk. Both research arms received identical medical care during the study period. Anthropometric measurements and blood samples were collected from the patients during each visit. After 12 weeks of supplementation, patients underwent either LSG or OAGB surgery. Subsequent follow-up visits were scheduled at 1 month (1 M PostOP), 3 months (3 M PostOP), and 6 months post-surgery (6 M PostOP). The patients followed a standardized diet under the supervision of a qualified dietitian. Upon recruitment, participants were provided with a balanced diet plan, which included a calorie deficit of 500–1000 kilocalories. Nutrient requirements were set at 25–30% for protein, 25–30% for fats, and 45–55% for carbohydrates of total daily energy intake, while mineral and vitamin requirements were based on the dietary standards for the Polish population [17]. Post-surgery, the dietary plan remained consistent, with 5–6 high-calorie-density meals per day. Fiber intake ranged from 10–30 g or 15 g/800–1000 kcal, depending on individual tolerance and time elapsed since the operation. All patients were prescribed vitamin supplements (WLS FitForMe, Rotterdam, The Netherlands).

2.4. Probiotic Intervention

The study product was a probiotic mixture contained nine strains of bacteria: Bifidobacterium bifidum W23, Bifidobacterium lactis W51 and W52, Lactobacillus acidophilus W37, Levilactobacillus brevis W63, Lacticaseibacillus casei W56, Ligilactobacillus salivarius W24, Lactococcus lactis W19, and Lactococcus lactis W58 in daily dose 2×10^9 CFU. This product is commercially sold in Poland under the name of Sanprobi Barrier (Sanprobi sp. z o. o. sp. k., Szczecin, Poland) and has been authorized by the appropriate health authorities regarding its composition and recommended dosage. Identical-looking placebo capsules contained maize starch and maltodextrin of maize origin. Patients were instructed to store the products in the refrigerator and take four capsules daily with meals (two capsules in the morning and two capsules in the evening) for 12 weeks. Patients were asked to continue supplementation until the last meal before the operation, within 24 h before the surgery.

2.5. Nutritional Status Assessment

Patients had their height and weight measured, and their BMI was calculated. The evaluation of the results of surgical treatment of obesity was based on the percentage of excess body weight loss (%EWL), the percentage of body weight loss (%WL), and the percentage of excess BMI loss (%EBMIL) [18]. In calculating %EWL, the ideal body weight was determined using the Deitel and Greenstein formula from 2003 [19]. The initial weight and BMI were measured during the first visit to the clinic.

2.6. Metabolic Parameters

All blood samples were collected following a 12 h fasting period and analyzed by a certified laboratory UCC in Gdańsk. The following parameters were determined: lipid panel, liver enzymes, anemia diagnostics, folic acid, vitamin B_{12}, glucose metabolism markers, and C-reactive protein (CRP). Insulin resistance was calculated using the homeostatic model assessment of insulin resistance (HOMA-IR) with the formula: HOMA-IR = [fasting blood glucose (mg/dL) $\times$ fasting insulin (mU/L)]/405.

2.7. Postoperative Complications

All postoperative complications were classified according to the 30 day postoperative Clavien–Dindo classification, which enables a standardized assessment of surgical complications. The complications were divided into five main grades (I–V), with grade I including the least severe complications that do not require intervention and grade V indicating the patient's death [20].

2.8. Statistical Methods

Statistical analysis involved using different methods based on the type and distribution of the data. For normally distributed data, measures like means and standard deviations (SDs) were employed, while non-normally distributed data were analyzed using medians and interquartile ranges (IQRs). The normality of the data was examined using the Shapiro–Wilk test and visually inspected through histograms. Categorical data were compared using contingency tables, chi-squared tests, or Fisher's exact test for limited observations (<5). Comparisons for normally distributed continuous data were done with *t*-tests or Welch's correction for unequal variances. To analyze the differences in continuous variables between treatment groups across multiple time points, repeated measures mixed ANOVA was conducted, followed by post hoc tests. Statistical significance was considered at a *p*-value of less than 0.05 for all two-sided tests. The statistical analyses and graphical representations were conducted using GraphPad Prism 10.2.1 and JASP statistical software version 0.18.1 and the Python version 3.9.16.

3. Results

3.1. Flow of Trial Participants and Comparison between Arms

Out of 174 patients interviewed for eligibility, 64 did not fulfill the criteria or declined participation. Given the increasing societal awareness of the importance of the intestinal microbiome, many prospective study candidates were already consuming probiotics, thus meeting one of the exclusion criteria. Consequently, 110 individuals were randomly assigned to either the placebo (n = 55) or probiotic (n = 55) group. Forty-eight patients (43.6%) completed the protocol and attended all four scheduled visits. To accomplish the 12-week intervention, patients were recruited 3 months before the surgery. Due to the individualized treatment approach, the time between recruitment and surgery, and consequently the duration of the intervention varied among patients. Therefore, only patients who underwent supplementation for at least 6 weeks were included in the study. Considering patients' treatment discontinuation (n = 19), withdrawals from the study (n = 6), supplementation durations less than 4 weeks (n = 1), non-adherence to the study protocol (n = 13), or absence at one of the follow-up visits (n = 13), a total of 48 individuals were included in the statistical analysis. Therefore, the study comprised 22 individuals in the probiotics and 26 in the placebo group.

One patient withdrew from the study due to abdominal pain and nausea after starting supplementation. After unblinding the study, it was revealed that he/she was taking a placebo. Another patient (with probiotics) reported a change in stool consistency after beginning supplementation, but the symptoms resolved within a week, and the patient remained in the study. This could have been a reaction to adaptation following the initiation of probiotic supplementation. According to Almutairi et al. [21], maltodextrin contained in the placebo may affect human gut physiology, but since both the placebo and the probiotics contained this substance, it should not have influenced the outcomes. The study flow is presented in Figure 1.

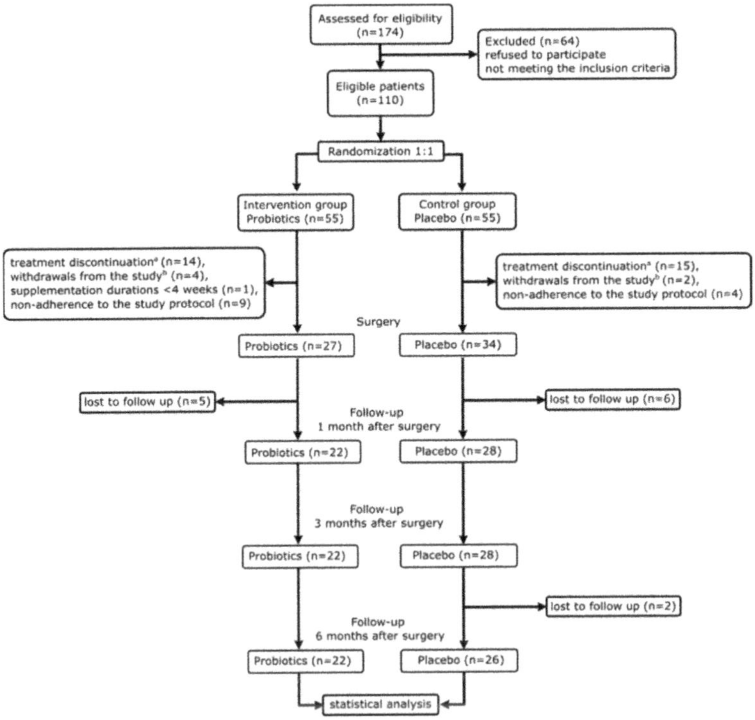

Figure 1. Study flow. [a] Treatment pathway was interrupted and participants did not proceed to surgery; [b] participants remained in the treatment cycle but opted out of participating in the research study. The absence of patients at the 1-month post-operation (1 M PostOP) visit was not due to non-compliance with the protocol but because some patients had a different treatment path that did not include a visit one month after surgery. To standardize the population, they were excluded from the statistical analysis in this publication.

All baseline characteristics were similar in both study arms, including age (42.2 $\pm$ 11.6 vs. 41.0 $\pm$ 11.2 years), initial BMI (43.6 $\pm$ 4.4 vs. 43.2 $\pm$ 7.1 kg/m^2), duration of supplementation (11.5 $\pm$ 1.9 vs. 11.5 $\pm$ 2 weeks) for the placebo and probiotics groups, respectively (Table 1). None of the assessed parameters showed significant differences between the groups before the intervention, except for folic acid, which was higher in the probiotic group (5.8 $\pm$ 1.6 vs. 7.2 $\pm$ 2.6; p = 0.028) (Table 2).

Table 1. Preintervention characteristic of groups.

	Placebo (n = 26)	Probiotics (n = 22)	p-Value
Sex (F/M) n	20/6	13/9	0.184
Age (years)	42.2 ± 11.6	41 ± 11.2	0.701
Duration of supplementation (weeks)	11.5 ± 1.9	11.5 ± 2	0.965 †
Max weight (kg)	135.9 ± 21.8	138.3 ± 27.1	0.733
Weight 6 M PreOP (kg)	129.2 ± 21.4	130.1 ± 31.0	0.907
Max BMI (kg/m^2)	45.9 ± 5.0	46.2 ± 6.2	0.885
BMI 6 M PreOP (kg/m^2)	43.6 ± 4.4	43.2 ± 7.1	0.825
Type of surgery (LSG/OAGB)	24/2	18/4	0.392 ‡
current-smokers n (%)	7 (26.9)	1 (4.5)	0.055 ‡
ever-smokers n (%)	9 (34.6)	9 (40.9)	0.584
DM1 n (%)	0	1 (4.5)	0.458 ‡
DM2 n (%)	6 (23.1)	6 (27.3)	0.738
HTN n (%)	14 (53.8)	12 (54.5)	0.961
DL n (%)	17 (65.4)	15 (68.2)	0.838
HT n (%)	9 (34.6)	7 (31.8)	0.838
fatty liver n (%)	21 (80.8)	19 (86.4)	0.604
OSAS (%)	17 (65.4)	17 (77.3)	0.367
Impaired fasting glucose n (%)	9 (34.6)	11 (0.5)	0.281

Abbreviations: BMI—body mass index; LSG—laparoscopic sleeve gastrectomy; F-female; M—male; OAGB—one anastomosis gastric bypass; DM1—diabetes mellitus type 1; DM2—diabetes mellitus type 2; HTN—hypertension; DL—dyslipidemia; HT—hypothyroidism; OSAS—obstructive sleep apnea syndrome; ‡—Fisher's exact test; †—U Mann–Whitney test.

Table 2. Preintervention laboratory parameters.

	Placebo (n = 26)	Probiotics (n = 22)	p-Value
Vit. D (pg/mL)	49.9 ± 15.1	52.5 ± 15.5	0.562
Folic Acid (ng/mL)	5.8 ± 1.6	7.2 ± 2.6	0.028
Vit. B_{12} (pg/mL)	349.8 ± 93.6	349.4 ± 113.6	0.99
Iron (ug/dL)	77.1 ± 30.8	82.5 ± 37.9	0.59
Insulin (uU/mL)	20.9 ± 14.9	22 ± 18.1	0.827
LDH (U/L)	192.5 ± 41.8	196.2 ± 32.7	0.738
ALT (U/L)	37.6 ± 18.3	34.7 ± 16.8	0.573
AST (U/L)	24.8 ± 10.9	24.2 ± 10.6	0.867
GGT (U/L)	46.4 ± 31.2	36.8 ± 18.6	0.212
ALP (U/L)	84.6 ± 26.1	75 ± 18.4	0.154
TG (mg/dL)	147.8 ± 67	140.5 ± 70.1	0.715
HDL (mg/dL)	43.5 ± 8.6	47.1 ± 13.1	0.262
LDL (mg/dL)	117.8 ± 39.3	115.1 ± 27.8	0.787
Cholesterol (mg/dL)	187.7 ± 45.3	188.5 ± 34.9	0.942
HbA1c%	5.7 ± 0.7	6.1 ± 1.3	0.287
HbA1c (mmol/mol)	39.2 ± 7.2	42.7 ± 14.4	0.272
Glucose (mg/dL)	102.3 ± 16.4	112.9 ± 41.3	0.238
Hemoglobin (g/dL)	13.8 ± 1.5	14.2 ± 1.8	0.45
HOMA-IR	5.6 ± 5.5	6.4 ± 6.4	0.633

Abbreviations: Vit. D—vitamin D; Vit. B_{12}—vitamin B_{12}; LDH—lactate dehydrogenase; ALT—alanine aminotransferase; AST—aspartate aminotransferase; GGT—gamma-glutamyl transferase; ALP—alkaline phosphatase; TG—triglycerides; HDL—high-density lipoprotein; LDL—low-density lipoprotein; HbA1c%—glycated hemoglobin percentage; HbA1c—glycated hemoglobin; HOMA-IR—homeostatic model assessment for insulin resistance.

3.2. Primary Outcomes

Patients' weights and BMIs were significantly improved at 1 M, 3 M, and 6 M post-op compared to baseline in both arms ($p < 0.001$ for all), with no difference between the groups. Similarly, no significant differences between the groups were observed in %WL, %EWL, and %EBMIL at any of the follow-up visits. Results are presented both in Table 3 and Figure 2.

Table 3. Primary outcomes.

	Placebo (n = 26)	Probiotics (n = 22)	Between Subjects Effects (Group)	Within Subjects Effects (Time)	Within Subjects Effects (Time × Group)
			Weight (kg)		
Max	135.9 ± 21.8	138.3 ± 27.1	0.749	<0.001	0.612
6 M PreOP	129.2 ± 21.4	130.1 ± 31			
3 M PreOP–PRO	122.5 ± 19.8	123.4 ± 27.4			
1 M PreOP	119.9 ± 20.4	120.9 ± 27.3			
OP	117.7 ± 19.5	119.5 ± 26.3			
1 M PostOP	107.5 ± 18.9	110.8 ± 26.6			
3 M PostOP	99.1 ± 16.9	102 ± 26.3			
6 M PostOP	92.1 ± 15.8	96 ± 24.7			
			BMI (kg/m^2)		
Max	45.9 ± 5	46.2 ± 6.2	0.966	<0.001	0.582
6 M PreOP	43.6 ± 4.4	43.2 ± 7.1			
3 M PreOP–PRO	41.4 ± 4.6	41.1 ± 6			
1 M PreOP	40.5 ± 4.6	40.2 ± 6			
OP	39.8 ± 4.6	39.7 ± 5.5			
1 M PostOP	36.3 ± 4.5	36.7 ± 5.4			
3 M PostOP	33.5 ± 4.4	33.8 ± 6			
6 M PostOP	31.2 ± 4.7	31.9 ± 6.1			
			%WL		
OP	8.7 ± 4.8	7.7 ± 4.5	0.229	<0.001	0.739
1 M PostOP	16.7 ± 4.9	14.8 ± 3.6			
3 M PostOP	23.2 ± 5.3	21.8 ± 5.2			
6 M PostOP	30.4 ± 11.5	26.5 ± 8.8			
			%EWL		
OP	17.5 ± 9.1	15.7 ± 9.1	0.636	<0.001	0.791
1 M PostOP	33.9 ± 10.2	31.3 ± 8.4			
3 M PostOP	47.3 ± 12.6	46.9 ± 16.3			
6 M PostOP	57.8 ± 16.7	56.8 ± 17.6			
			%EBMIL		
OP	20.9 ± 11	18.8 ± 10.8	0.803	<0.001	0.7
1 M PostOP	40.7 ± 13.3	38 ± 12			
3 M PostOP	56.7 ± 17.1	57.4 ± 23.9			
6 M PostOP	72.6 ± 34.6	62 ± 40.4			

Abbreviations: BMI—body mass index; %WL—percentage of weight loss; %EWL—percentage of excess weight loss; %EBMIL—percentage of excess BMI loss.

3.3. *Secondary Outcomes*

In this section, we present the secondary outcomes of the study. The data in Tables 4 and 5 provide detailed results on these outcomes.

3.3.1. Glycemic Parameters

Table 4 illustrates that all glycemic parameters—glucose, insulin, HbA1c%, HbA1c, and HOMA-IR—were significantly improved at 1 M, 3 M, and 6 M PostOP compared to baseline in both arms ($p < 0.001$ for all), with no difference between the groups.

3.3.2. Lipid Profile

As shown in Table 4, triglycerides were significantly improved at 1 M, 3 M, and 6 M PostOP compared to the initial value ($p < 0.001$ for all). High-density lipoprotein (HDL) significantly decreased in 1 M PostOP but then increased at 6 M PostOP compared to baseline ($p < 0.001$ for both). There was no improvement in low-density lipoprotein (LDL) concentration after BS. The concentration of total cholesterol decreased compared to the baseline value at 1 ($p < 0.001$) and 3 M PostOP ($p = 0.01$), but the effect did not persist at the 6-month post-surgery check-in. No statistically significant differences were observed in the concentrations of triglycerides, HDL, LDL, and total cholesterol between the groups at any time point.

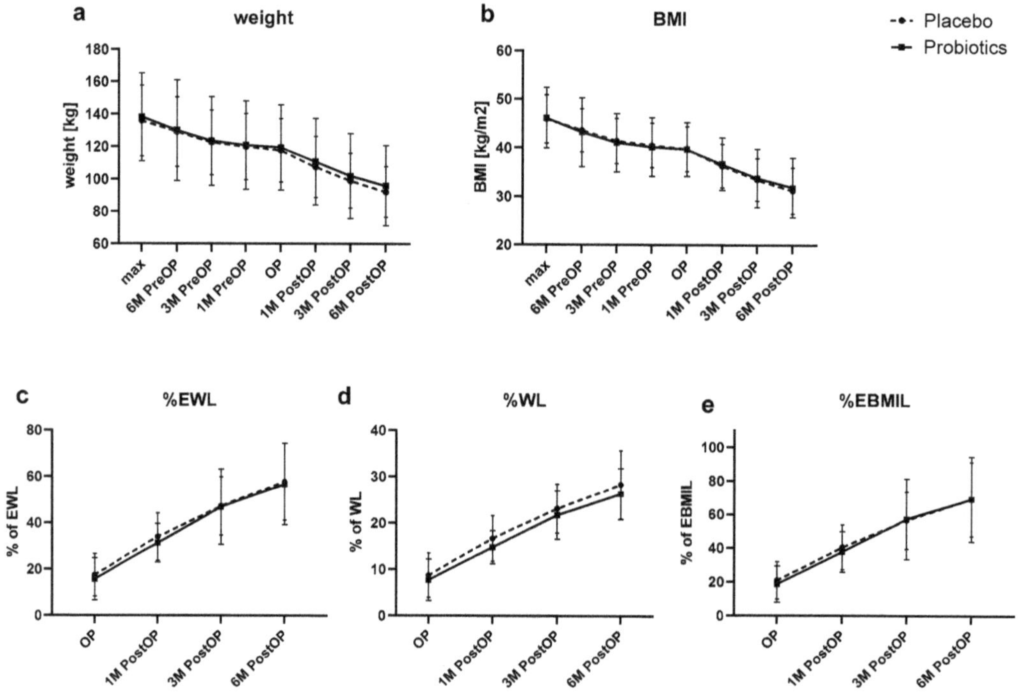

Figure 2. Comparison of primary outcomes between two groups at various time points. BMI—body mass index; %EWL—percentage of excess weight loss, %WL—percentage of weight loss; %EBMIL—percentage of excess body mass index loss. (**a**) Comparison of Weight Over Time Between Groups; (**b**) Comparison of BMI Over Time Between Groups; (**c**) Comparison of %EWL Over Time Between Groups; (**d**) Comparison of %WL Over Time Between Groups; (**e**) Comparison of %EBMIL Over Time Between Groups.

3.3.3. Liver Enzymes

Lactate dehydrogenase (LDH) and gamma-glutamyl transferase (GGT) were significantly reduced in all time points in comparison to baseline ($p < 0.013$ for all time points for both parameters). The concentration of alkaline phosphatase (ALP) improved compared to the baseline value at 1 ($p < 0.009$), but the effect did not persist over time. There was no change in aspartate aminotransferase (AST) after surgery compared to initial value. No differences were noted between the groups in the concentrations of any liver enzymes at any time point (Table 4).

3.3.4. Iron Parameters

As indicated in Table 4, iron was increased at 6 M PostOP in comparison to baseline ($p < 0.008$) but with no differences at other time points. There was no change in hemoglobin concentration after BS. No statistically significant differences were observed in the concentrations of iron and hemoglobin between the groups.

Table 4. Comparison of Study Secondary Outcomes Between Groups.

	Baseline		1 M PostOP		3 M PostOP		6 M PostOP		Between Subjects Effects (Group)	Within Subjects Effects (Time)	Within Subjects Effects (Time × Group)
	Placebo $n = 26$	Probiotics $n = 22$	Placebo $n = 26$	Probiotics $n = 22$	Placebo $n = 26$	Probiotics $n = 22$	Placebo $n = 26$	Probiotics $n = 22$	p-Value	p-Value	p-Value
Vit. D (pg/mL)	49.9 ± 15.1	52.5 ± 15.5	51.5 ± 12.6	58.7 ± 18.5	52.4 ± 15.5	63.5 ± 18.6	57.8 ± 21.3	60.1 ± 18.2	0.132	0.018	0.276
Folic Acid (ng/mL)	5.8 ± 1.6	7.2 ± 2.6	8.7 ± 3.2	8.7 ± 2.9	8.9 ± 3.7	8.6 ± 3.3	11.8 ± 8.3	8.8 ± 4.1	0.517	0.002	0.097
Vit. B_{12} (pg/mL)	349.8 ± 93.6	349.4 ± 113.6	483.2 ± 169.3	472.3 ± 147.4	455.4 ± 202	422.1 ± 182.1	411 ± 142.6	397.6 ± 163.1	0.694	<0.001	0.866
Iron (ug/dL)	77.1 ± 30.8	82.5 ± 37.9	72.5 ± 20.9	72.4 ± 26.1	79.2 ± 25.5	86.7 ± 32.3	85.7 ± 27.1	92.8 ± 36.4	0.408	0.016	0.845
Insulin (uU/mL)	20.9 ± 14.9	22 ± 18.1	8.5 ± 3.8	13.5 ± 9.1	7.8 ± 3.4	9.3 ± 5.4	7.3 ± 2.4	9.3 ± 8	0.168	<0.001	0.527
LDH (U/L)	192.5 ± 41.8	196.2 ± 32.7	179.5 ± 38.1	175.7 ± 34.2	160.9 ± 46.8	176.7 ± 44.6	160.7 ± 33.6	163.2 ± 36.1	0.618	<0.001	0.35
ALT (U/L)	37.6 ± 18.3	34.7 ± 16.8	35.6 ± 18.7	44 ± 25.5	24.1 ± 23.1	27.5 ± 14.5	17.9 ± 7.4	20 ± 8.8	0.421	<0.001	0.34
AST (U/L)	24.8 ± 10.9	24.2 ± 10.6	21.3 ± 7.5	24.9 ± 8.8	22.2 ± 24.5	25.2 ± 20.7	17.7 ± 5.6	17.8 ± 6.7	0.536	0.072	0.795
GGT (Ul)	46.4 ± 31.2	36.8 ± 18.6	28.3 ± 21.1	28.2 ± 15.4	25.5 ± 18	28.7 ± 32	24.5 ± 23.3	34.3 ± 54.3	0.907	0.006	0.132
ALP (U/L)	84.6 ± 26.1	75 ± 18.4	72.1 ± 22.2	69.6 ± 15.9	74 ± 24.2	77.6 ± 22.7	79.7 ± 25.2	82.7 ± 25.5	0.811	0.001	0.065
TG (mg/dL)	147.8 ± 67	140.5 ± 70.1	111.6 ± 52	110.6 ± 29.8	105.1 ± 56.1	99.2 ± 27.4	99.6 ± 41.3	99.1 ± 39.9	0.756	<0.001	0.901
HDL (mg/dL)	43.5 ± 8.6	47.1 ± 13.1	35.8 ± 6.2	39.2 ± 8.1	40.8 ± 5.6	45.3 ± 8.7	47.5 ± 6.9	51.9 ± 10.3	0.061	<0.001	0.906
LDL (mg/dL)	117.8 ± 39.3	115.1 ± 27.8	109.2 ± 40.3	105.6 ± 29	112.5 ± 40.4	114.5 ± 29.3	112.5 ± 34.1	117.7 ± 36	0.981	0.194	0.697
Cholesterol (mg/dL)	187.7 ± 45.3	188.5 ± 34.9	160.7 ± 41.9	162.7 ± 34.6	168.6 ± 47.9	173.3 ± 33.4	169.5 ± 43.1	182 ± 41	0.613	<0.001	0.665
HbA1c%	5.7 ± 0.7	6.1 ± 1.3	5.2 ± 0.5	5.4 ± 0.8	5.3 ± 0.4	5.3 ± 0.7	5.3 ± 0.5	5.5 ± 1.1	0.301	<0.001	0.5
HbA1c (mmol/mol)	39.2 ± 7.2	42.7 ± 14.4	33.2 ± 4.8	36 ± 9.3	34 ± 4.7	34.5 ± 8.2	34.3 ± 4.9	36.3 ± 11.5	0.293	<0.001	0.47
Glucose (mg/dL)	102.3 ± 16.4	112.9 ± 41.3	90.8 ± 8.1	98.9 ± 13.5	87.9 ± 9.1	89.2 ± 8.1	89.2 ± 11.2	90.6 ± 11.9	0.098	<0.001	0.341
Hemoglobin (g/dL)	13.8 ± 1.5	14.2 ± 1.8	13.6 ± 1.2	14.1 ± 1.3	13.8 ± 1.5	14.2 ± 1.2	13.7 ± 1.4	14.2 ± 1.3	0.271	0.726	0.907
HOMA-IR	5.6 ± 5.5	6.4 ± 6.4	2 ± 1	3.5 ± 2.7	1.7 ± 0.9	2.1 ± 1.4	1.6 ± 0.6	2.2 ± 2.2	0.167	<0.001	0.607

Abbreviations: Vit. D—vitamin D; Vit. B_{12}—vitamin B_{12}; LDH—lactate dehydrogenase; ALT—alanine aminotransferase; AST—aspartate aminotransferase; GGT—gamma-glutamyl transferase; ALP—alkaline phosphatase; TG—triglycerides; HDL—high-density lipoprotein; LDL—low-density lipoprotein; HbA1c%—glycated hemoglobin percentage; HbA1c—glycated hemoglobin; HOMA-IR—homeostatic model assessment for insulin resistance.

Table 5. Comparison of Clavien–Dindo classification outcomes between groups.

Clavien–Dindo Grade	Placebo *n* (%)	Probiotics *n* (%)	*p*-Value
all	2 (7.7)	3 (13.6)	0.649
I	0	1 (4.5)	0.458
II	2 (7.7)	0	0.493
IIIa	0	1 (4.5)	0.458
IIIb	0	1 (4.5)	0.458
IVa	0	0	1
IVb	0	0	1
V	0	0	1

Types of complications occurring according to the Clavien–Dindo classification: Grade I—vomiting; Grade II—abdominal pain and excessive drainage of the surgical wound; Grade IIIa—gastrointestinal bleeding; Grade IIIb—wound dehiscence accompanied by surgical site infection; Grade IV and V—no complications.

3.3.5. Vitamins

Foliate and vit. B_{12} were significantly increased in all time points in comparison to baseline ($p < 0.036$ for all time points for both parameters). Vitamin D was increased 6 months post-op in comparison to baseline ($p < 0.019$). No significant differences were observed in the concentrations of vitamins between the groups. The comparison of concentrations of all examined parameters is presented in Table 4.

3.3.6. Postoperative Complications

During the 30-day postoperative period, complications classified according to the Clavien–Dindo scale occurred in two patients (7.7%) in the placebo group and in three patients (13.6%) in the probiotics group. In the probiotics group, single cases of Grade I, IIIA, and IIIB complications were noted, while in the placebo group, only Grade II complications occurred (7.7%). No Grade IVA, IVB, or V complications were observed in either group. There were no statistically significant differences in the incidence of complications between the groups (Table 5).

4. Discussion

In the presented study, we have observed that probiotic supplementation before BS did not affect body weight, BMI, or any of the recommended tools for assessing the anthropometric effects of bariatric surgery, i.e., %WL, %EWL, %EBMIL at any time point, nor did it improve the metabolic profile of patients at any time point after surgery. To the best of our knowledge, this is the first randomized, double-blind, placebo-controlled clinical trial assessing the impact of probiotic therapy on the effects of surgical treatment of obesity in which all supplementation occurs before surgery.

In a meta-analysis conducted by Mohamed Aziz Daghmouri et al., parameters corresponding to our main goals, such as BMI change, absolute and percentage weight change from baseline, %EWL, fat mass change, and waist circumference change did not differ between the placebo and probiotics groups 3 months after surgery [22]. In another meta-analysis, Wang et al. observed that individuals supplementing with probiotics exhibited lower body weight three months after BS compared to those receiving a placebo. However, other anthropometric measurements, such as %EWL, BMI, or waist circumference, showed no differences between the two groups [23].

The gut microbiome plays a significant role in glucose metabolism, liver function, lipid profile, vitamins levels, and iron metabolism. Microbiota influences glucose metabolism through modulation of insulin sensitivity and secretion, as well as impacting glucose absorption and utilization [24]. The link between probiotics and the liver's function involves the direct transport of gut-derived products to the liver via the portal vein. Metabolites from the gut microbiota can directly affect the liver's functions, influencing its susceptibility to metabolical changes [25]. The gut microbiota may influence plasma cholesterol levels through bile acid metabolism and the production of dehydrogenase enzymes (ismA), which transform cholesterol into poorly absorbed sterol coprostanol, reducing serum total cholesterol levels [26]. The intestinal microbiome can influence iron metabolism by increasing the acidity of the environment, producing enzymes that convert ferric iron (Fe^{3+}) to ferrous iron (Fe^{2+}), or by producing chelating substances that hinder its absorption [27,28]. Moreover, the interaction between host and microbiota metabolism affects vitamin levels [29].

Research on the effects of probiotic supplementation before BS is inconsistent. In a meta-analysis by Mohamed Aziz Daghmouri et al., insulin concentrations were lower in the probiotics group, with no differences in HbA1c levels [22]. Meanwhile, in a meta-analysis conducted by Wang et al., no differences were observed in any of the assessed glycemic parameters—glucose, insulin, HbA1c, HOMA-IR, and quantitative insulin sensitivity check index (QUICKI) [23]. In the work of Sherf-Dagan et al., a 6-month supplementation was carried out before BS in non-alcoholic fatty liver disease patients. It shows that the differences in AST, ALT, and GGT concentrations before 3, 6, and 12 months after the intervention did not differ between the probiotics and placebo groups [30]. Conversely, in the meta-analysis conducted by Wang et al., probiotics showed significant effects on regulating AST levels [23]. The meta-analysis conducted by Wang et al. revealed that while probiotic supplementation did not impact total cholesterol, LDL, or HDL cholesterol levels, there was a greater reduction in triglyceride levels among the probiotics group compared to the placebo 3 M postoperatively [23]. Daghmouri et al. revealed that no significant difference was found in HDL-cholesterol levels between the groups three months post-surgery. However, a significantly greater reduction in triglyceride and LDL levels was observed in the probiotic group compared to the placebo [22]. Regarding iron metabolism, studies indicate that probiotic therapy before BS does not significantly affect iron parameters such as ferritin and hemoglobin levels [23]. Some studies showed that probiotics supplementation increased the concentration of vitamin D in serum after surgery compared to the placebo group [31,32]. In our study, we did not observe any impact of multistrain probiotic supplementation on the metabolic profile after BS. However, it is worth noting that all the above-described publications referred to studies in which probiotic therapy was introduced after surgery. We did not find any other studies that examined the impact of probiotic therapy as a preparatory element before surgery on the outcomes of surgical treatment for obesity.

The multi-strain probiotic was used in this study because in earlier examinations, it demonstrated a positive impact on anthropometric and metabolic risk factors. It also enhanced the integrity of the gut barrier [33–35] and altered the effects of microbiota on biochemical, physiological, and immunological factors associated with obesity and inflammation [36]. A possible explanation for the lack of the expected favorable results in the group with probiotics is the fact that prehabilitation, as well as the surgery itself, have a significant impact on the host–microbiome metabolism [37]. Other studies in patients undergoing BS have also failed to demonstrate the efficacy of this multi-strain probiotic in reducing the severity of depressive symptoms, with the surgery itself leading to a significant reduction in both the probiotic and placebo groups [38]. The effect of probiotic therapy may be overshadowed by the substantial impact of prehabilitation and surgery on the microbiome, anthropometry, and metabolic status of patients. BS significantly affects gut microbiota [39]. Additionally, the perioperative preparation of the patient for surgery also contributes to the depletion of the intestinal microbiota. Surgical interventions disrupt the integrity of the intestinal barrier, potentially leading to increased bacterial translocation and systemic inflammation. Moreover, these interventions result in the reconstruction of the digestive tract and alterations in environmental conditions for microorganisms, which may cause significant changes in the local microbiome [40]. Consequently, this may decrease the effects of modifying the intestinal microbiota before surgery. Probiotic therapy appears to directly affect the patient's metabolism during its administration. This implies that the timing of probiotic supplementation—before and after BS—may cause different effects. Supplementation before surgery focuses on optimizing patients' health before BS, which may alleviate early postoperative gut dysbiosis caused by microbiome changes during surgery, reduce inflammation, improve metabolic profile, and promote recovery [41]. Postoperative probiotics therapy emphasizes maintaining a balanced microbiome after surgery, which can potentially directly influence patients' weight, low-grade inflammation, and metabolic profile as well as mitigate gastrointestinal symptoms caused by the surgical intervention [32,42]. In addition, the effects of probiotics are strain-dependent; it is still not fully understood which strains, in what amounts, and at what time will be effective in modeling the intestinal microbiota to optimally influence the host's metabolism and body weight. Currently, we have scientific evidence that the state of the intestinal microbiome is related to the development, progression, and therapeutic options in obesity and its consequences. Still, the full potential of this knowledge is not yet used in practice. The composition and activity of the gut microbiota vary individually, thus, there is no universal method of microbiota modification that would bring health benefits. Therefore, it is crucial to focus on performing thorough microbiota research in individual disease entities and to try to target microbiota modifications in narrow groups of patients. The strong point of the presented study is its design as a randomized, double-blind, and placebo-controlled research in which randomization was successful; both demogeographic data and assessed parameters in baseline did not differ between presented groups. One of the limitations of our study is the low number of patients. Despite recruiting the planned number of participants, less than 50% of patients qualified for statistical analysis, which reduced the power of the study. Therefore, it is possible that we did not detect existing differences between the groups. However, this sample size was sufficient to confirm the impact of the intervention on numerous anthropometric and biochemical parameters. It is likely that the effect of the probiotic is not sufficient to influence these parameters significantly. Therefore, caution should be exercised when interpreting the data and comparing it with the literature. Additionally, bariatric patients are a specific group whose diet, both before and after surgery, is low-calorie and possibly insufficient to ensure optimal nutrition for the microorganisms inhabiting the digestive tract. It would be valuable to repeat the presented study on a larger number of patients, but also with a changed methodology, where patients would receive both probiotics and prebiotics. Moreover, microbiota analysis would shed more light on the obtained results.

5. Conclusions

In conclusion, it seems that preoperative probiotic administration does not affect weight loss and clinically significant metabolic parameters in patients treated with BS. However, due to the limited population of participants, it is possible that we may underestimate the existing differences between the groups. Therefore, caution should be exercised in the interpretation and comparison of our findings with other literature. Additional high-quality randomized controlled trials will be necessary in the future to further explore the potential therapeutic effects of probiotics in patients with morbid obesity undergoing bariatric treatment.

Author Contributions: Conceptualization, M.P., M.S. (Marta Stankiewicz), M.S. (Michał Szymański) and Ł.K.; methodology, M.P., M.S. (Marta Stankiewicz), M.S. (Michał Szymański) and Ł.K.; validation, M.P. and M.P.-S.; formal analysis, M.P.; investigation, M.P. and M.S. (Marta Stankiewicz); resources, M.P. and Ł.K.; data curation, M.P.; writing—original draft preparation, M.P. and S.C.-S.; writing—review and editing, M.P., S.C.-S., I.Ł. and M.P.-S.; visualization, M.P.; supervision, M.S. (Marta Stankiewicz), M.S. (Michał Szymański), Ł.K. and M.P.-S. All authors have read and agreed to the published version of the manuscript.

Funding: This research received no external funding.

Institutional Review Board Statement: The study was conducted in accordance with the Declaration of Helsinki and approved by the Bioethics Committee for Scientific Research at the Medical University of Gdansk (No. NKNNB/447/2021, 21 May 2021).

Informed Consent Statement: Informed consent was obtained from all subjects involved in the study.

Data Availability Statement: The data sets used and/or analyzed during the current study are available from the corresponding author upon reasonable request as we are currently working on additional publications from this project, and some of the data will be used in these forthcoming studies.

Conflicts of Interest: I.Ł. is a shareholder of the company Sanprobi, a manufacturer of probiotics. However, the content of this study was not constrained by this fact. The remaining authors declare that the research was conducted in the absence of any commercial or financial relationships that could be construed as a potential conflict of interest.

References

1. Tomé-Castro, X.M.; Rodriguez-Arrastia, M.; Cardona, D.; Rueda-Ruzafa, L.; Molina-Torres, G.; Roman, P. Probiotics as a Therapeutic Strategy in Obesity and Overweight: A Systematic Review. *Benef. Microbes* **2021**, *12*, 5–15. [CrossRef] [PubMed]
2. Available online: https://www.who.int/news-room/fact-sheets/detail/obesity-and-overweight (accessed on 1 June 2024).
3. Murray, C.J.L.; Aravkin, A.Y.; Zheng, P.; Abbafati, C.; Abbas, K.M.; Abbasi-Kangevari, M.; Abd-Allah, F.; Abdelalim, A.; Abdollahi, M.; Abdollahpour, I.; et al. Global Burden of 87 Risk Factors in 204 Countries and Territories, 1990–2019: A Systematic Analysis for the Global Burden of Disease Study 2019. *Lancet* **2020**, *396*, 1223–1249. [CrossRef] [PubMed]
4. Wiggins, T.; Guidozzi, N.; Welbourn, R.; Ahmed, A.R.; Markar, S.R. Association of Bariatric Surgery with All-Cause Mortality and Incidence of Obesity-Related Disease at a Population Level: A Systematic Review and Meta-Analysis. *PLoS Med.* **2020**, *17*, e1003206. [CrossRef] [PubMed]
5. Kim, M.-H.; Yun, K.E.; Kim, J.; Park, E.; Chang, Y.; Ryu, S.; Kim, H.-L.; Kim, H.-N. Gut Microbiota and Metabolic Health among Overweight and Obese Individuals. *Sci. Rep.* **2020**, *10*, 19417. [CrossRef] [PubMed]
6. Duan, M.; Wang, Y.; Zhang, Q.; Zou, R.; Guo, M.; Zheng, H. Characteristics of Gut Microbiota in People with Obesity. *PLoS ONE* **2021**, *16*, e0255446. [CrossRef]
7. Kotzampassi, K. Bacteria and Obesity: The Proportion Makes the Difference. *Surgery* **2013**, *3*, 152. [CrossRef]
8. Wagner, N.R.F.; Zaparolli, M.R.; Cruz, M.R.R.; Schieferdecker, M.E.M.; Campos, A.C.L. Postoperative changes in intestinal microbiota and use of probiotics in roux-en-y gastric bypass and sleeve vertical gastrectomy: An integrative review. *ABCD Arq. Bras. Cir. Dig.* **2018**, *31*, e1400. [CrossRef] [PubMed]
9. Aron-Wisnewsky, J.; Warmbrunn, M.V.; Nieuwdorp, M.; Clément, K. Metabolism and Metabolic Disorders and the Microbiome: The Intestinal Microbiota Associated With Obesity, Lipid Metabolism, and Metabolic Health—Pathophysiology and Therapeutic Strategies. *Gastroenterology* **2021**, *160*, 573–599. [CrossRef]
10. Sun, L.-J.; Li, J.-N.; Nie, Y.-Z. Gut Hormones in Microbiota-Gut-Brain Cross-Talk. *Chin. Med. J.* **2020**, *133*, 826–833. [CrossRef]
11. Liu, Y.; Wang, J.; Wu, C. Modulation of Gut Microbiota and Immune System by Probiotics, Pre-Biotics, and Post-Biotics. *Front. Nutr.* **2022**, *8*, 634897. [CrossRef]
12. Kwok, K.O.; Fries, L.R.; Silva-Zolezzi, I.; Thakkar, S.K.; Iroz, A.; Blanchard, C. Effects of Probiotic Intervention on Markers of Inflammation and Health Outcomes in Women of Reproductive Age and Their Children. *Front. Nutr.* **2022**, *9*, 889040. [CrossRef] [PubMed]
13. Cristofori, F.; Dargenio, V.N.; Dargenio, C.; Miniello, V.L.; Barone, M.; Francavilla, R. Anti-Inflammatory and Immunomodulatory Effects of Probiotics in Gut Inflammation: A Door to the Body. *Front. Immunol.* **2021**, *12*, 578386. [CrossRef] [PubMed]
14. Sanchez, M.; Darimont, C.; Panahi, S.; Drapeau, V.; Marette, A.; Taylor, V.; Doré, J.; Tremblay, A. Effects of a Diet-Based Weight-Reducing Program with Probiotic Supplementation on Satiety Efficiency, Eating Behaviour Traits, and Psychosocial Behaviours in Obese Individuals. *Nutrients* **2017**, *9*, 284. [CrossRef]
15. Kasama, K.; Mui, W.; Lee, W.J.; Lakdawala, M.; Naitoh, T.; Seki, Y.; Sasaki, A.; Wakabayashi, G.; Sasaki, I.; Kawamura, I.; et al. IFSO-APC Consensus Statements 2011. *Obes. Surg.* **2012**, *22*, 677–684. [CrossRef]
16. Mannaerts, G.H.H.; Van Mil, S.R.; Stepaniak, P.S.; Dunkelgrün, M.; De Quelerij, M.; Verbrugge, S.J.; Zengerink, H.F.; Biter, L.U. Results of Implementing an Enhanced Recovery After Bariatric Surgery (ERABS) Protocol. *Obes. Surg.* **2016**, *26*, 303–312. [CrossRef] [PubMed]
17. Jarosz, M.; Rychlik, E.; Stoś, K.; Charzewska, J. *Normy Żywienia dla Populacji Polski i ich Zastosowanie*; Narodowy Instytut Zdrowia Publicznego—Państwowy Zakład Higieny: Warszawa, Poland, 2020; ISBN 978-83-65870-28-5.
18. Budzyński, A.; Major, P.; Głuszek, S.; Kaseja, K.; Koszutski, T.; Leśniak, S.; Lewandowski, T.; Lipka, M.; Lisik, W.; Makarewicz, W. Polskie Rekomendacje w Zakresie Chirurgii Bariatrycznej i Metabolicznej. *Medycyna Praktyczna. Chirurgia* **2017**, 13–26.
19. Deitel, M.; Greenstein, R.J. Recommendations for Reporting Weight Loss. *Obes. Surg.* **2003**, *13*, 159–160. [CrossRef]
20. Dindo, D.; Demartines, N.; Clavien, P.-A. Classification of Surgical Complications: A New Proposal With Evaluation in a Cohort of 6336 Patients and Results of a Survey. *Ann. Surg.* **2004**, *240*, 205–213. [CrossRef]
21. Almutairi, R.; Basson, A.R.; Wearsh, P.; Cominelli, F.; Rodriguez-Palacios, A. Validity of Food Additive Maltodextrin as Placebo and Effects on Human Gut Physiology: Systematic Review of Placebo-Controlled Clinical Trials. *Eur. J. Nutr.* **2022**, *61*, 2853–2871. [CrossRef]

22. Daghmouri, M.A.; Chaouch, M.A.; Yang, W.; Akremi, S.; Jaoua, H.; Fadhel, K.B.; Gouader, A.; Reissfelder, C.; Elhadedy, H.; Rahbari, N.; et al. Probiotics in Bariatric Surgery Ensure Greater Lipids and Glycemic Profile with No Effect on Anthropometric Measurements and Inflammatory Markers: A Systematic Review and Meta-Analysis of RCT. *Surg. Open Dig. Adv.* **2022**, *7*, 100061. [CrossRef]
23. Wang, Y.; Zheng, Y.; Kuang, L.; Yang, K.; Xie, J.; Liu, X.; Shen, S.; Li, X.; Wu, S.; Yang, Y.; et al. Effects of Probiotics in Patients with Morbid Obesity Undergoing Bariatric Surgery: A Systematic Review and Meta-Analysis. *Int. J. Obes.* **2023**, *47*, 1029–1042. [CrossRef] [PubMed]
24. Utzschneider, K.M.; Kratz, M.; Damman, C.J.; Hullarg, M. Mechanisms Linking the Gut Microbiome and Glucose Metabolism. *J. Clin. Endocrinol. Metab.* **2016**, *101*, 1445–1454. [CrossRef] [PubMed]
25. Albillos, A.; De Gottardi, A.; Rescigno, M. The Gut-Liver Axis in Liver Disease: Pathophysiological Basis for Therapy. *J. Hepatol.* **2020**, *72*, 558–577. [CrossRef] [PubMed]
26. Kenny, D.J.; Plichta, D.R.; Shungin, D.; Koppel, N.; Hall, A.B.; Fu, B.; Vasan, R.S.; Shaw, S.Y.; Vlamakis, H.; Balskus, E.P.; et al. Cholesterol Metabolism by Uncultured Human Gut Bacteria Influences Host Cholesterol Level. *Cell Host Microbe* **2020**, *28*, 245–257.e6. [CrossRef] [PubMed]
27. Sargun, A.; Gerner, R.R.; Raffatellu, M.; Nolan, E.M. Harnessing Iron Acquisition Machinery to Target *Enterobacteriaceae*. *J. Infect. Dis.* **2021**, *223*, S307–S313. [CrossRef] [PubMed]
28. Xiao, L.; Tang, R.; Wang, J.; Wan, D.; Yin, Y.; Xie, L. Gut Microbiota Bridges the Iron Homeostasis and Host Health. *Sci. China Life Sci.* **2023**, *66*, 1952–1975. [CrossRef] [PubMed]
29. Rossi, M.; Amaretti, A.; Raimondi, S. Folate Production by Probiotic Bacteria. *Nutrients* **2011**, *3*, 118–134. [CrossRef] [PubMed]
30. Sherf-Dagan, S.; Zelber-Sagi, S.; Zilberman-Schapira, G.; Webb, M.; Buch, A.; Keidar, A.; Raziel, A.; Sakran, N.; Goitein, D.; Goldenberg, N.; et al. Probiotics Administration Following Sleeve Gastrectomy Surgery: A Randomized Double-Blind Trial. *Int. J. Obes.* **2018**, *42*, 147–155. [CrossRef] [PubMed]
31. Karbaschian, Z.; Mokhtari, Z.; Pazouki, A.; Kabir, A.; Hedayati, M.; Moghadam, S.S.; Mirmiran, P.; Hekmatdoost, A. Probiotic Supplementation in Morbid Obese Patients Undergoing One Anastomosis Gastric Bypass-Mini Gastric Bypass (OAGB-MGB) Surgery: A Randomized, Double-Blind, Placebo-Controlled, Clinical Trial. *Obes. Surg.* **2018**, *28*, 2874–2885. [CrossRef]
32. Mokhtari, Z.; Karbaschian, Z.; Pazouki, A.; Kabir, A.; Hedayati, M.; Mirmiran, P.; Hekmatdoost, A. The Effects of Probiotic Supplements on Blood Markers of Endotoxin and Lipid Peroxidation in Patients Undergoing Gastric Bypass Surgery; a Randomized, Double-Blind, Placebo-Controlled, Clinical Trial with 13 Months Follow-Up. *Obes. Surg.* **2019**, *29*, 1248–1258. [CrossRef]
33. Sabico, S.; Al-Mashharawi, A.; Al-Daghri, N.M.; Wani, K.; Amer, O.E.; Hussain, D.S.; Ahmed Ansari, M.G.; Masoud, M.S.; Alokail, M.S.; McTernan, P.G. Effects of a 6-Month Multi-Strain Probiotics Supplementation in Endotoxemic, Inflammatory and Cardiometabolic Status of T2DM Patients: A Randomized, Double-Blind, Placebo-Controlled Trial. *Clin. Nutr.* **2019**, *38*, 1561–1569. [CrossRef] [PubMed]
34. Szulińska, M.; Łoniewski, I.; Van Hemert, S.; Sobieska, M.; Bogdański, P. Dose-Dependent Effects of Multispecies Probiotic Supplementation on the Lipopolysaccharide (LPS) Level and Cardiometabolic Profile in Obese Postmenopausal Women: A 12-Week Randomized Clinical Trial. *Nutrients* **2018**, *10*, 773. [CrossRef] [PubMed]
35. Sabico, S.; Al-Mashharawi, A.; Al-Daghri, N.M.; Yakout, S.; Alnaami, A.M.; Alokail, M.S.; McTernan, P.G. Effects of a Multi-Strain Probiotic Supplement for 12 Weeks in Circulating Endotoxin Levels and Cardiometabolic Profiles of Medication Naïve T2DM Patients: A Randomized Clinical Trial. *J. Transl. Med.* **2017**, *15*, 249. [CrossRef] [PubMed]
36. Kaczmarczyk, M.; Szulińska, M.; Łoniewski, I.; Kręgielska-Narożna, M.; Skonieczna-Żydecka, K.; Kosciolek, T.; Bezshapkin, V.; Bogdański, P. Treatment With Multi-Species Probiotics Changes the Functions, Not the Composition of Gut Microbiota in Postmenopausal Women With Obesity: A Randomized, Double-Blind, Placebo-Controlled Study. *Front. Cell. Infect. Microbiol.* **2022**, *12*, 815798. [CrossRef] [PubMed]
37. Ulker, İ.; Yildiran, H. The Effects of Bariatric Surgery on Gut Microbiota in Patients with Obesity: A Review of the Literature. *Biosci. Microbiota Food Health* **2019**, *38*, 3–9. [CrossRef] [PubMed]
38. Komorniak, N.; Kaczmarczyk, M.; Łoniewski, I.; Martynova-Van Kley, A.; Nalian, A.; Wroński, M.; Kaseja, K.; Kowalewski, B.; Folwarski, M.; Stachowska, E. Analysis of the Efficacy of Diet and Short-Term Probiotic Intervention on Depressive Symptoms in Patients after Bariatric Surgery: A Randomized Double-Blind Placebo Controlled Pilot Study. *Nutrients* **2023**, *15*, 4905. [CrossRef] [PubMed]
39. Komorniak, N.; Martynova-Van Kley, A.; Nalian, A.; Wroński, M.; Kaseja, K.; Kowalewski, B.; Kaźmierczak-Siedlecka, K.; Łoniewski, I.; Kaczmarczyk, M.; Podsiadło, K.; et al. Association between Fecal Microbiota, SCFA, Gut Integrity Markers and Depressive Symptoms in Patients Treated in the Past with Bariatric Surgery—The Cross-Sectional Study. *Nutrients* **2022**, *14*, 5372. [CrossRef] [PubMed]
40. Zheng, Z.; Hu, Y.; Tang, J.; Xu, W.; Zhu, W.; Zhang, W. The Implication of Gut Microbiota in Recovery from Gastrointestinal Surgery. *Front. Cell. Infect. Microbiol.* **2023**, *13*, 1110787. [CrossRef] [PubMed]

41. Liu, W.; Zheng, C.; Li, Q.; Xu, T.; Cao, W.; Shi, M.; Huang, F.; Liu, L.; Luo, Y.; Zhang, W.; et al. Preoperative Oral Probiotics Relieve Insulin Resistance and Gut Dysbacteriosis in Patients with Gastric Cancer after Gastrectomy. *J. Funct. Foods* **2023**, *101*, 105426. [CrossRef]
42. Melali, H.; Abdolahi, A.; Sheikhbahaei, E.; Vakili, K.; Mahmoudieh, M.; Keleidari, B.; Shahabi, S. Impact of Probiotics on Gastrointestinal Function and Metabolic Status After Roux-En-Y Gastric Bypass: A Double-Blind, Randomized Trial. *Obes. Surg.* **2024**, *34*, 2033–2041. [CrossRef]

nutrients

MDPI

Article

Low Zinc Alleviates the Progression of Thoracic Aortic Dissection by Inhibiting Inflammation

Lin Zhu [1,2,†], Peng An [1,†], Wenting Zhao [1], Yi Xia [1], Jingyi Qi [1,2], Junjie Luo [1,2,*] and Yongting Luo [1,*]

1 Department of Nutrition and Health, China Agricultural University, Beijing 100193, China
2 Food Laboratory of Zhongyuan, Luohe 462300, China
* Correspondence: luojj@cau.edu.cn (J.L.); luo.yongting@cau.edu.cn (Y.L.)
† These authors contributed equally to this work.

Abstract: Vascular inflammation triggers the development of thoracic aortic dissection (TAD). Zinc deficiency could dampen tissue inflammation. However, the role of zinc as a nutritional intervention in the progression of TAD remains elusive. In this study, we employed a classical β-aminopropionitrile monofumarate (BAPN)-induced TAD model in mice treated with low zinc and observed that the TAD progression was greatly ameliorated under low zinc conditions. Our results showed that low zinc could significantly improve aortic dissection and rupture (BAPN + low zinc vs. BAPN, 36% vs. 100%) and reduce mortality (BAPN + low zinc vs. BAPN, 22% vs. 57%). Mechanically, low zinc attenuated the infiltration of macrophages and inhibited the expression of inflammatory cytokines, suppressed the phenotype switch of vascular smooth muscle cells from contractile to synthetic types, and eventually alleviated the development of TAD. In conclusion, this study suggested that low zinc may serve as a potential nutritional intervention approach for TAD prevention.

Keywords: thoracic aortic dissection; low zinc; inflammation; vascular smooth muscle cells; phenotypic transition

1. Introduction

Aortic dissection (AD) is a life-threatening condition caused by a tear in the intimal layer of the aorta or bleeding within the aortic wall, resulting in the separation (dissection) of the layers of the aortic wall [1]. This disease progresses rapidly and has a high fatality rate [2]. The fatality rate reaches 50.0% within 24 h after the onset of AD and rises to 68.2% after 48 h [3]. Currently, there are no clinically effective drugs to prevent or delay AD progression, which underscores the urgent need for developing effective treatment strategies.

Several clinical and epidemiological studies have indicated a tight association between low serum zinc concentration and the occurrence and mortality of cardiovascular diseases [4–6]. One study analyzed the clinical data of 108 patients with aortic aneurysm and found that the zinc content of aortic wall tissue in patients with thoracic aortic aneurysm (TAA) was lower than that in the control group [7]. Consistently, other studies have confirmed that zinc deficiency exists in the aortic wall of patients with aortic aneurysm [8,9]. It was also found that the concentrations of Zn in serum and tissue of AD patients were significantly lower than that of the healthy group [10]. These studies suggested a strong association between reduced zinc levels and the occurrence of AD. However, the role of zinc in the progression of AD remains unclear.

Diet and lifestyle manipulation have become key steps for the primary and secondary prevention of cardiovascular diseases, and nutritional intervention can effectively improve physical condition by maintaining cardiovascular health [11]. As an essential trace element, zinc has a variety of physiological effects on the human body [12]. Notably, animal models of zinc deficiency have confirmed that low levels of zinc induced lymphopenia and compromised cell- and antibody-mediated immune responses in several studies [13,14]. For instance, zinc deficiency can affect the shift of the Th cells' response to a Th2 predominance, decrease the killing activity of natural killer cells, reduce levels of phagocytosis and intracellular killing in granulocytes, monocytes and macrophages, and diminish the total number of neutrophils [13–17]. Consistently, another study demonstrated that zinc deficiency reduced the production of interferon-gamma, interleukin-2 (IL-2), and tumor necrosis factor-alpha (TNF-α) [18]. The pathogenesis of TAD includes vascular smooth muscle cells (VSMCs) phenotypic transformation and apoptosis, extracellular matrix (ECM) degradation, endothelial dysfunction and immune cell infiltration [19]. In recent years, a large number of clinical and basic studies have demonstrated that inflammatory response is involved in the formation of the TAD [20–22]. The AD patients with serious clinical symptoms and developed progression showed higher activities of inflammatory cells in the aortic wall compared with asymptomatic and clinically stable patients [22]. The infiltration of inflammatory cells increases with aggravation during the AD process, and macrophages are the main inflammatory cells in the dissected aorta [23]. Infiltration of macrophages into the aortic wall recruits subsequent immune cells, increases inflammatory response and promotes the development of the AD [24]. Since the accumulation and activation of inflammatory cells within the vascular wall promote aortic weakening and extracellular matrix degeneration [25], and zinc deficiency dampens tissue inflammation; we speculate that low zinc may ameliorate AD by down-regulating inflammation.

Given the potential association between low zinc and AD pathology, this study investigated the effects of low zinc on β-aminopropionitrile monofumarate (BAPN)-induced TAD model to explore whether low zinc could alleviate the process of TAD and be used as a potential nutritional intervention approach.

2. Methods and Material

2.1. Animals

Three-week-old male C57BL/6N mice were purchased from Beijing Vital River Laboratory Animal Technology (Beijing, China). The animals were kept in individually ventilated cages pathogen-free and allowed to eat food and drink water freely. Weight loss, behavioral changes and feeding or drinking habits were used to assess the health of mice. All animal procedures were approved by the China Agricultural University Laboratory Animal Welfare and Animal Experimental Ethical Inspection.

2.2. Experimental Design

Three-week-old male C57BL/6N mice were administrated with BAPN (2 g/kg/day; A3134, Sigma-Aldrich, St. Louis, MO, USA) in the drinking water for 30 days to induce TAD (n = 14 per group). The mice in the BAPN group (n = 14) were given a normal diet (30 mg Zn/kg; Beijing HFK Bioscience, Beijing, China). The mice in BAPN + low zinc group (n = 14) were given a low zinc diet (1 mg Zn/kg; Beijing HFK Bioscience) after BAPN induced one week. The mice in the control group (n = 14) were given water without BAPN and a normal diet (30 mg Zn/kg; Beijing HFK Bioscience) for 30 days. The animal experiment ended after BAPN-induced 30 days, followed by the collection of ultrasound images, blood and aortic tissue of mice in each group.

2.3. Echocardiography Analysis

Echocardiography analysis was performed using the Vevo 2100 high-resolution imaging system (FUJIFILM Visual Sonics, Toronto, ON, Canada) equipped with an 18- to 38-MHz (MS400, mouse cardiovascular) scan head. The mouse chest was depilated before echocardiography analysis. Then mice were anesthetized with 0.5–1.5% isoflurane in an anesthesia induction chamber. After anesthesia, mice were placed on a homeothermic plate and applied ultrasonic coupling agent to the chest. The left margin of the sternum, the right margin of the sternum, the apex of the heart and the suprasternal fossa of mice were scanned by the scan head, and ultrasound images of the heart were collected after

BAPN-induced 30 days. The maximal diameters of the aorta were measured at the level of the aortic outflow tract of the innominate artery.

2.4. Enzyme-Linked Immunosorbent Assay (ELISA)

After the animal experiment ended, the whole blood was collected, left at room temperature for 3 h, centrifuged at 3000 rpm for 10 min, and the upper serum was taken for the ELISA experiment. The levels of TNF-α were estimated with Mouse TNF-α ELISA Kit (EK282/4-01, Multi Sciences, Shanghai, China) according to the manufacturer's instructions. Briefly, the standards and samples were added into holes of the enzyme label plate, respectively. The TNF-α in the sample was bound to the solid antibody after incubation. Then unbound biotinylated antibody was washed and removed, and horseradish peroxidase-labeled streptavidin (Streptavidin-HRP) solution, TMB substrate solution, and stop solution were gradually added. Absorbance at 450 nm was estimated within 30 min.

2.5. Immunofluorescence Staining

Mouse aortic tissues were stored at 4% paraformaldehyde after the animal experiment ended and divided into 5-µm-thick serial sections. Tissue paraffin sections were dewaxed first, and microwave antigen repair was performed. Seal with 5% goat serum (dilute with 1× PBS) after several washes with PBS. Then paraffin sections were incubated overnight at 4 °C with the specific primary antibody Mac-3 (1:100 dilutions; 108501, BioLegend, San Diego, CA, USA). After several washes with PBS, the paraffin sections were incubated with fluorescent secondary antibody Alexa Fluor 488 goat Anti-Mouse IgG (1:1000 dilution; ab150113, Abcam, Cambridge, UK) for 1–2 h at 4 °C. Antifade mounting medium with DAPI (S2110, Solarbio, Beijing, China) was used for the paraffin section's seal. Immunofluorescence was visualized using a confocal microscope (Zeiss, Jena, Germany).

2.6. Hematoxylin and Eosin (HE), Elastic Van Gieson (EVG), Masson's Trichrome and Alcian Blue Staining

Mouse aortic tissues were divided into 5-µm-thick serial sections, and the paraffin sections were stained after deparaffinized. Aortic sections were stained with hematoxylin and eosin (G1120, Solarbio), elastic Van Gieson (G1593, Solarbio), Masson's trichrome (G1340, Solarbio), alcian blue (G1560, Solarbio) according to the manufacturer's instructions. Images were acquired by a fluorescence microscope bright field camera (Leica, Wetzlar, Germany).

2.7. Real-Time Quantitative PCR (Q-PCR)

Frozen aortic tissues were homogenized using an automatic bead homogenizer. Total RNA was extracted from aortic tissue using TRIzol (15596026, Thermo, Waltham, MA, USA) according to the manufacturer's instructions. RNA samples (1 µg) were reverse-transcribed into cDNA with a HiScript III RT SuperMix for qPCR kit (R323-01, Vazyme, Nanjing, China), and the cDNA was amplified by real-time quantitative PCR using SYBR qPCR Master Mix (Q711-02, Vazyme). The amount of target mRNA in samples was estimated by the $2^{-\Delta\Delta CT}$ relative quantification method. All samples were amplified using at least 3 technical replicates per sample. The primers used for Q-PCR are shown in Supplementary Table S1.

2.8. Western Blot

Frozen aortic tissues were homogenized using an automatic bead homogenizer. Total proteins were obtained from aortic tissues using a RIPA buffer containing a stop protease and phosphatase inhibitor (9806, Cell Signaling Technology, Danvers, MA, USA). The whole protein samples of each group were heated at 95 °C for 5 min, then equal amounts of protein were loaded and separated into 15%, 10% or 8% sodium dodecyl sulfate-polyacrylamide gels. Subsequently, all proteins were transferred onto the polyvinylidene fluoride membrane. The membrane was incubated overnight at 4 °C with the specific primary antibody;

then, they were incubated with the corresponding secondary antibodies. Protein bands were visualized by using a chemiluminescent reagent (Thermo, Pierce, MA, USA) and ChemiScope 3600 MINI (Clinx Scientific Instrument, Shanghai, China). All antibodies used for the western blot are shown in Supplementary Table S2.

2.9. Statistical Analysis

Data presented were expressed as the mean of three or more biological replicates/ biologically independent experiments. Results are analyzed in GraphPad Prism 8.0 (GraphPad Software, San Diego, CA, USA). Differences were analyzed by one-way, two-way analysis of variance (ANOVA) and Tukey's post hoc test (experiments with ≥3 groups) as appropriate. For survival curves, differences were analyzed with the log-rank (Mantel-Cox) test. Statistical significance was assigned at * $p < 0.05$, ** $p < 0.01$ and *** $p < 0.001$.

3. Results

3.1. Low Zinc Significantly Mitigates BAPN-Induced TAD Development in Mice

Previous studies have shown that TAD models can be established by administering BAPN to mice [26–28]. The mechanism of the BAPN-induced TAD model was that BAPN inhibits the activity of lysyl oxidase (LOX), which catalyzes the cross-linking of lysine residues in elastin and collagen, thereby increasing the degradation of ECM proteins as crucial components of aortic integrity, eventually resulting in the occurrence of AD [29]. To investigate the role of zinc in AD, we performed in vivo experiments using a BAPN-induced TAD mouse model [26–28]. The normal zinc (BAPN group) and the low zinc (BAPN + low zinc group) mice were treated with BAPN for 30 days, while the control mice (control group) were treated without BAPN ($n = 14$ per group) (Figure 1A). The BAPN + low zinc group was given a special diet after BAPN was induced for one week. The survival curve showed that low zinc treatment could significantly increase the survival rate compared with the BAPN group ($p = 0.0249$, Figure 1B). During the 30 days of BAPN administration, 57% ($n = 8$) of the BAPN group mice and 22% ($n = 3$) of the BAPN + low zinc group mice died from AD and rupture (Figure 1B,C). In addition, 43% ($n = 6$) of the BAPN group mice and 14% ($n = 2$) of the BAPN + low zinc group mice experienced AD without rupture (Figure 1C). The BAPN group also presented a great difference in aortic diameter and TAD occurrence compared with the BAPN + low zinc group (Figure 1D).

Furthermore, vascular ultrasound images and maximal aortic diameter measurement after 30 days of modeling demonstrated that the BAPN + low zinc group mitigated BAPN-induced aortic dilation and reduced the average maximal aortic diameter in comparison with the BAPN group (Figure 2A,B).

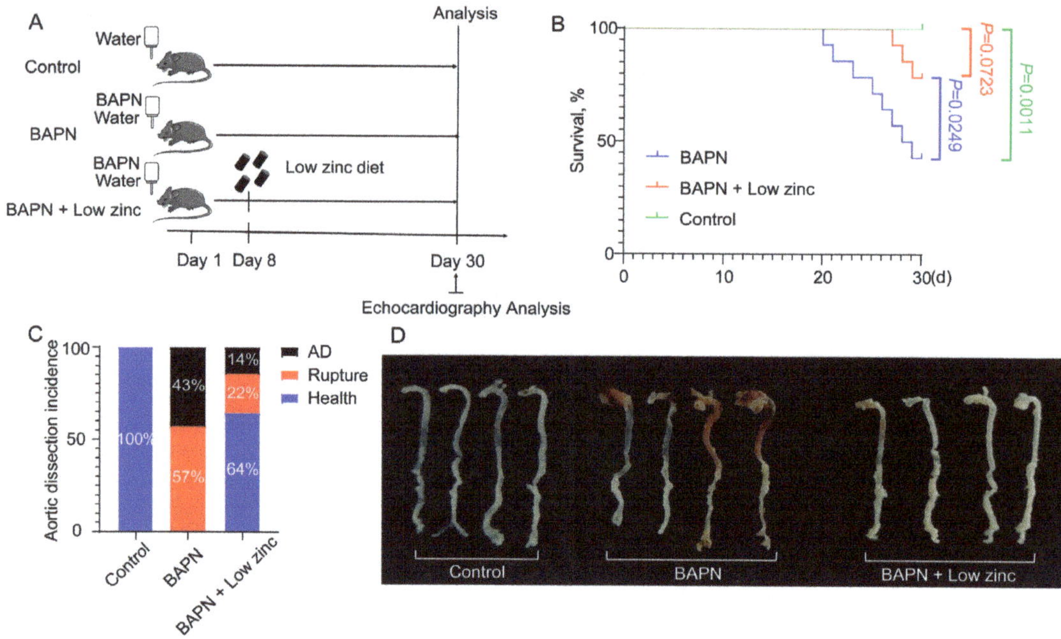

Figure 1. Low zinc represses TAD progression. (**A**) Experimental design diagram. (**B**) The survival rate was estimated by the Kaplan-Meier method and compared by log-rank test (n = 14 per group). (**C**) TAD incidence. (**D**) Representative macrographs of the aorta.

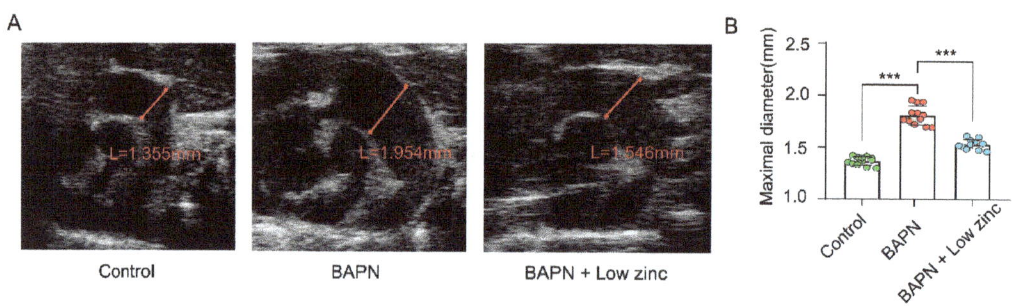

Figure 2. Echocardiography analysis at the end of the animal experiment (BAPN-induced 30 days). (**A**) Representative ultrasound images of thoracic aortas. (**B**) Measurements of maximum aortic diameter, green blots represent control group, red blots represent BAPN group and blue blots represent BAPN + Low zinc group, n = 12 per group, by one-way ANOVA (*** $p < 0.001$).

The degradation of ECM during AD progression results in VSMC loss and contributes to rupture and dilation of the aortic wall [30]. Elastic fibers and collagen fibers are two major macromolecules within the arterial ECM. We found that total elastin content and elastic fiber cross-links were reduced during the occurrence of AD, and the collagen expression was increased, and disorderly deposition may correspond to a slow reparative process triggered by elastic fiber fragmentation and depletion [31]. In addition, proteoglycan content is minimal in normal vascular tissue while significantly increasing in diseased vascular tissue [32]. Therefore, we performed a pathological staining analysis. HE staining showed that BAPN-induced dissecting aneurysm formation was alleviated in the BAPN + low zinc group compared with the BAPN group (Figure 3A). EVG staining demonstrated that BAPN-induced elastic fiber fragmentation and disarray were also mitigated in the low zinc treatment group (Figure 3A). BAPN-induced mice caused the characteristic features of ECM degradation, including excessive collagen deposition and proteoglycan accumulation. Masson's trichrome and Alcian blue staining showed that these features were alleviated by low zinc treatment (Figure 3A). Consistently, the quantitative statistics of elastin breaks and collagen content also indicated that low zinc could mitigate TAD development (Figure 3B,C).

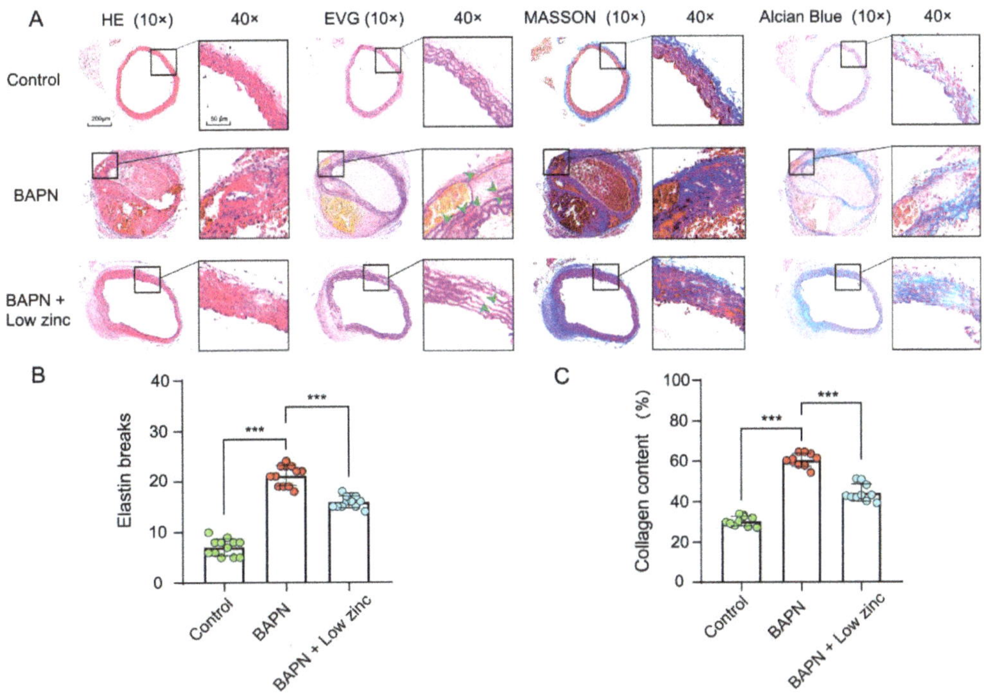

Figure 3. Pathological staining analysis after animal experiment end (BAPN-induced 30 days). (**A**) Representative images showing hematoxylin and eosin (HE) (first column), elastic van Gieson (EVG) (second column), Masson's trichrome (MASSON) (third column) and Alcian blue (final column) staining in paraffin sections from the indicated mice (top for the control group, middle for the BAPN group, bottom for the BAPN + low zinc group). Green arrowheads indicate elastin breaks. Scale bar, 200 μm for 10 magnifications, 50 μm for 40 magnifications. (**B**) Quantification of elastin breaks in paraffin sections from the mouse cohorts shown in (**A**), $n = 12$per group, by one-way ANOVA (*** $p < 0.001$). (**C**) Quantification of collagen content in paraffin sections from the mouse cohorts shown in (**A**), $n = 10$ per group, by one-way ANOVA (*** $p < 0.001$). Green blots represent control group, red blots represent BAPN group and blue blots represent BAPN + Low zinc group.

3.2. Low Zinc Inhibits the Transition of Contractile VSMCs to Synthetic VSMCs

The characteristic plasticity of VSMCs is that they can adapt to environmental stimuli and mechanical stresses, thereby switching between contractile and synthetic types [33]. During AD progression, the balance between contractile and synthetic VSMCs is shifted towards synthetic VSMCs, and the proteolytic enzyme production is increased [30]. In fact, the phenotypic switch of VSMCs is the key to AD and rupture [34,35]. Thus, the real-time Q-PCR was performed to discern differently expressed genes in the aortic tissues of each group and revealed that VSMC phenotypic switch was inhibited in the BAPN + low zinc group.

The VSMC contractile genes, including *Myh11* (myosin heavy polypeptide 11), *Acta2* (actin alpha 2), *Myl9* (myosin light polypeptide 9), *Ccn1* (calponin 1) and *Ramp1* (receptor activity modifying protein 1) were up-regulated in low zinc aortas compared with the BAPN group (Figure 4A). Meanwhile, the VSMC synthetic genes, including *Col1A1* (collagen type I alpha 1), *Cxcl2* (C-X-C motif chemokine ligand 2) and *Fn1* (fibronectin 1), were down-regulated in low zinc aortas compared with the BAPN group (Figure 4B). Furthermore, the expression levels of selected typical VSMC contractile proteins (ACTA2, CCN1 and MYH11) were also rescued with low zinc treatment (Figure 4C). Taken together, these results demonstrated the critical role of low zinc in VSMC phenotypic switch in TAD pathogenesis.

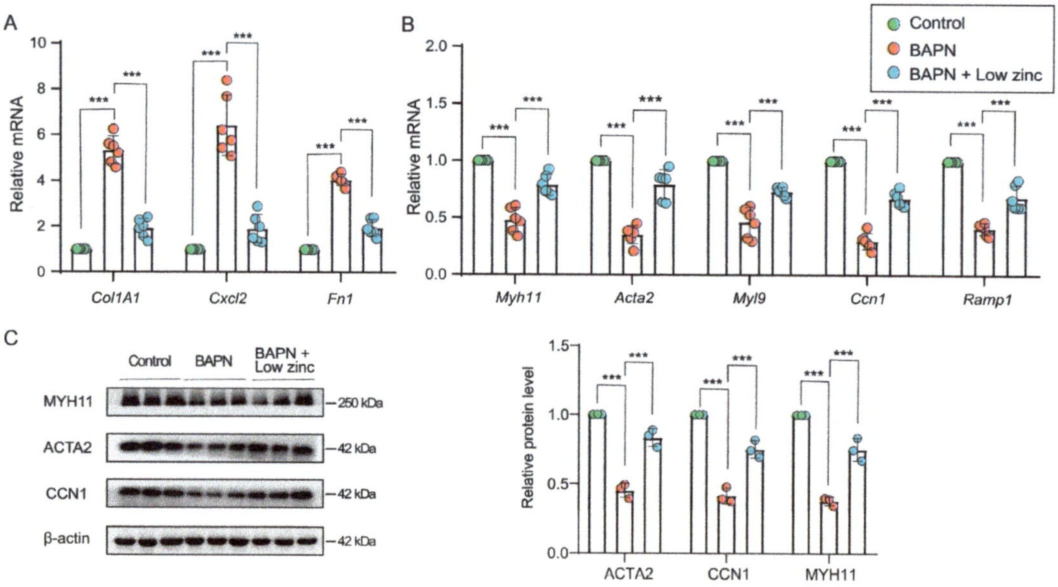

Figure 4. Low zinc suppressed the phenotype switch of vascular smooth muscle cells. (**A**) Relative mRNA levels of selected VSMC synthetic genes (*Col1A1*, *Cxcl2* and *Fn1*) in mice aorta ($n = 6$ per group); by two-way ANOVA (*** $p < 0.001$). (**B**) Relative mRNA levels of selected VSMC contractile genes (*Myh11*, *Acta2*, *Myl9*, *Ccn1* and *Ramp1*) in mice aorta ($n = 6$ per group); by two-way ANOVA (*** $p < 0.001$). (**C**) The protein levels (left column is western blot result, right column is quantitative analysis) of selected VSMC contractile markers (MYH11, ACTA2 and CCN1) in mice aorta ($n = 3$ per group); by two-way ANOVA (*** $p < 0.001$). All samples were collected after the animal experiment ended (BAPN-induced 30 days).

3.3. *Low Zinc Alleviates TAD Development by Reducing Inflammation*

Inflammation was involved in the occurrence of TAD by regulating the homeostasis of the aortic wall, and the increase of inflammatory response resulted in VSMCs apoptosis and ECM destruction in the aortic wall [24]. The characteristic of inflammatory response is the presence of T lymphocytes, macrophages, mast cells, and neutrophils. At the onset of AD, there is a large number of infiltrated macrophages into the aortic wall lesions [23]. In our results, the immunofluorescence staining demonstrated that the green fluorescence signal intensity (Mac-3, biomarker of macrophages) decreased significantly undergo low zinc, suggesting low zinc countered BAPN-induced inflammatory cell infiltration of macrophages (Figure 5A,B).

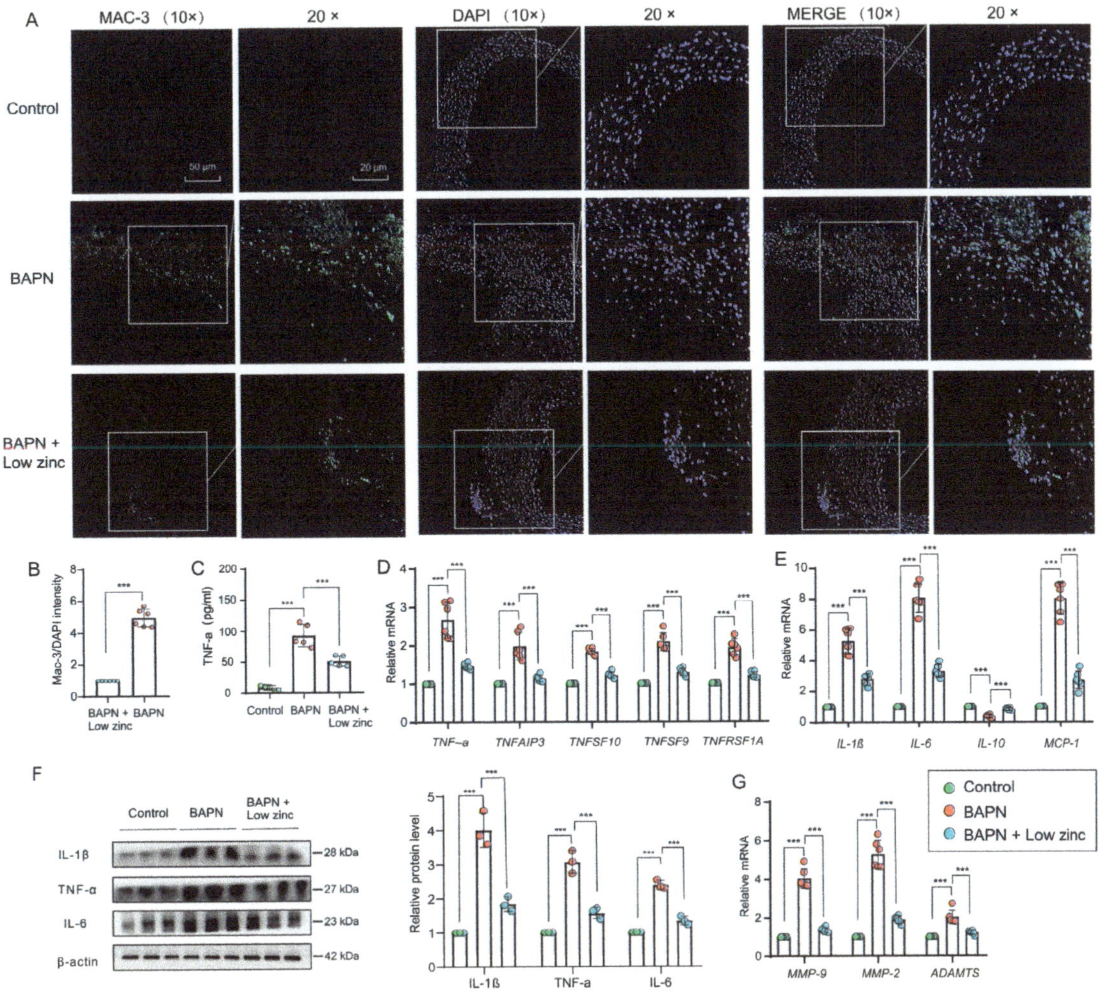

Figure 5. Low zinc inhibited TAD by down-regulating inflammation. (**A**) Representative confocal images of mice aorta stained with Mac-3 (green) and DAPI (blue) (scale bars, 50 μm for 10 magnifications; 20 μm for 20 magnifications). (**B**) Quantification of Mac-3 levels ($n = 6$ per group); by one-way ANOVA (*** $p < 0.001$). (**C**) The expression level of TNF-α in mice serum ($n = 5$ per group), by one-way ANOVA (*** $p < 0.001$). (**D**) Relative mRNA levels of *TNF-α*, *TNFAIP3*, *TNFSF10*, *TNFSF9* and *TNFSF1A* of tumor necrosis factors in mice aorta ($n = 6$ per group); by two-way ANOVA (*** $p < 0.001$). (**E**) Relative mRNA levels of *IL-1β*, *IL-6*, *IL-10* and *MCP-1* of interleukin and chemokines in mice aorta ($n = 6$ per group); by two-way ANOVA (*** $p < 0.001$). (**F**) The protein levels (left column is western blot result, right column is quantitative analysis) of selected typical proinflammatory factors (IL-1β, TNF-α and IL-6) in mice aorta ($n = 3$ per group); by two-way ANOVA (*** $p < 0.001$). (**G**) Relative mRNA levels of *MMP-9*, *MMP-2* and *ADAMTS* of extracellular matrix enzymes in mice aorta ($n = 6$ per group); by two-way ANOVA (*** $p < 0.001$). All samples were collected after the animal experiment ended (BAPN-induced 30 days).

Multiple inflammatory factors, such as tumor necrosis factor-α (TNF-α) and interleukin-6 (IL-6), are released during the occurrence of AD [36]. Enzyme-linked immunosorbent assay (ELISA) showed that TNF-α expression was significantly decreased in aortic tissues of the BAPN + low zinc group compared with the BAPN group (Figure 5C). Q-PCR indicated that transcriptional levels of the tumor necrosis factors, including *TNF-α*, *TNFAIP3*, *TNFSF10*, *TNFSF9* and *TNFSF1A*, were down-regulated in aortas of the BAPN + low zinc group compared with the BAPN group (Figure 5D).

Specific cytokines and chemokines can promote the recruitment of inflammatory cells in the aortic media. As previously reported, the expression of *TNF-α*, *CRP*, *IL-2*, *IL-1β*, *IL-6*, *IL-8* and *MCP-1* (monocyte chemotactic protein-1) is up-regulated in AD, while the expression of *IL-10* is down-regulated [23,37–39]. Our data demonstrated that the interleukin and chemokines, including *IL-1β*, *IL-6* and *MCP-1*, were down-regulated in the aortas of the BAPN + low zinc group compared with the BAPN group, while the *IL-10* was on the reverse trend (Figure 5E). Furthermore, the protein levels of selected typical proinflammatory factors (IL-1β, TNF-α and IL-6) were also down-regulated with low zinc treatment (Figure 5F).

In addition, ECM enzymes can promote the degradation of ECM. According to previous studies, the expression of *MMP-2* and *MMP-9* (MMP, matrix metalloproteinase) is up-regulated in AD, and the ADAMTS degrades ECM components in the cardiovascular system [40,41]. Our results showed that the ECM enzymes, including *MMP-2*, *MMP-9* and *ADAMTS*, were down-regulated in the aortas of the BAPN + low zinc group compared with the BAPN group (Figure 5G). Taken together, these results indicated that low zinc significantly reduced transcriptional levels of representative biomarkers during the process of TAD, such as tumor necrosis factors, interleukin and chemokines, and ECM enzymes, eventually leading to alleviating the development of TAD.

In conclusion, low zinc treatment down-regulated the degree of the inflammatory response by decreasing the infiltration of macrophage, reduced the expression of cytokines and chemokines from these inflammatory cells, and inhibited the phenotype switch from contractile VSMCs to synthetic VSMCs, eventually alleviating TAD development (Figure 6).

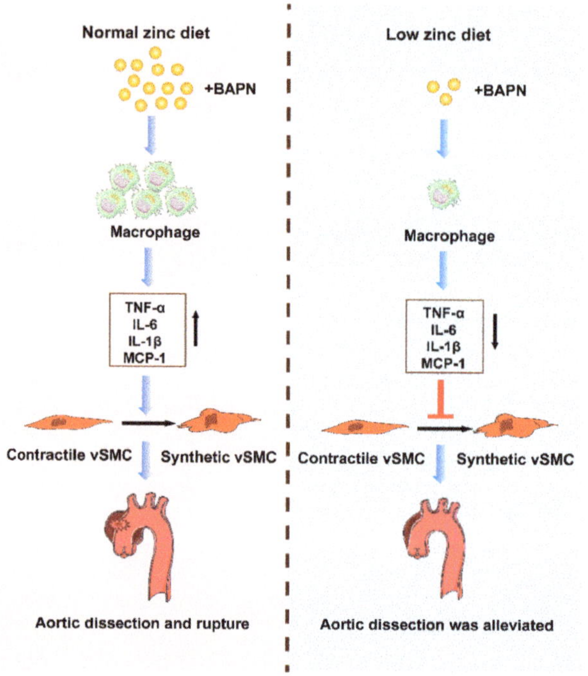

Figure 6. Schematic illustration of low zinc alleviated the progression of TAD. In BAPN-treated mice, compared with a normal zinc diet, low zinc treatment reduces the infiltration of macrophage, decreases

the expression of cytokines and chemokines, and inhibits the phenotype switch from contractile VSMCs to synthetic VSMCs, eventually alleviating TAD development. Part of the elements in this figure uses resources from Servier Medical Art under a Creative Commons Attribution license. TAD indicates thoracic aortic dissection, and BAPN indicates β-aminopropionitrile monofumarate.

4. Discussion

Our findings suggest that low zinc treatment can alleviate TAD progression, which is supported by a BAPN-induced TAD model treated with low zinc. To our knowledge, this study is the first to investigate the role of low zinc in TAD progression through nutritional intervention. The evidence, such as the survival curve, the vascular ultrasound and pathological images, and the markers of the VSMC phenotypic switch, indicates a successful construction of the TAD model. Strikingly, it was observed that low zinc significantly improved the formation and rupture of AD and reduced mortality. Further analysis reveals that low zinc down-regulates aortic inflammation by attenuating the infiltration of macrophages, suppressing the switch of VSMCs from contractile to synthetic phenotypes, and eventually inhibiting TAD development. This study not only delineates the critical role of low zinc in TAD progression but also identifies a potential nutritional intervention strategy for TAD prevention through low zinc.

Zinc is an essential trace element of the human body and plays an irreplaceable role in the physiological and biochemical processes [42]. This micronutrient has to be supplied with food on a daily basis to maintain zinc homeostasis and proper function [43]. A zinc-deficient mouse model can be established by feeding mice with a low zinc diet [44,45]. Functional studies have indicated that abnormal trace elements may be involved in the occurrence and development of aortic diseases [10,46–48]. For instance, zinc levels were dysregulated in the VSMCs of hypertensive patients [12]. The results of the meta-analysis support the conclusion of zinc reduction in aortic aneurysm patients, although this conclusion still needs to be supported by high-quality evidence [48]. In addition, this study also found that plasma zinc concentrations in patients with an aneurysm were reduced [48]. Therefore, the potential role of low zinc in TAD progression is noteworthy.

There are two main steps during the formation of AD: (1) aortic intima tear or ulceration, aortic intima rupture, and blood entering the tunica media; (2) rupture of the nourishing vessels in the aortic media, and the blood in the vessels spills into the media. After the formation of dissection, aortic inflammation triggers the dilation and subsequent rupture of the aorta [49]. The inflammatory cells infiltrate into the adventitia of the aortic wall, where they produce enzymes, cytokines and chemokines that can degrade the ECM of the aorta and directly interact with VSMCs [20,50–52]. Eventually, the inflammatory response resulted in vascular remodeling and progressive degeneration of the aortic wall, which may finally lead to AD and rupture [53]. We demonstrated that low zinc treatment dramatically decreased the infiltration of inflammatory cells, reduced the expression of inflammatory markers, and mitigated TAD progression. These results suggested low zinc prevented the development of AD by mitigating inflammatory response in the aortic wall.

VSMCs play an indispensable role in vascular homeostasis and contractility [30]. During AD progression, VSMCs convert from a contractile to a synthetic phenotype [34,54], leading to the degradation of ECM, thereby promoting SMC detachment from ECMs and accelerating SMC migration and apoptosis [30]. Here, we demonstrated that low zinc significantly reduced the expression of VSMCs synthetic markers while upregulated the expression of contractile markers, which alleviated the vascular malfunction caused by BAPN induction. Taken together, these data suggest that low zinc-reduced tissue inflammation might alleviate TAD progression partially by inhibiting the synthetic phenotype of VSMCs. However, the molecular mechanism of how low zinc inhibits the phenotypic transition of VSMCs remains unclear.

Apart from the indispensable role of VSMCs in vascular homeostasis, the ECM is critical for the maintenance of the structure and function of the arterial wall by providing elasticity and distensibility. In addition, the ECM also provides critical signals, both directly by interacting with adhesion molecules and indirectly as a reservoir for signaling factors [55]. The ECM degradation and the expression of ECM enzymes such as MMP-2, MMP-9 and ADAMTs are elevated during the development of the AD [39,40,51]. In our study, low zinc down-regulated the expression of some representative ECM enzymes (MMP-2, MMP-9 and ADAMTs) and alleviated the characteristic features of ECM degradation (less fragmentation of elastin fibers, collagen deposition and proteoglycan accumulation). In line with these studies, our results suggested that low zinc intervention inhibited the degradation of ECM in the BAPN-induced TAD model. However, it still needs more studies to explore the potential mechanism.

Although our study reveals the role of low zinc in the process of TAD through in vivo experiments, it is still unclear whether low zinc plays the same role in cell experiments in vitro. In fact, our results suggest that it is difficult to conduct in vitro experiments because the regulation of low zinc on AD is complex, involving immune cells, inflammation and related factors, and SMCs. In the body, zinc homeostasis depends on three important protein families: zinc transporters (ZnTs), zinc importers (ZiPs) and metallothionein (MT) [56]. Whether the constructed conditional zinc transporter/zinc storage protein gene knockout mice have a more positive inhibitory effect on TAD development than low zinc treatment alone needs further experimental exploration. It has been found that zinc levels are reduced in the arteries and serum/plasma of patients with AD based on available clinical data [7–10]. However, it is unclear whether the incidence of AD in zinc deficiency patients is lower than that in the general population, which warrants further investigation in the future.

Collectively, this study demonstrated the protective effects of low zinc on the development of TAD. Low zinc treatment robustly reduced the infiltration of macrophages and down-regulated aortic inflammation, thereby inhibiting the phenotype switch of VSMCs and the degradation of ECM, leading to diminished TAD progression. In conclusion, our findings suggest that low zinc may be an effective and promising strategy for the prevention and treatment of TAD.

Supplementary Materials: The following supporting information can be downloaded at: https://www.mdpi.com/article/10.3390/nu15071640/s1, Table S1: Primers for Q-PCR analysis; Table S2: Antibodies for western blot.

Author Contributions: Conceptualization, J.L., Y.L. and P.A.; investigation, J.L. and Y.L.; writing—original draft preparation, L.Z. and P.A.; writing—review and editing, J.L. and Y.L.; visualization, W.Z., Y.X. and J.Q.; supervision, J.L. and Y.L.; project administration, L.Z. and P.A.; funding acquisition, Y.L. All authors have read and agreed to the published version of the manuscript.

Funding: This work was supported by the National Natural Science Foundation of China (31970717, 82170429), the Chinese Universities Scientific Fund (2020TC015), and the Beijing Municipal Natural Science Foundation (7222111).

Institutional Review Board Statement: The animal study protocol was approved by the Committee on the Ethics of Animal Experiments of China Agricultural University (Approval Code: AW32902202-5-1; Approval Date: 23 September 2022).

Informed Consent Statement: Not applicable.

Data Availability Statement: The data presented in this study are available in the article or supplementary material.

Acknowledgments: We thank the support of the experimental platform of the Beijing Advanced Innovation Center for Food Nutrition and Human Health.

Conflicts of Interest: The authors declare no conflict of interest.

Abbreviations

TAD, thoracic aortic dissection; VSMCs, vascular smooth muscle cells; ECM, extracellular matrix; ELISA, enzyme-linked immunosorbent assay; HE, hematoxylin and eosin; EVG, Elastic-Van Gieson; Q-PCR, quantitative PCR; BAPN, β-aminopropionitrile monofumarate; Myh11, myosin heavy polypeptide 11; Acta2, actin alpha 2; Myl9, myosin light polypeptide 9; Ccn1, calponin 1; Ramp1, receptor activity modifying protein 1; Col1A1, collagen type I alpha 1; Cxcl2, C-X-C motif chemokine ligand 2; Fn1, fibronectin 1; TNF-α, tumor necrosis factor-α; IL, interleukin; MMP, matrix metalloproteinase; MCP-1, monocyte chemotactic protein-1.

References

1. Nienaber, C.A.; Clough, R.E.; Sakalihasan, N.; Suzuki, T.; Gibbs, R.; Mussa, F.; Jenkins, M.P.; Thompson, M.M.; Evangelista, A.; Yeh, J.S.; et al. Aortic dissection. *Nat. Rev. Dis. Prim.* **2016**, *2*, 16053. [CrossRef] [PubMed]
2. Hagan, P.G.; Nienaber, C.A.; Isselbacher, E.M.; Bruckman, D.; Karavite, D.J.; Russman, P.L.; Evangelista, A.; Fattori, R.; Suzuki, T.; Oh, J.K.; et al. The International Registry of Acute Aortic Dissection (IRAD): New insights into an old disease. *JAMA* **2000**, *283*, 897–903. [CrossRef]
3. Clough, R.E.; Nienaber, C.A. Management of acute aortic syndrome. *Nat. Rev. Cardiol.* **2015**, *12*, 103–114. [CrossRef] [PubMed]
4. Pilz, S.; Dobnig, H.; Winklhofer-Roob, B.M.; Renner, W.; Seelhorst, U.; Wellnitz, B.; Boehm, B.O.; März, W. Low serum zinc concentrations predict mortality in patients referred to coronary angiography. *Br. J. Nutr.* **2009**, *101*, 1534–1540. [CrossRef] [PubMed]
5. Singh, R.B.; Gupta, U.C.; Mittal, N.; Niaz, M.A.; Ghosh, S.; Rastogi, V. Epidemiologic study of trace elements and magnesium on risk of coronary artery disease in rural and urban Indian populations. *J. Am. Coll. Nutr.* **1997**, *16*, 62–67. [CrossRef]
6. Giacconi, R.; Caruso, C.; Malavolta, M.; Lio, D.; Balistreri, C.R.; Scola, L.; Candore, G.; Muti, E.; Mocchegiani, E. Pro-inflammatory genetic background and zinc status in old atherosclerotic subjects. *Ageing Res. Rev.* **2008**, *7*, 306–318. [CrossRef]
7. Socha, K.; Karwowska, A.; Kurianiuk, A.; Markiewicz-Żukowska, R.; Guzowski, A.; Gacko, M.; Hirnle, T.; Borawska, M.H. Estimation of Selected Minerals in Aortic Aneurysms-Impaired Ratio of Zinc to Lead May Predispose? *Biol. Trace Elem. Res.* **2021**, *199*, 2811–2818. [CrossRef]
8. Pincemail, J.; Defraigne, J.O.; Cheramy-Bien, J.P.; Dardenne, N.; Donneau, A.F.; Albert, A.; Labropoulos, N.; Sakalihasan, N. On the potential increase of the oxidative stress status in patients with abdominal aortic aneurysm. *Redox Rep.* **2012**, *17*, 139–144. [CrossRef]
9. Kurianiuk, A.; Socha, K.; Gacko, M.; Błachnio-Zabielska, A.; Karwowska, A. The Relationship between the Concentration of Cathepsin A, D, and E and the Concentration of Copper and Zinc, and the Size of the Aneurysmal Enlargement in the Wall of the Abdominal Aortic Aneurysm. *Ann. Vasc. Surg.* **2019**, *55*, 182–188. [CrossRef]
10. Edvinsson, M.; Ilbäck, N.G.; Frisk, P.; Thelin, S.; Nyström-Rosander, C. Trace Element Changes in Thoracic Aortic Dissection. *Biol. Trace Elem. Res.* **2016**, *169*, 159–163. [CrossRef]
11. Gać, P.; Czerwińska, K.; Macek, P.; Jaremków, A.; Mazur, G.; Pawlas, K.; Poręba, R. The importance of selenium and zinc deficiency in cardiovascular disorders. *Environ. Toxicol. Pharmacol.* **2021**, *82*, 103553. [CrossRef]
12. Zhao, L.; Oliver, E.; Maratou, K.; Atanur, S.S.; Dubois, O.D.; Cotroneo, E.; Chen, C.N.; Wang, L.; Arce, C.; Chabosseau, P.L.; et al. The zinc transporter ZIP12 regulates the pulmonary vascular response to chronic hypoxia. *Nature* **2015**, *524*, 356–360. [CrossRef]
13. Rink, L.; Haase, H. Zinc homeostasis and immunity. *Trends Immunol.* **2007**, *28*, 1–4. [CrossRef] [PubMed]
14. Murakami, M.; Hirano, T. Intracellular zinc homeostasis and zinc signaling. *Cancer Sci.* **2008**, *99*, 1515–1522. [CrossRef] [PubMed]
15. Wellinghausen, N.; Kirchner, H.; Rink, L. The immunobiology of zinc. *Immunol. Today* **1997**, *18*, 519–521. [CrossRef]
16. Ibs, K.H.; Rink, L. Zinc-altered immune function. *J. Nutr.* **2003**, *133*, 1452s–1456s. [CrossRef] [PubMed]
17. Prasad, A.S. Effects of zinc deficiency on Th1 and Th2 cytokine shifts. *J. Infect. Dis.* **2000**, *182* (Suppl. S1), S62–S68. [CrossRef]
18. Beck, F.W.; Prasad, A.S.; Kaplan, J.; Fitzgerald, J.T.; Brewer, G.J. Changes in cytokine production and T cell subpopulations in experimentally induced zinc-deficient humans. *Am. J. Physiol.* **1997**, *272*, E1002–E1007. [CrossRef]
19. Yin, Z.Q.; Han, H.; Yan, X.; Zheng, Q.J. Research Progress on the Pathogenesis of Aortic Dissection. *Curr. Probl. Cardiol.* **2022**, 101249. [CrossRef]
20. He, R.; Guo, D.C.; Estrera, A.L.; Safi, H.J.; Huynh, T.T.; Yin, Z.; Cao, S.N.; Lin, J.; Kurian, T.; Buja, L.M.; et al. Characterization of the inflammatory and apoptotic cells in the aortas of patients with ascending thoracic aortic aneurysms and dissections. *J. Thorac. Cardiovasc. Surg.* **2006**, *131*, 671–678. [CrossRef]
21. Schillinger, M.; Domanovits, H.; Bayegan, K.; Hölzenbein, T.; Grabenwöger, M.; Thoenissen, J.; Röggla, M.; Müllner, M. C-reactive protein and mortality in patients with acute aortic disease. *Intensive Care Med.* **2002**, *28*, 740–745. [CrossRef] [PubMed]
22. Kuehl, H.; Eggebrecht, H.; Boes, T.; Antoch, G.; Rosenbaum, S.; Ladd, S.; Bockisch, A.; Barkhausen, J.; Erbel, R. Detection of inflammation in patients with acute aortic syndrome: Comparison of FDG-PET/CT imaging and serological markers of inflammation. *Heart* **2008**, *94*, 1472–1477. [CrossRef] [PubMed]
23. del Porto, F.; Proietta, M.; Tritapepe, L.; Miraldi, F.; Koverech, A.; Cardelli, P.; Tabacco, F.; de Santis, V.; Vecchione, A.; Mitterhofer, A.P.; et al. Inflammation and immune response in acute aortic dissection. *Ann. Med.* **2010**, *42*, 622–629. [CrossRef] [PubMed]

24. He, R.; Guo, D.C.; Sun, W.; Papke, C.L.; Duraisamy, S.; Estrera, A.L.; Safi, H.J.; Ahn, C.; Buja, L.M.; Arnett, F.C.; et al. Characterization of the inflammatory cells in ascending thoracic aortic aneurysms in patients with Marfan syndrome, familial thoracic aortic aneurysms, and sporadic aneurysms. *J. Thorac. Cardiovasc. Surg.* **2008**, *136*, 922–929.e1. [CrossRef]
25. Schulz, E.; Gori, T.; Münzel, T. Oxidative stress and endothelial dysfunction in hypertension. *Hypertens. Res.* **2011**, *34*, 665–673. [CrossRef]
26. Pan, L.; Bai, P.; Weng, X.; Liu, J.; Chen, Y.; Chen, S.; Ma, X.; Hu, K.; Sun, A.; Ge, J. Legumain Is an Endogenous Modulator of Integrin αvβ3 Triggering Vascular Degeneration, Dissection, and Rupture. *Circulation* **2022**, *145*, 659–674. [CrossRef]
27. Yang, Y.Y.; Li, L.Y.; Jiao, X.L.; Jia, L.X.; Zhang, X.P.; Wang, Y.L.; Yang, S.; Li, J.; Du, J.; Wei, Y.X.; et al. Intermittent Hypoxia Alleviates β-Aminopropionitrile Monofumarate Induced Thoracic Aortic Dissection in C57BL/6 Mice. *Eur. J. Vasc. Endovasc. Surg.* **2020**, *59*, 1000–1010. [CrossRef]
28. Yang, H.; Yang, F.; Luo, M.; Chen, Q.; Liu, X.; Zhang, Y.; Zhu, G.; Chen, W.; Li, T.; Shu, C.; et al. Metabolomic Profile Reveals That Ceramide Metabolic Disturbance Plays an Important Role in Thoracic Aortic Dissection. *Front. Cardiovasc. Med.* **2022**, *9*, 826861. [CrossRef]
29. Sawada, H.; Beckner, Z.A.; Ito, S.; Daugherty, A.; Lu, H.S. β-Aminopropionitrile-induced aortic aneurysm and dissection in mice. *JVS Vasc. Sci.* **2022**, *3*, 64–72. [CrossRef]
30. Rombouts, K.B.; van Merrienboer, T.A.R.; Ket, J.C.F.; Bogunovic, N.; van der Velden, J.; Yeung, K.K. The role of vascular smooth muscle cells in the development of aortic aneurysms and dissections. *Eur. J. Clin. Investig.* **2022**, *52*, e13697. [CrossRef]
31. Wu, D.; Shen, Y.H.; Russell, L.; Coselli, J.S.; LeMaire, S.A. Molecular mechanisms of thoracic aortic dissection. *J. Surg. Res.* **2013**, *184*, 907–924. [CrossRef] [PubMed]
32. Wight, T.N. A role for proteoglycans in vascular disease. *Matrix Biol.* **2018**, *71–72*, 396–420. [CrossRef] [PubMed]
33. Ailawadi, G.; Moehle, C.W.; Pei, H.; Walton, S.P.; Yang, Z.; Kron, I.L.; Lau, C.L.; Owens, G.K. Smooth muscle phenotypic modulation is an early event in aortic aneurysms. *J. Thorac. Cardiovasc. Surg.* **2009**, *138*, 1392–1399. [CrossRef]
34. Frismantiene, A.; Philippova, M.; Erne, P.; Resink, T.J. Smooth muscle cell-driven vascular diseases and molecular mechanisms of VSMC plasticity. *Cell Signal.* **2018**, *52*, 48–64. [CrossRef]
35. Lacolley, P.; Regnault, V.; Nicoletti, A.; Li, Z.; Michel, J.B. The vascular smooth muscle cell in arterial pathology: A cell that can take on multiple roles. *Cardiovasc. Res.* **2012**, *95*, 194–204. [CrossRef]
36. Cai, Y.L.; Wang, Z.W. The expression and significance of IL-6, IFN-γ, SM22α, and MMP-2 in rat model of aortic dissection. *Eur. Rev. Med. Pharmacol. Sci.* **2017**, *21*, 560–568. [PubMed]
37. Zhang, L.; Liao, M.F.; Tian, L.; Zou, S.L.; Lu, Q.S.; Bao, J.M.; Pei, Y.F.; Jing, Z.P. Overexpression of interleukin-1β and interferon-γ in type I thoracic aortic dissections and ascending thoracic aortic aneurysms: Possible correlation with matrix metalloproteinase-9 expression and apoptosis of aortic media cells. *Eur. J. Cardiothorac. Surg.* **2011**, *40*, 17–22. [CrossRef] [PubMed]
38. Liu, X.; Liu, J.; Li, Y.; Zhang, H. The Correlation between the Inflammatory Effects of Activated Macrophages in Atherosclerosis and Aortic Dissection. *Ann. Vasc. Surg.* **2022**, *85*, 341–346. [CrossRef] [PubMed]
39. Adam, M.; Kooreman, N.G.; Jagger, A.; Wagenhäuser, M.U.; Mehrkens, D.; Wang, Y.; Kayama, Y.; Toyama, K.; Raaz, U.; Schellinger, I.N.; et al. Systemic Upregulation of IL-10 (Interleukin-10) Using a Nonimmunogenic Vector Reduces Growth and Rate of Dissecting Abdominal Aortic Aneurysm. *Arterioscler. Thromb. Vasc. Biol.* **2018**, *38*, 1796–1805. [CrossRef]
40. Wu, X.; Ye, J.; Cai, W.; Yang, X.; Zou, Q.; Lin, J.; Zheng, H.; Wang, C.; Chen, L.; Li, Y. LDHA mediated degradation of extracellular matrix is a potential target for the treatment of aortic dissection. *Pharmacol. Res.* **2022**, *176*, 106051. [CrossRef]
41. Worley, J.R.; Baugh, M.D.; Hughes, D.A.; Edwards, D.R.; Hogan, A.; Sampson, M.J.; Gavrilovic, J. Metalloproteinase expression in PMA-stimulated THP-1 cells. Effects of peroxisome proliferator-activated receptor-gamma (PPAR gamma) agonists and 9-cis-retinoic acid. *J. Biol. Chem.* **2003**, *278*, 51340–51346. [CrossRef] [PubMed]
42. Taheri, S.; Asadi, S.; Nilashi, M.; Ali Abumalloh, R.; Ghabban, N.M.A.; Mohd Yusuf, S.Y.; Supriyanto, E.; Samad, S. A literature review on beneficial role of vitamins and trace elements: Evidence from published clinical studies. *J. Trace Elem. Med. Biol.* **2021**, *67*, 126789. [CrossRef] [PubMed]
43. Krebs, N.F. Overview of zinc absorption and excretion in the human gastrointestinal tract. *J. Nutr.* **2000**, *130*, 1374s–1377s. [CrossRef] [PubMed]
44. Ayton, S.; Lei, P.; Appukuttan, A.T.; Renoir, T.; Foliaki, S.; Chen, F.; Adlard, P.A.; Hannan, A.J.; Bush, A.I. Brain Zinc Deficiency Exacerbates Cognitive Decline in the R6/1 Model of Huntington's Disease. *Neurotherapeutics* **2020**, *17*, 243–251. [CrossRef]
45. Knoell, D.L.; Julian, M.W.; Bao, S.; Besecker, B.; Macre, J.E.; Leikauf, G.D.; DiSilvestro, R.A.; Crouser, E.D. Zinc deficiency increases organ damage and mortality in a murine model of polymicrobial sepsis. *Crit. Care Med.* **2009**, *37*, 1380–1388. [CrossRef]
46. Li, B.; Wang, Z.; Hong, J.; Che, Y.; Chen, R.; Hu, Z.; Hu, X.; Wu, Q.; Hu, J.; Zhang, M. Iron deficiency promotes aortic medial degeneration via destructing cytoskeleton of vascular smooth muscle cells. *Clin. Transl. Med.* **2021**, *11*, e276. [CrossRef]
47. Socha, K.; Borawska, M.H.; Gacko, M.; Guzowski, A. Diet and the content of selenium and lead in patients with abdominal aortic aneurysm. *Vasa* **2011**, *40*, 381–389. [CrossRef]
48. Talebi, S.; Ghaedi, E.; Sadeghi, E.; Mohammadi, H.; Hadi, A.; Clark, C.C.T.; Askari, G. Trace Element Status and Hypothyroidism: A Systematic Review and Meta-analysis. *Biol. Trace Elem. Res.* **2020**, *197*, 1–14. [CrossRef]

49. Erbel, R.; Aboyans, V.; Boileau, C.; Bossone, E.; Bartolomeo, R.D.; Eggebrecht, H.; Evangelista, A.; Falk, V.; Frank, H.; Gaemperli, O.; et al. 2014 ESC Guidelines on the diagnosis and treatment of aortic diseases: Document covering acute and chronic aortic diseases of the thoracic and abdominal aorta of the adult. The Task Force for the Diagnosis and Treatment of Aortic Diseases of the European Society of Cardiology (ESC). *Eur. Heart J.* **2014**, *35*, 2873–2926. [CrossRef]
50. Schachner, T.; Golderer, G.; Sarg, B.; Lindner, H.H.; Bonaros, N.; Mikuz, G.; Laufer, G.; Werner, E.R. The amounts of alpha 1 antitrypsin protein are reduced in the vascular wall of the acutely dissected human ascending aorta. *Eur. J. Cardiothorac. Surg.* **2010**, *37*, 684–690. [CrossRef]
51. Allaire, E.; Schneider, F.; Saucy, F.; Dai, J.; Cochennec, F.; Michineau, S.; Zidi, M.; Becquemin, J.P.; Kirsch, M.; Gervais, M. New insight in aetiopathogenesis of aortic diseases. *Eur. J. Vasc. Endovasc. Surg.* **2009**, *37*, 531–537. [CrossRef] [PubMed]
52. Wang, X.L.; Liu, O.; Qin, Y.W.; Zhang, H.J.; Lv, Y. Association of the polymorphisms of MMP-9 and TIMP-3 genes with thoracic aortic dissection in Chinese Han population. *Acta Pharmacol. Sin.* **2014**, *35*, 351–355. [CrossRef] [PubMed]
53. Wortmann, M.; Peters, A.S.; Erhart, P.; Körfer, D.; Böckler, D.; Dihlmann, S. Inflammasomes in the Pathophysiology of Aortic Disease. *Cells* **2021**, *10*, 2433. [CrossRef] [PubMed]
54. Li, G.; Wang, M.; Caulk, A.W.; Cilfone, N.A.; Gujja, S.; Qin, L.; Chen, P.Y.; Chen, Z.; Yousef, S.; Jiao, Y.; et al. Chronic mTOR activation induces a degradative smooth muscle cell phenotype. *J. Clin. Investig.* **2020**, *130*, 1233–1251. [CrossRef]
55. Bax, M.; Romanov, V.; Junday, K.; Giannoulatou, E.; Martinac, B.; Kovacic, J.C.; Liu, R.; Iismaa, S.E.; Graham, R.M. Arterial dissections: Common features and new perspectives. *Front. Cardiovasc. Med.* **2022**, *9*, 1055862. [CrossRef]
56. Zhao, T.; Huang, Q.; Su, Y.; Sun, W.; Huang, Q.; Wei, W. Zinc and its regulators in pancreas. *Inflammopharmacology* **2019**, *27*, 453–464. [CrossRef]

nutrients

MDPI

Article

Positive Association of Serum Vitamin B6 Levels with Intrapulmonary Lymph Node and/or Localized Pleural Metastases in Non-Small Cell Lung Cancer: A Retrospective Study

Lu Liu [1,†], Hang Yu [2,†], Jingmin Bai [3,†], Qing Xu [1], Yong Zhang [1], Xinsheng Zhang [1], Zhimeng Yu [1] and Yinghua Liu [1,4,*]

1 Department of Nutrition, The First Medical Center of Chinese PLA General Hospital, Beijing 100853, China; deer_3016@163.com (L.L.); aqing_930@163.com (Q.X.); zhangyong301@126.com (Y.Z.); zhangxinsheng198431@126.com (X.Z.); yzm18701180993@163.com (Z.Y.)

2 Department of Respiratory and Critical Medicine, Medical School of Chinese People's Liberation Army, Beijing 100853, China; yuhang_301@126.com

3 Department of Radiotherapy, The First Medical Center of Chinese PLA General Hospital, Beijing 100853, China; dr_bai@foxmail.com

4 National Clinical Research Center for Geriatric Diseases, Chinese PLA General Hospital, Beijing 100853, China

* Correspondence: liuyinghua77@163.com; Tel.: +86-010-66937785

† These authors contributed equally to this work.

Abstract: The relationship between vitamin B levels and the development and progression of lung cancer remains inconclusive. We aimed to investigate the relationship between B vitamins and intrapulmonary lymph nodes as well as localized pleural metastases in patients with non-small cell lung cancer (NSCLC). This was a retrospective study including patients who underwent lung surgery for suspected NSCLC at our institution from January 2016 to December 2018. Logistic regression models were used to evaluate the associations between serum B vitamin levels and intrapulmonary lymph node and/or localized pleural metastases. Stratified analysis was performed according to different clinical characteristics and tumor types. A total of 1498 patients were included in the analyses. Serum vitamin B_6 levels showed a positive association with intrapulmonary metastasis in a multivariate logistic regression (odds ratio (OR) of 1.016, 95% confidence interval (CI) of 1.002–1.031, $p = 0.021$). After multivariable adjustment, we found a high risk of intrapulmonary metastasis in patients with high serum vitamin B_6 levels (fourth quartile (Q4) vs. Q1, OR of 1.676, 95%CI of 1.092 to 2.574, $p = 0.018$, p for trend of 0.030). Stratified analyses showed that the positive association between serum vitamin B_6 and lymph node metastasis appeared to be stronger in females, current smokers, current drinkers, and those with a family history of cancer, squamous cell carcinoma, a tumor of 1–3 cm in diameter, or a solitary tumor. Even though serum vitamin B_6 levels were associated with preoperative NSCLC upstaging, B_6 did not qualify as a useful biomarker due to weak association and wide confidence intervals. Thus, it would be appropriate to prospectively investigate the relationship between serum vitamin B_6 levels and lung cancer further.

Keywords: vitamin B_6; non-small cell lung cancer (NSCLC); TNM stage; lymph node metastasis; localized pleural metastasis

1. Introduction

Lung cancer is one of the most prevalent malignancies and remains the leading cause of cancer death worldwide [1]. Non-small cell lung cancer (NSCLC) accounts for approximately 85% of lung cancers and represents a significant economic and social burden [2,3]. Tumor–nodes–metastasis (TNM) staging is commonly used to clarify the staging of NSCLC and plays an important role in the treatment and prognosis [4]. However, it is difficult to accurately assess tumor staging preoperatively, as the results are mainly obtained by computed tomography, positron emission tomography, and local biopsy, and they are often incomplete and differ from the final pathological results [4–6]. This is mainly due to the challenge of carrying out a comprehensive and accurate preoperative assessment of lymph nodes and localized pleural metastases [7–11].

The B vitamins (including vitamin B_1, B_2, B_6, B_9, and B_{12}) play important roles as co-factors in various biological processes, such as tissue metabolism, cellular stress responses, signal transduction pathways, and gene expression regulation [12–14]. The relationship between B vitamin levels and the development and progression of lung cancer has been a popular topic, but the results remain inconclusive [15–22]. B vitamins were reported as tumor promoters [15,23–26], tumor suppressors [19], or being unrelated to carcinogenesis [27,28] in various studies. Meanwhile, there have been few reports on the association of B vitamins with different stages of lung cancer. The present study aimed to investigate the association between B vitamins and intrapulmonary lymph nodes as well as localized pleural metastases in NSCLC patients, and to clarify the association in different populations by stratified analysis.

2. Materials and Methods

2.1. Study Population

This retrospective study was approved by the Ethics Committee of Chinese PLA General Hospital (No. S2022-615-01) and was conducted in accordance with the Declaration of Helsinki (as revised in 2013). The study was registered in the Chinese Clinical Trial Registry (chictr.org.cn, ChiCTR2300069309). Informed consent was waived for this retrospective analysis. From January 2016 to December 2018, patients who underwent lung surgery in our hospital for suspected NSCLC were screened for inclusion. The inclusion criteria were as follows: (1) age $\geq$ eighteen years old; (2) preoperatively evaluated for the absence of distant metastasis; (3) lung nodule(s) or mass(es) treated by surgical resection for suspected NSCLC; (4) no chemotherapy, radiotherapy, targeted drug therapy, or immunotherapy prior to surgery; (5) received serum B vitamin testing (fasting for more than eight hours) within three days before surgery; (6) the diets of patients were arranged by the Nutrition Department, and the daily vitamin B_6 intake was about 2 mg, which met the Chinese Daily Reference Intake (DRI) recommendations and ensured the uniformity of dietary intake; and (7) no nutritional support therapy or additional nutritional supplements in the past year. The exclusion criteria included: (1) nutritional status score ≥ 1 or total score ≥ 3 in the Nutrition Risk Screening 2002; (2) comorbidities such as uncontrolled diabetes, autoimmune disease, extrapulmonary malignancy, or severe renal or hepatic insufficiency; (3) pregnant female patients during; (4) taking antiepileptics, non-steroidal anti-inflammatory drugs, or oral contraceptives within six months; and/or (5) meeting conditions that the investigator believed may influence vitamin B metabolism. In total, 1498 patients were enrolled in this study.

2.2. Data Collection

Clinical data were collected using the medical record system of our institute, and included age, sex, body mass index (BMI), family history of cancer, marital status, smoking history, alcohol consumption, the season of blood sampling for vitamin testing, educational level, surgical records, pathological findings including diameter and number of tumor(s), lung computed tomography report for the density of tumor(s), and serum levels of vitamins B_1, B_2, B_6, B_9, and B_{12}.

2.3. Serum Vitamin Level Testing

We used a vitamin analyzer approved by the Chinese National Medical Products Administration (LK3000V, Tianjin Lanbiao Electronic Technology Development Co., Ltd., Tianjin, China) to detect the serum content of vitamin B_1, vitamin B_2, vitamin B_6, vitamin B_9, and vitamin B_{12} in the form of thionine, riboflavin, pyridoxal $5'$ phosphate (PLP),

L-5,6,7,8-tetrahydrofolic acid, and cobalamin, respectively. The analyzer enabled the use of an electrochemiluminescence method to deposit the measured substance on the sensor surface; then, the reverse voltage was applied to dissolve the substance accumulated on the sensor and the content was analyzed based on the polarization curve of the dissolution process. The normal thresholds were as follows: vitamin B_1, 50–150 nmol/L, vitamin B_2, 4.26–18.42 mg/L; vitamin B_6, 14.6–72.9 nmol/L; vitamin B_9, 6.8–36.3 nmol/L; and vitamin B_{12}, 200–900 pg/mL.

2.4. *Intrapulmonary Metastasis Status Classification*

We evaluated intrapulmonary lymph nodes and pleural metastases using surgical records and pathology reports. The location and number of metastases were recorded. All the metastatic findings were pathologically confirmed according to the World Health Organization Classification of Thoracic Tumors 2021 [29] and the 8th edition of the Pathological Tumor–Node–Metastasis (pTNM) Staging from the Union for International Cancer Control [4]. Patients were then divided into two groups based on the presence or absence of intrapulmonary metastases.

2.5. *Covariates*

Based on previous experience and studies [18,23,27,30], clinical characteristics were evaluated as potential confounders of the association between serum vitamin levels and intrapulmonary metastasis status, including age, sex, BMI, family history of cancer, smoking history, alcohol consumption, the season of blood collection for vitamin testing, educational level, and tumor type (pathology, diameter, number, and density).

2.6. *Statistical Analyses*

Continuous variables are presented as mean ± standard deviation (normal distribution) or median [interquartile range] (non-normal distribution). Categorical variables are presented as numbers and percentages. Quantitative variables were compared between groups using Student's *t*-test, analysis of variance, or non-parametric tests, while comparisons of categorical variables between groups were made using chi-squared tests.

Univariate and multivariate logistic regression analyses were used to evaluate the associations between serum vitamin levels and the presence of lung cancer or intrapulmonary metastases. Patients were then divided into four groups by quartiles of the serum vitamins selected by multivariate logistic regression analysis. A stratified analysis was used to examine the vitamin–metastasis association for different levels of factors including: age (<40, 40–60, or >60 years), sex, BMI (<18.5, 18.5–24, or >24 kg/m^2), family history of tumors (yes or no), smoking history (never a smoker, ex-smoker, or current smoker), alcohol consumption (yes or no), and the pathology (adenocarcinoma or squamous cell carcinoma), diameter (<1, 1–3, or >3 cm), number (solitary or multiple), and density (solid or subsolid) of the tumor(s). Estimated effects were reported as odds ratios (OR) and 95% confidence intervals (95% CI). The last three quartiles of serum vitamins were each compared to the first quartile with the lowest concentration. Tests for linear trends across serum vitamin quartiles were performed by assigning medians to each quartile and calculating coefficients for the quartile variables. *p*-values for interactions were also assessed by likelihood ratio tests comparing regression models with and without the cross-product terms for each assessed factor and serum vitamin levels (quartiles).

All analyses were performed in R software (version 4.2.2, The Free Software Foundation, Boston, MA, USA) and IBM SPSS Statistics for Windows, version 26.0 (IBM Corp., Armonk, NY, USA). A two-sided p-value < 0.05 was considered statistically significant for all tests.

3. Results

3.1. Participant Characteristics

A total of 1498 patients with suspected NSCLC who underwent lung surgery were enrolled, of whom 1283 patients had postoperative pathologically confirmed NSCLC and 215 patients had benign pulmonary nodules (Table 1). Compared to patients with benign nodules, NSCLC patients were older (59 years, $p < 0.001$), had more male patients (49.6%, $p = 0.001$), larger nodule diameters ($p = 0.018$), more subsolid nodules (47.4%, $p < 0.001$), and higher vitamin B_6 levels (35.6 nmol/L vs. 32.4 nmol/L, $p = 0.023$).

Table 1. Basic characteristics of all patients enrolled in this study.

Characteristics	All Patients (n = 1498)	Patients with Non-Small Cell Lung Cancer (n = 1283)	Patients with Benign Lung Nodule (n = 215)	p-Value
Age (year), median [IQR]	58 [53, 64]	59 [51, 65]	52 [48, 55]	<0.001 †
Sex				
Male, N (%)	717 (47.9)	636 (49.6)	81 (37.7)	0.001 ‡
Female, N (%)	781 (52.1)	647 (50.4)	134 (62.3)	
BMI (kg/m^2), median [IQR]	24.4 [22.3, 26.8]	24.4 [22.5, 26.6]	24.9 [22.7, 27.3]	0.323 †
Family history of cancer				
No, N (%)	1188 (79.3)	1018 (79.3)	170 (79.1)	0.926 ‡
Yes, N (%)	310 (20.7)	265 (20.7)	45 (20.9)	
Marital status				
Married, N (%)	1466 (97.9)	1256 (97.9)	210 (97.7)	0.514 ‡
Never married, N (%)	8 (0.5)	6 (0.5)	2 (0.9)	
Divorced or widowed, N (%)	24 (1.6)	21 (1.6)	3 (1.4)	
Smoking history				
Never a smoker, N (%)	937 (62.6)	807 (62.9)	130 (60.5)	0.308 ‡
Ex-smoker, N (%)	207 (13.8)	182 (14.2)	25 (11.6)	
Current smoker, N (%)	354 (23.6)	294 (22.9)	60 (27.9)	
Alcohol consumption				
No, N (%)	1042 (69.6)	904 (70.5)	138 (64.2)	0.064 ‡
Yes, N (%)	456 (30.4)	379 (29.5)	77 (35.8)	
Season of blood sampling for vitamin testing				
June–September, N (%)	616 (41.1)	529 (41.2)	87 (40.5)	0.833 ‡
Other, N (%)	882 (58.9)	754 (58.8)	128 (59.5)	
Educational level				
No greater than elementary school, N (%)	203 (13.5)	179 (14.0)	24 (11.2)	0.985 ‡
High school graduation, N (%)	693 (46.3)	585 (45.6)	108 (50.2)	
University or postgraduate graduation, N (%)	602 (40.2)	519 (40.5)	83 (38.6)	
Diameter of tumor (cm), median [IQR]	1.5 [1.0, 2.4]	1.6 [1.0, 2.5]	1.5 [0.9, 2.4]	0.018 †
Number of tumor(s)				
Solitary, N (%)	1405 (93.8)	1197 (93.3)	208 (96.7)	0.053 ‡
Multiple, N (%)	93 (6.2)	86 (6.7)	7 (3.3)	
Density of tumor				
Solid, N (%)	854 (57.0)	675 (52.6)	179 (83.3)	<0.001 ‡
Subsolid, N (%)	644 (43.0)	608 (47.4)	3 6(16.7)	
Serum vitamin levels				
Vitamin B_1, nmol/L	88.3 [75.2, 108.2]	88.3 [77.9, 104.1]	88.8 [73.5, 108.6]	0.685 †
Vitamin B_2, mg/L	4.5 [4.0, 5.1]	4.5 [4.1, 5.1]	4.6 [4.1, 5.3]	0.538 †
Vitamin B_6, nmol/L	35.1 [29.3, 39.8]	35.6 [30.2, 40.4]	32.4 [25.8, 38.5]	0.023 †
Vitamin B_9, nmol/L	20.4 [16.6, 24.5]	20.4 [17.4, 24.0]	20.8 [17.5, 24.2]	0.643 †
Vitamin B_{12}, pg/mL	432.4 [348.2, 519.5]	434.8 [360.4, 529.3]	423.7 [326.6, 537.2]	0.688 †

IQR, interquartile range; BMI, body mass index. † p-value based on non-parametric test (continuous variable). ‡ p-value based on chi-squared test (categorical variable).

In 1283 NSCLC patients, 276 patients had intrapulmonary metastases, including 223 (80.8%) patients with lymph node metastases (metastatic group) and 53 (19.2%) patients with localized pleural metastases (non-metastatic group) (Table 2). Age, BMI, marital status, and the season of blood sampling were similar in both groups. Compared to the non-metastatic group, the metastatic group had more female patients (62.3%, $p < 0.001$), more patients with no family history of cancer (83.7%, $p = 0.044$), more current smokers (32.6%, $p < 0.001$) and current drinkers (35.5%, $p = 0.014$), more squamous cell carcinoma (21.0%, $p < 0.001$), a larger tumor size (2.5 [1.8, 3.5] cm vs. 1.5 [1.0, 2.2] cm, $p < 0.001$), more multiple tumors (19.9%, $p < 0.001$), and more solid tumors (79.3%, $p < 0.001$). For serum vitamins, the metastatic group had a higher vitamin B_6 level (36.7 nmol/L vs. 35.1 nmol/L, $p = 0.037$) and a lower vitamin B_{12} level ($p = 0.039$) than the non-metastatic group. There were no significant differences in the serum vitamin B_1, B_2, and B_9 levels between the two groups (Table 2).

Table 2. Basic characteristics of NSCLC patients in this study.

Characteristics	Total (n = 1283)	Patients with Intrapulmonary Metastases (n = 276)	Patients without Intrapulmonary Metastases (n = 1007)	*p*-Value
Age (year), median [IQR]	59 [51, 65]	59 [52, 65]	59 [51, 65]	0.800 †
Sex				
Male, N (%)	636 (49.6)	104 (37.7)	532 (52.8)	<0.001 ‡
Female, N (%)	647 (50.4)	172 (62.3)	475 (47.2)	
BMI (kg/m^2), median [IQR]	24.4 [22.5, 26.6]	24.4 [22.1, 26.9]	24.4 [22.5, 26.5]	0.909 †
Family history of cancer				
No, N (%)	1018 (79.3)	231 (83.7)	787 (78.2)	0.044 ‡
Yes, N (%)	265 (20.7)	45 (16.3)	220 (21.8)	
Marital status				
Married, N (%)	1256 (97.9)	270 (97.8)	985 (97.9)	0.919 ‡
Never married, N (%)	6 (0.5)	1 (0.4)	5 (0.5)	
Divorced or widowed, N (%)	21 (1.6)	5 (1.8)	16 (1.6)	
Smoking history				
Never a smoker, N (%)	807 (62.9)	134 (48.6)	673 (66.8)	<0.001 ‡
Ex-smoker, N (%)	182 (14.2)	52 (18.8)	130 (12.9)	
Current smoker, N (%)	294 (22.9)	90 (32.6)	204 (20.3)	
Alcohol consumption				
No, N (%)	904 (70.5)	178 (64.5)	726 (72.1)	0.014 ‡
Yes, N (%)	379 (29.5)	98 (35.5)	281 (27.9)	
Season of blood sampling for vitamin testing				
June–September, N (%)	529 (41.2)	126 (45.7)	403 (40.0)	0.092 ‡
Other, N (%)	754 (58.8)	150 (54.3)	604 (60.0)	
Educational level				
No greater than elementary school, N (%)	179 (14.0)	42 (15.2)	137 (13.6)	0.007 ‡
High school graduation, N (%)	585 (45.6)	145 (52.5)	440 (43.7)	
University or postgraduate graduation, N (%)	519 (40.5)	89 (32.2)	430 (42.7)	
Pathology of tumor				
Adenocarcinoma, N (%)	1125 (87.7)	218 (79.0)	907 (90.1)	<0.001 ‡
Squamous cell carcinoma, N (%)	158 (12.3)	58 (21.0)	100 (9.9)	
Intrapulmonary metastasis				
Lymph node, N (%)	223 (17.5)	223 (80.8)		NA §
Localized pleura, N (%)	53 (4.1)	53 (19.2)		
None, N (%)	1007 (78.4)		1007 (100)	
Diameter of tumor (cm), median [IQR]	1.6 [1.0, 2.5]	2.5 [1.8, 3.5]	1.5 [1.0, 2.2]	<0.001 †
Number of tumor(s)				
Solitary, N (%)	1197 (93.3)	221 (80.1)	976 (96.9)	<0.001 ‡
Multiple, N (%)	86 (6.7)	55 (19.9)	31 (3.1)	

Table 2. *Cont.*

Characteristics	Total (n = 1283)	Patients with Intrapulmonary Metastases (n = 276)	Patients without Intrapulmonary Metastases (n = 1007)	*p*-Value
Density of tumor				
Solid, N (%)	675 (52.6)	219 (79.3)	456 (45.3)	<0.001 ‡
Subsolid, N (%)	608 (47.4)	57 (20.7)	551 (54.7)	
Serum vitamin levels				
Vitamin B_1, nmol/L	88.3 [77.9, 104.1]	89.3 [77.7, 108.6]	88.1 [78.0, 102.7]	0.237 †
Vitamin B_2, mg/L	4.5 [4.1, 5.1]	4.6 [4.2, 5.2]	4.5 [4.1, 5.1]	0.162 †
Vitamin B_6, nmol/L	35.6 [30.2, 40.4]	36.7 [30.5, 42.0]	35.1 [30.2, 40.2]	0.037 †
Vitamin B_9, nmol/L	20.4 [17.4, 24.0]	20.2 [17.1, 24.5]	20.5 [17.5, 23.9]	0.929 †
Vitamin B_{12}, pg/mL	434.8 [360.4, 529.3]	418.2 [340.6, 532.3]	437.8 [365.7, 527.4]	0.039 †

IQR, interquartile range; BMI, body mass index. † *p*-value based on non-parametric test (continuous variable). ‡ *p*-value based on chi-squared test (categorical variable). § used for grouping, not for comparison between groups.

3.2. Association of Serum B Vitamin Levels with Presence of Lung Cancer

None of the serum B vitamins showed a significant association with the presence of lung cancer in the univariate logistic regression (Table 3). In multivariate analysis, age and a subsolid tumor were positively associated with the presence of lung cancer.

Table 3. Association between clinical characteristics and presence of lung cancer in all patients.

Characteristics	Univariate Analysis		Multivariate Analysis	
	OR (95% CI)	*p*-Value	OR (95% CI)	*p*-Value
Age, year (continuous)	1.060 (1.044, 1.076)	<0.001	1.073 (1.056, 1.090)	<0.001
Female (vs. male)	0.615 (0.457, 0.827)	0.001		
BMI, kg/m^2 (continuous)	0.976 (0.931, 1.023)	0.305		
Family history of cancer (vs. none)	0.983 (0.689, 1.403)	0.926		
Married (vs. other)	1.419 (0.499, 4.041)	0.512		
Current smoker (vs. never a smoker and ex-smoker)	0.903 (0.764, 1.068)	0.232		
Current drinker (vs. not)	0.751 (0.555, 1.018)	0.065		
Blood sampling in Jun–Sep (vs. other)	0.969 (0.722, 1.300)	0.833		
High educational level (vs. low)	0.980 (0.793, 1.211)	0.852		
Diameter of tumor, cm (continuous)	1.086 (0.973, 1.212)	0.143		
Multiple tumors (vs. solitary tumor)	2.135 (0.974, 4.677)	0.058		
Subsolid tumor (vs. solid tumor)	4.479 (3.080, 6.513)	<0.001	5.690 (3.850, 8.408)	<0.001
Serum vitamin levels				
Vitamin B_1 (continuous)	0.999 (0.992, 1.005)	0.728		
Vitamin B_2 (continuous)	0.985 (0.911, 1.065)	0.711		
Vitamin B_6 (continuous)	1.009 (0.944, 1.024)	0.251		
Vitamin B_9 (continuous)	0.995 (0.968, 1.023)	0.731		
Vitamin B_{12} (continuous)	1.000 (0.999, 1.001)	0.759		

OR, odds ratio; 95% CI, 95% confidence interval; BMI: body mass index.

3.3. Association of Serum B Vitamin Levels with Intrapulmonary Metastases

Among the serum B vitamins, only vitamin B_6 levels showed a positive association with intrapulmonary metastases in a multivariate logistic regression (OR: 1.016; 95%CI: 1.002–1.031) (Table 4). Other significantly associated factors included: female gender, the diameter and number of the tumors as risk factors, and the density of the tumor as a protective factor. Meanwhile, there were no significant differences in the demographic, clinical, or tumor characteristics of patients in different quartiles for serum vitamin B_6, except for those with different smoking histories ($p < 0.032$) (Table 5).

Table 4. Association between clinical characteristics and presence of intrapulmonary metastases in NSCLC patients.

Characteristics	Univariate Analysis		Multivariate Analysis	
	OR (95% CI)	*p*-Value	OR (95% CI)	*p*-Value
Age, year (continuous)	1.003 (0.989, 1.017)	0.703		
Female (vs. male)	1.852 (1.410, 2.434)	<0.001	1.439 (1.039, 1.993)	0.028
BMI, kg/m^2 (continuous)	1.006 (0.963, 1.051)	0.786		
Family history of cancer (vs. none)	0.697 (0.490, 0.991)	0.045		
Married (vs. other)	1.181 (0.481, 2.903)	0.716		
Current smoker (vs. never a smoker and ex-smoker)	1.511 (1.298, 1.759)	<0.001		
Current drinker (vs. not)	1.422 (1.073, 1.887)	0.014		
Blood sampling in Jun–Sep (vs. other)	0.794 (0.607, 1.039)	0.093		
High educational level (vs. low)	0.778 (0.643, 0.942)	0.010		
Squamous cell carcinoma (vs. adenocarcinoma)	2.413 (1.691, 3.444)	<0.001		
Diameter of tumor, cm (continuous)	1.686 (1.530, 1.859)	<0.001	1.495 (1.337, 1.672)	<0.001
Multiple tumors (vs. solitary tumor)	7.835 (4.928, 12.459)	<0.001	26.004 (14.517, 46.580)	<0.001
Subsolid tumor (vs. solid tumor)	0.215 (0.157, 0.296)	<0.001	0.220 (0.142, 0.342)	<0.001
Serum vitamin levels				
Vitamin B_1 (continuous)	1.004 (0.999, 1.010)	0.134		
Vitamin B_2 (continuous)	1.013 (0.943, 1.088)	0.725		
Vitamin B_6 (continuous)	1.016 (1.004, 1.028)	0.010	1.016 (1.002, 1.031)	0.021
Vitamin B_9 (continuous)	1.004 (0.979, 1.030)	0.729		
Vitamin B_{12} (continuous)	0.999 (0.998, 1.000)	0.074		

OR, odds ratio; 95% CI, 95% confidence interval; BMI: body mass index.

Table 5. Characteristics of NSCLC patients by quartile of serum vitamin B_6 in this study.

Characteristics	Serum Vitamin B_6 Quartile				*p*-Value
	Q1 (n = 322)	Q2 (n = 320)	Q3 (n = 321)	Q4 (n = 320)	
Age (year), median [IQR]	59 [51, 64]	59 [51, 66]	58 [50, 64]	59 [53, 66]	0.369 †
Sex					
Male, N (%)	162 (50.3)	165 (51.6)	158 (49.2)	151 (47.2)	0.724 ‡
Female, N (%)	160 (49.7)	155 (48.4)	163 (50.8)	169 (52.8)	
BMI (kg/m^2), median [IQR]	24.5 [22.2, 26.5]	24.5 [22.6, 26.6]	24.3 [22.7, 26.5]	24.3 [22.3, 26.6]	0.835 †
Family history of cancer					
No, N (%)	245 (76.1)	254 (79.4)	257 (80.1)	262 (81.9)	0.329 ‡
Yes, N (%)	77 (23.9)	66 (20.6)	64 (19.9)	58 (18.1)	
Smoking history					
Never a smoker, N (%)	198 (61.5)	207 (64.7)	209 (65.1)	193 (60.3)	0.032 ‡
Ex-smoker, N (%)	47 (14.6)	39 (12.2)	33 (10.3)	63 (19.7)	
Current smoker, N (%)	77 (23.9)	74 (23.1)	79 (24.6)	64 (20.0)	
Alcohol consumption					
No, N (%)	228 (70.8)	222 (69.4)	242 (75.4)	212 (66.3)	0.083 ‡
Yes, N (%)	94 (29.2)	98 (30.6)	79 (24.6)	108 (33.8)	
Pathology of tumor					
Adenocarcinoma, N (%)	282 (87.6)	282 (88.1)	285 (88.8)	276 (86.3)	0.794 ‡
Squamous cell carcinoma, N (%)	40 (12.4)	38 (11.9)	36 (11.2)	44 (13.8)	
Diameter of tumor (cm), median [IQR]	1.6 [1.0, 2.5]	1.5 [1.0, 2.5]	1.5 [1.0, 2.5]	1.8 [1.0, 2.7]	0.277 †
Number of tumor(s)					
Solitary, N (%)	297 (92.2)	305 (95.3)	304 (94.7)	291 (90.9)	0.089 ‡
Multiple, N (%)	25 (7.8)	15 (4.7)	17 (5.3)	29 (9.1)	
Density of the tumor					
Solid, N (%)	176 (54.7)	166 (51.9)	166 (51.7)	167 (52.2)	0.864 ‡
Subsolid, N (%)	146 (45.3)	154 (48.1)	155 (48.3)	153 (47.8)	

IQR, interquartile range; BMI, body mass index; Q, quartile of vitamin B_6. † *p*-value based on non-parametric test (continuous variable). ‡ *p*-value based on chi-squared test (categorical variable).

After multivariable adjustment, the highest quartile (Q4) of serum vitamin B_6 was significantly associated with a 67.6% higher risk of metastasis compared with those in the lowest quartile (Q1) (OR = 1.676, 95% CI = 1.092–2.574, p = 0.018), with a p for trend of 0.030 (Table 6). We also evaluated the effect modification of the association between serum vitamin B_6 and metastases by age, sex, BMI, family history of cancer, smoking history, alcohol consumption, and the pathology, diameter, number, and density of the tumor(s) (Table 6). The risk association appeared stronger for women (Q4 vs. Q1: OR of 1.968, 95% CI of 1.144 to 3.386, p = 0.014, p for trend = 0.014). Patients with a family history of cancer also appeared to have experienced a stronger association between vitamin B_6 and metastasis (Q4 vs. Q1: OR of 5.337, 95% CI of 1.492 to 19.093, p = 0.010, p for trend = 0.010). The association between serum vitamin B_6 and intrapulmonary metastasis also appeared to be stronger for current smokers, current drinkers, and patients with squamous cell carcinoma, a tumor of 1–3 cm in diameter, or a solitary tumor (Table 6). Meanwhile, age, sex, smoking history, alcohol consumption, and tumor type (pathology, diameter, number, and density) showed significant interactions with vitamin B_6.

Table 6. Multivariable-adjusted odds ratios and 95% confidence intervals of intrapulmonary metastases by quartile of serum vitamin B_6, stratified by age, sex, BMI, family history of cancer, smoking history, alcohol consumption, tumor pathology and characteristics in NSCLC patients in this study *.

Stratified Characteristics			Vit B_6 (μmol/L) (in Quartiles)				*p* for Trend ‡	*p* for Interaction §
			Q1 (n = 322)	Q2 (n = 320)	Q3 (n = 321)	Q4 (n = 320)		
All patients	(n = 1283)	OR	1.0 (Ref)	1.208 (0.775, 1.885)	1.123 (0.717, 1.759)	1.676 (1.092, 2.574)	0.030	
		p-value †		0.404	0.612	0.018		
Age, y	<40 (n = 43)	OR	1.0 (Ref)	NA ¶	NA ¶	NA ¶	NA ¶	0.032
		p-value †						
	40 to 60 (n = 693)	OR	1.0 (Ref)	1.432 (0.769, 2.669)	1.130 (0.593, 2.152)	1.803 (0.978, 3.325)	0.112	
		p-value †		0.258	0.711	0.059		
	>60 (n = 547)	OR	1.0 (Ref)	1.172 (0.602, 2.283)	1.084 (0.549, 2.137)	1.738 (0.914, 3.305)	0.119	
		p-value †		0.640	0.817	0.092		
Sex	Male (n = 636)	OR	1.0 (Ref)	0.966 (0.473, 1.946)	0.731 (0.338, 1.579)	1.172 (0.569, 2.414)	0.838	<0.001
		p-value †		0.926	0.425	0.667		
	Female (n = 647)	OR	1.0 (Ref)	1.252 (0.704, 2.229)	1.404 (0.799, 2.466)	1.968 (1.144, 3.386)	0.014	
		p-value †		0.444	0.238	0.014		
BMI, kg/m^2	<18.5 (n = 11)	OR	1.0 (Ref)	NA ¶	NA ¶	NA ¶	NA ¶	0.527
		p-value †						
	18.5 to 24.0 (n = 553)	OR	1.0 (Ref)	1.478 (0.749, 2.917)	0.949 (0.472, 1.909)	1.947 (0.999, 3.793)	0.137	
		p-value †		0.260	0.884	0.050		
	>24.0 (n = 719)	OR	1.0 (Ref)	1.025 (0.560, 1.873)	1.245 (0.683, 2.271)	1.633 (0.920, 2.898)	0.069	
		p-value †		0.937	0.474	0.094		
Family history of cancer	No (n = 1018)	OR	1.0 (Ref)	0.997 (0.614, 1.618)	0.847 (0.515, 1.393)	1.375 (0.865, 2.185)	0.252	0.846
		p-value †		0.989	0.513	0.179		
	Yes (n = 265)	OR	1.0 (Ref)	4.176 (1.151, 15.146)	4.646 (1.377, 15.674)	5.337 (1.492, 19.093)	0.010	
		p-value †		0.030	0.013	0.010		
Smoking history	Never a smoker (n = 807)	OR	1.0 (Ref)	1.428 (0.754, 2.704)	1.257 (0.653, 2.421)	1.356 (0.709, 2.593)	0.476	<0.001
		p-value †		0.274	0.494	0.357		
	Ex-smoker (n = 182)	OR	1.0 (Ref)	1.684 (0.564, 5.026)	0.528 (0.138, 2.022)	1.810 (0.694, 4.722)	0.393	
		p-value †		0.350	0.351	0.225		
	Current smoker (n = 294)	OR	1.0 (Ref)	0.697 (0.298, 1.630)	1.211 (0.555, 2.642)	2.462 (1.104, 5.491)	0.016	
		p-value †		0.405	0.631	0.028		

Table 6. *Cont.*

Stratified Characteristics			Vit B_6 (μmol/L) (in Quartiles)				*p* for Trend ‡	*p* for Interaction §
			Q1 (n = 322)	Q2 (n = 320)	Q3 (n = 321)	Q4 (n = 320)		
Alcohol consumption	Never a drinker (n = 904)	OR	1.0 (Ref)	1.441 (0.837, 2.483)	0.818 (0.463, 1.445)	1.371 (0.797, 2.358)	0.642	<0.001
		p-value †		0.188	0.488	0.254		
	Current drinker (n = 379)	OR	1.0 (Ref)	0.800 (0.357, 1.793)	2.159 (1.008, 4.628)	2.163 (1.041, 4.492)	0.006	
		p-value †		0.588	0.048	0.039		
Pathology of tumor	Adenocarcinoma (n = 1125)	OR	1.0 (Ref)	1.124 (0.682, 1.853)	1.193 (0.725, 1.962)	1.360 (0.836, 2.214)	0.211	<0.001
		p-value †		0.645	0.487	0.216		
	Squamous cell carcinoma (n = 158)	OR	1.0 (Ref)	1.523 (0.519, 4.470)	0.761 (0.248, 2.333)	3.933 (1.421, 10.888)	0.024	
		p-value †		0.444	0.633	0.008		
Diameter of tumor, cm	<1 (n = 370)	OR	1.0 (Ref)	0.339 (0.031, 3.656)	0.450 (0.055, 3.659)	1.069 (0.183, 6.262)	0.898	<0.001
		p-value †		0.373	0.455	0.941		
	1–3 (n = 731)	OR	1.0 (Ref)	1.661 (0.944, 2.923)	1.759 (1.000, 3.094)	2.152 (1.233, 3.755)	0.009	
		p-value †		0.078	0.050	0.007		
	>3 (n = 182)	OR	1.0 (Ref)	0.684 (0.279, 1.679)	0.455 (0.180, 1.149)	1.406 (0.605, 3.265)	0.645	
		p-value †		0.408	0.096	0.429		
Number of tumor(s)	Solitary (n = 1197)	OR	1.0 (Ref)	1.205 (0.752, 1.932)	1.156 (0.719, 1.859)	1.664 (1.051, 2.636)	0.043	<0.001
		p-value †		0.439	0.548	0.030		
	Multiple (n = 86)	OR	1.0 (Ref)	1.058 (0.225, 4.985)	0.578 (0.118, 2.826)	1.319 (0.327, 5.323)	0.776	
		p-value †		0.943	0.499	0.698		
Density of tumor	Solid (n = 675)	OR	1.0 (Ref)	1.251 (0.760, 2.059)	1.048 (0.634, 1.730)	1.519 (0.932, 2.477)	0.167	<0.001
		p-value †		0.379	0.856	0.094		
	Subsolid (n = 608)	OR	1.0 (Ref)	1.113 (0.388, 3.191)	1.628 (0.559, 4.743)	2.468 (0.963, 6.325)	0.038	
		p-value †		0.842	0.372	0.060		

OR, odds ratio; Q, quartile of vitamin B_6; BMI, body mass index. * Adjusted for factors including age, sex, BMI, family history of cancer, smoking history, alcohol consumption, season of blood sampling for serum vitamin testing, educational level, pathology, and tumor type (diameter, number, and density), unless the factor is used for stratification. † Q2–Q4 of serum vitamin B_6 are each compared with Q1. ‡ *p* for trend is based on the statistical significance of the coefficient of the quartile variable (median value within each quartile). § *p* for interaction is based on the statistical significance of the cross-product term added to multivariable models. ¶ not enough data for stratified analysis.

4. Discussion

In this retrospective study, we found that serum vitamin B_6 levels might be positively associated with intrapulmonary lymph nodes and/or localized pleural metastases in NSCLC patients, and the risk association was stronger for women, current smokers, current drinkers, and patients with squamous cell carcinoma, tumors 1–3 cm in diameter, or a solitary tumor. However, even though serum vitamin B_6 levels were associated with preoperative NSCLC upstaging, B_6 did not qualify as a useful biomarker due to weak associations and wide confidence intervals. Preoperative vitamin B_6 levels might have some value in the preoperative evaluation of intrapulmonary lymph nodes and/or localized pleural metastases in NSCLC; thus, it would be appropriate to prospectively investigate the relationship between serum vitamin B_6 levels and lung cancer further.

Vitamin B_6 promotes cell growth, differentiation, proliferation, and metastasis [31] and has adjuvant anti-inflammatory and antioxidant effects [32]. Although large cohort studies have been conducted, the association between vitamin B_6 intake, blood levels, and catabolic levels with lung cancer remains inconclusive. Vitamin B_6 has been implicated as a tumor promoter [15,23–26], tumor suppressor [19], or being unrelated to carcinogenesis [27,28] in various studies. This contradiction may be attributed to the significant variation in vitamin B_6 among populations of different races, diets, lifestyles, and vitamin supplementation habits [33,34]. In our study, we found that patients with lung cancer had higher serum vitamin B_6 levels than patients with benign lung nodules, while patients with intrapulmonary metastases had higher serum vitamin B_6 levels than non-metastatic patients, i.e., serum vitamin B_6 levels increased with increasing tumor status. Theoretically, vitamin B_6 could promote tumor cell growth, differentiation, and proliferation, as well as be a risk factor for lung carcinogenesis [35,36]. On the other hand, it could act as an antitumor factor with regard to the inflammatory response caused by tumor cells [37–39]. Several studies have shown that vitamin B_6 can act as a promotor in tumors by affecting DNA stability [40,41] and the activation of antioxidant enzymes [42–45], which are involved in the regulation of post-translational modifications of activated proteins. The relationship of vitamin B_6 with post-translational modifications of key proteins such as NF-κB [46,47], as well as inflammasomes such as NLRP3 [48,49] and receptor-interacting protein 140 (RIP140) [47,50], has received significant attention. Although there are no specific findings related to the mechanism of vitamin B_6 and lung cancer metastasis, we speculated that these two aspects mentioned above together determine the effect of vitamin B_6 on tumors. Factors such as demographics and tumor type may play different roles in both aspects, leading to different conclusions. In our study, the positive relationship between vitamin B_6 and intrapulmonary metastasis suggests that vitamin B_6 may contribute to tumor metastasis in NSCLC patients.

We measured serum PLP as an assessment of vitamin B_6 levels. Vitamin B_6 consists of pyridoxal (PN), pyridoxamine (PM), pyridoxal (PL), and their phosphorylated derivatives pyridoxal 5′-phosphate (PNP), pyridoxamine 5′-phosphate (PMP), and PLP [51]. PLP is the bioactive form of vitamin B_6 in vivo and has been the common measure of vitamin B_6 status testing in previous studies [19,38,51–54]. However, PLP is considered unstable because it may be influenced by inflammatory status, alkaline phosphatase levels, serum albumin, and inorganic phosphate [55]. Recent studies have used plasma vitamer ratios (PAr), calculated as PA:(PLP + PL), to eliminate the influence of the above factors [55,56]. However, PAr requires the simultaneous measurement of three indices, and mainly reflects the catabolism of vitamin B_6 in the inflammatory state. In contrast, PLP serves as a representation of the true vitamin B_6 levels and can directly reflect the relationship between vitamin B_6 and lung cancer. PLP is also more compatible with clinical applications because it requires less blood sampling and is less expensive.

A stratified analysis was performed to clarify the association of vitamin B_6 with intrapulmonary metastasis in different populations. We found that the risk association was much stronger in some situations. Vitamin B_6 served as a strong risk factor in females, current smokers, current drinkers, and those with a family history of cancer. The study by Fanidi et al. also found a positive trend for elevated PLP levels and lung cancer risk in their cohort of Asian women [19]. In addition, an elevated serum vitamin B_6 level, even within the normal range, was a risk factor for those with a family history of cancer, suggesting a possible genetic link might exist between them. Meanwhile, smoking and alcohol consumption are well-known risk factors for lung cancer [15,19]. Vitamin B_6 may be associated with smoking-induced inflammation and immune activation, which was also one of the mechanisms related to smoking in lung cancer development [30,57,58].

Interestingly, pathology, tumor size, tumor number, and morphology all seemed to influence the strength of vitamin B_6 as a risk factor for intrapulmonary metastasis. Previous studies showed that increased vitamin B_6 catabolism was positively associated with the risk of lung carcinogenesis, especially in squamous cell carcinoma [15]. This finding was confirmed in our study. In addition, we found a stronger risk association in patients with a solitary tumor or a tumor 1–3 cm in diameter. A consistent trend toward an increased risk of metastasis with increasing vitamin B_6 levels was also found in the subsolid tumor population. These associations have not been previously studied, and the theoretical basis for them remains unclear. In clinical practice, patients with a solitary, subsolid tumor or a tumor 1–3 cm in diameter without metastases are good candidates for surgery. If the vitamin–metastasis association could be confirmed by future studies, vitamin B_6 could be of great value in supporting surgical treatment as a preoperative predictor for metastasis assessment.

In this study, we found that age, sex, smoking history, alcohol consumption, and several characteristics of tumors had significant interactions with vitamin B_6, respectively. That is, different degrees of the above factors could significantly affect the strength of the association between vitamin B_6 and intrapulmonary metastasis. The results of the interaction and stratified analysis further confirmed that women, current smokers, current drinkers, patients with squamous cell carcinoma, those with tumors 1–3 cm in size, and those with a solitary tumor may be a part of the special population whose vitamin B_6 levels should be of great concern. In addition, although there was a significant interaction between age and vitamin B_6, the p for trend was found to be statistically insignificant (ranging from 0.112 to 0.119), which might be caused by the sample size. Furthermore, there was no significant interaction between family history and vitamin B_6, suggesting that the effect of family history on the association should be further investigated.

Tumor staging is crucial in cancer treatment and determines the outcome. The pTNM staging results could not be obtained comprehensively before surgery. Clinical TNM staging might be relatively accurate in evaluating the tumor stage, but are not precise in the evaluation of the nodule and metastasis stage, especially in the early stage of lung cancer. In our study, we found 53 patients (53/1283) who underwent surgery had postoperative confirmation of localized pleural metastases, suggesting that surgical treatment may not be appropriate for them. Vitamin B_6 testing may have the potential to improve preoperative TNM staging. Further studies with larger sample sizes are needed to verify the value of vitamin B_6 in surgical management.

Notably, the results obtained in this study should be treated with caution. On one hand, the association between lung cancer and vitamins is very complex. Many factors may affect serum vitamin levels, including dietary habits, vitamin supplements, body metabolism, and a variety of complications. In this study, we collected as much nutritional information as possible and excluded conditions that could affect serum vitamins. However, more rigorous prospective studies are necessary to properly research the pathogenetic relationship between vitamin levels in the blood and the occurrence and progression of lung cancer. On the other hand, even though vitamin B_6 levels showed positive association with intrapulmonary metastases in NSCLC patients, the relationship was weak, and the confidence intervals overlapped hugely. Thus, the statistically significant difference between groups of patients could not be translated into a predictor on the level of individual patients based on the results of this study. Vitamin B_6 levels might have some value in the preoperative evaluation of intrapulmonary metastases in NSCLC, but more research is needed before conclusions can be drawn.

This study had several limitations. First, the sample size of this study was limited. Studies with larger sample sizes are needed for further validation. Second, there may be an interaction between vitamin B_6 and tumor metastasis status. The study identified a positive association between vitamin B_6 and intrapulmonary metastases, but the cause-and-effect relationship between them was not clear. Third, this study was retrospective; therefore, prospective cohort studies are needed to explore the mechanism of action of vitamin B_6 levels and lung cancer. Fourth, we collected as much information as possible about patients' dietary intake, nutritional status, and nutritional supplementation, but as a retrospective study, nutrition-related clinical information was not sufficiently detailed and might influence the results.

5. Conclusions

In conclusion, our study demonstrated a possible positive association between serum vitamin B_6 levels and intrapulmonary lymph nodes and/or localized pleural metastases in NSCLC patients, and the association was stronger in specific populations including women, current smokers, current drinkers, patients with squamous cell carcinoma, those with tumors 1–3 cm in diameter, and those with a solitary tumor. However, B_6 did not qualify as a useful biomarker due to weak associations and wide confidence intervals. Preoperative vitamin B_6 levels might have some value in the preoperative evaluation of intrapulmonary lymph nodes and/or localized pleural metastases in NSCLC, and thus the relationship between serum vitamin B_6 levels and lung cancer should be prospectively investigated in the future.

Author Contributions: Conceptualization, design, supervision, and project administration, Y.L. and L.L.; resources, Q.X., Y.Z. and X.Z.; methodology and investigation, J.B., Z.Y. and L.L.; data analysis, interpretation, and writing—original draft preparation, H.Y. and L.L.; writing—review and editing, Y.L., Q.X., Y.Z., X.Z., J.B. and Z.Y. All authors have read and agreed to the published version of the manuscript.

Funding: This research was funded by the Key Project of Chinese Military Health Care Projects, grant number 22BJZ20.

Institutional Review Board Statement: The study was conducted in accordance with the Declaration of Helsinki and approved by the Ethics Committee of Chinese PLA General Hospital (protocol code: No. S2022-615-01, and date of approval: 26 October 2022).

Informed Consent Statement: Patient consent was waived by the Ethics Committee of Chinese PLA General Hospital due to the following reasons: (1) the medical records and biological specimens used were obtained in previous clinical consultations; (2) the risk to the subject of the study was no greater than the minimal risk; (3) subjects' privacy and personally identifiable information was protected; (4) waiving informed consent or some elements of informed consent did not affect the rights and health of the subject; and (5) no further follow-up of subject information was required.

Data Availability Statement: The raw data supporting the conclusions of this article will be made available by the authors, without undue reservation.

Conflicts of Interest: The authors declare no conflict of interest.

References

1. Siegel, R.L.; Miller, K.D.; Jemal, A. Cancer Statistics, 2017. *CA Cancer J. Clin.* **2017**, *67*, 7–30. [CrossRef] [PubMed]
2. Miller, K.D.; Siegel, R.L.; Lin, C.C.; Mariotto, A.B.; Kramer, J.L.; Rowland, J.H.; Stein, K.D.; Alteri, R.; Jemal, A. Cancer treatment and survivorship statistics, 2016. *CA Cancer J. Clin.* **2016**, *66*, 271–289. [CrossRef] [PubMed]
3. Minguet, J.; Smith, K.H.; Bramlage, P. Targeted therapies for treatment of non-small cell lung cancer–Recent advances and future perspectives. *Int. J. Cancer* **2016**, *138*, 2549–2561. [CrossRef] [PubMed]
4. Goldstraw, P.; Chansky, K.; Crowley, J.; Rami-Porta, R.; Asamura, H.; Eberhardt, W.E.; Nicholson, A.G.; Groome, P.; Mitchell, A.; Bolejack, V.; et al. The IASLC Lung Cancer Staging Project: Proposals for Revision of the TNM Stage Groupings in the Forthcoming (Eighth) Edition of the TNM Classification for Lung Cancer. *J. Thorac. Oncol.* **2016**, *11*, 39–51. [CrossRef] [PubMed]

5. Musika, W.; Kamsa-Ard, S.; Jirapornkul, C.; Santong, C.; Phunmanee, A. Lung Cancer Survival with Current Therapies and New Targeted Treatments: A Comprehensive Update from the Srinagarind Hospital-Based Cancer Registry from (2013 to 2017). *Asian Pac. J. Cancer Prev.* **2021**, *22*, 2501–2507. [CrossRef] [PubMed]
6. MacMahon, H.; Naidich, D.P.; Goo, J.M.; Lee, K.S.; Leung, A.N.C.; Mayo, J.R.; Mehta, A.C.; Ohno, Y.; Powell, C.A.; Prokop, M.; et al. Guidelines for Management of Incidental Pulmonary Nodules Detected on CT Images: From the Fleischner Society 2017. *Radiology* **2017**, *284*, 228–243. [CrossRef] [PubMed]
7. Bitenc, M.; Cufer, T.; Kern, I.; Miklavcic, M.; Petrovic, S.; Groznik, V.; Sadikov, A. Real-life long-term outcomes of upfront surgery in patients with resectable stage I–IIIA non-small cell lung cancer. *Radiol. Oncol.* **2022**, *56*, 346–354. [CrossRef]
8. Solberg, S.; Nilssen, Y.; Terje Brustugun, O.; Magnus Haram, P.; Helland, A.; Moller, B.; Strand, T.E.; Gyrid Freim Wahl, S.; Fjellbirkeland, L. Concordance between clinical and pathology TNM-staging in lung cancer. *Lung Cancer* **2022**, *171*, 65–69. [CrossRef]
9. Navani, N.; Fisher, D.J.; Tierney, J.F.; Stephens, R.J.; Burdett, S.; Group, N.M.-a.C. The Accuracy of Clinical Staging of Stage I-IIIa Non-Small Cell Lung Cancer: An Analysis Based on Individual Participant Data. *Chest* **2019**, *155*, 502–509. [CrossRef]
10. Zheng, X.; He, B.; Hu, Y.; Ren, M.; Chen, Z.; Zhang, Z.; Ma, J.; Ouyang, L.; Chu, H.; Gao, H.; et al. Diagnostic Accuracy of Deep Learning and Radiomics in Lung Cancer Staging: A Systematic Review and Meta-Analysis. *Front. Public Health* **2022**, *10*, 938113. [CrossRef]
11. Zhu, M.; Yang, Z.; Wang, M.; Zhao, W.; Zhu, Q.; Shi, W.; Yu, H.; Liang, Z.; Chen, L. A computerized tomography-based radiomic model for assessing the invasiveness of lung adenocarcinoma manifesting as ground-glass opacity nodules. *Respir. Res.* **2022**, *23*, 96. [CrossRef] [PubMed]
12. Kurzius-Spencer, M.; da Silva, V.; Thomson, C.A.; Hartz, V.; Hsu, C.H.; Burgess, J.L.; O'Rourke, M.K.; Harris, R.B. Nutrients in one-carbon metabolism and urinary arsenic methylation in the National Health and Nutrition Examination Survey (NHANES) 2003–2004. *Sci. Total Environ.* **2017**, *607–608*, 381–390. [CrossRef] [PubMed]
13. Islam, A.; Shaukat, Z.; Hussain, R.; Gregory, S.L. One-Carbon and Polyamine Metabolism as Cancer Therapy Targets. *Biomolecules* **2022**, *12*, 1902. [CrossRef] [PubMed]
14. Lyon, P.; Strippoli, V.; Fang, B.; Cimmino, L. B Vitamins and One-Carbon Metabolism: Implications in Human Health and Disease. *Nutrients* **2020**, *12*, 2867. [CrossRef]
15. Brasky, T.M.; White, E.; Chen, C.L. Long-Term, Supplemental, One-Carbon Metabolism-Related Vitamin B Use in Relation to Lung Cancer Risk in the Vitamins and Lifestyle (VITAL) Cohort. *J. Clin. Oncol.* **2017**, *35*, 3440–3448. [CrossRef]
16. Vollset, S.E.; Clarke, R.; Lewington, S.; Ebbing, M.; Halsey, J.; Lonn, E.; Armitage, J.; Manson, J.E.; Hankey, G.J.; Spence, J.D.; et al. Effects of folic acid supplementation on overall and site-specific cancer incidence during the randomised trials: Meta-analyses of data on 50,000 individuals. *Lancet* **2013**, *381*, 1029–1036. [CrossRef]
17. Fanidi, A.; Carreras-Torres, R.; Larose, T.L.; Yuan, J.M.; Stevens, V.L.; Weinstein, S.J.; Albanes, D.; Prentice, R.; Pettinger, M.; Cai, Q.; et al. Is high vitamin B12 status a cause of lung cancer? *Int. J. Cancer* **2019**, *145*, 1499–1503. [CrossRef]
18. Ebbing, M.; Bonaa, K.H.; Nygard, O.; Arnesen, E.; Ueland, P.M.; Nordrehaug, J.E.; Rasmussen, K.; Njolstad, I.; Refsum, H.; Nilsen, D.W.; et al. Cancer incidence and mortality after treatment with folic acid and vitamin B12. *JAMA* **2009**, *302*, 2119–2126. [CrossRef]
19. Fanidi, A.; Muller, D.C.; Yuan, J.M.; Stevens, V.L.; Weinstein, S.J.; Albanes, D.; Prentice, R.; Thomsen, C.A.; Pettinger, M.; Cai, Q.; et al. Circulating Folate, Vitamin B6, and Methionine in Relation to Lung Cancer Risk in the Lung Cancer Cohort Consortium (LC3). *J. Natl. Cancer Inst.* **2018**, *110*, 57–67.
20. Yang, J.; Li, H.; Deng, H.; Wang, Z. Association of One-Carbon Metabolism-Related Vitamins (Folate, B6, B12), Homocysteine and Methionine with the Risk of Lung Cancer: Systematic Review and Meta-Analysis. *Front. Oncol.* **2018**, *8*, 493. [CrossRef]
21. Yan, H.; Jin, X.; Yin, L.; Zhu, C.; Feng, G. Investigating Causal Associations of Circulating Micronutrients Concentrations with the Risk of Lung Cancer: A Mendelian Randomization Study. *Nutrients* **2022**, *14*, 4569. [CrossRef] [PubMed]
22. O'Connor, E.A.; Evans, C.V.; Ivlev, I.; Rushkin, M.C.; Thomas, R.G.; Martin, A.; Lin, J.S. Vitamin and Mineral Supplements for the Primary Prevention of Cardiovascular Disease and Cancer: Updated Evidence Report and Systematic Review for the US Preventive Services Task Force. *JAMA* **2022**, *327*, 2334–2347. [CrossRef] [PubMed]
23. Zuo, H.; Ueland, P.M.; Midttun, O.; Tell, G.S.; Fanidi, A.; Zheng, W.; Shu, X.; Xiang, Y.; Wu, J.; Prentice, R.; et al. Vitamin B6 catabolism and lung cancer risk: Results from the Lung Cancer Cohort Consortium (LC3). *Ann. Oncol.* **2019**, *30*, 478–485. [CrossRef] [PubMed]
24. Zuo, H.; Ueland, P.M.; Eussen, S.J.; Tell, G.S.; Vollset, S.E.; Nygard, O.; Midttun, O.; Meyer, K.; Ulvik, A. Markers of vitamin B6 status and metabolism as predictors of incident cancer: The Hordaland Health Study. *Int. J. Cancer* **2015**, *136*, 2932–2939. [CrossRef]
25. Zuo, H.; Ueland, P.M.; Midttun, O.; Vollset, S.E.; Tell, G.S.; Theofylaktopoulou, D.; Travis, R.C.; Boutron-Ruault, M.C.; Fournier, A.; Severi, G.; et al. Results from the European Prospective Investigation into Cancer and Nutrition Link Vitamin B6 Catabolism and Lung Cancer Risk. *Cancer Res.* **2018**, *78*, 302–308. [CrossRef]
26. Meyer, H.E.; Willett, W.C.; Fung, T.T.; Holvik, K.; Feskanich, D. Association of High Intakes of Vitamins B6 and B12 from Food and Supplements with Risk of Hip Fracture Among Postmenopausal Women in the Nurses' Health Study. *JAMA Netw. Open* **2019**, *2*, e193591. [CrossRef]

27. Takata, Y.; Shu, X.O.; Buchowski, M.S.; Munro, H.M.; Wen, W.; Steinwandel, M.D.; Hargreaves, M.K.; Blot, W.J.; Cai, Q. Food intake of folate, folic acid and other B vitamins with lung cancer risk in a low-income population in the Southeastern United States. *Eur. J. Nutr.* **2020**, *59*, 671–683. [CrossRef]
28. Obeid, R.; Pietrzik, K.; Smoking, B. Vitamins, and Lung Cancer: The Chicken or the Egg Causality Dilemma. *J. Clin. Oncol.* **2018**, *36*, 626–627. [CrossRef]
29. Board WCoTE. *World Health Organization Classification of Tumours, Volume 5: Thoracic Tumours*, 5th ed.; IARC Press: Lyon, France, 2021; Available online: https://tumourclassification.iarc.who.int/ (accessed on 15 April 2023).
30. Lu, X.; Ma, L.; Yin, X.; Ji, H.; Qian, Y.; Zhong, S.; Yan, A.; Zhang, Y. The impact of tobacco exposure on tumor microenvironment and prognosis in lung adenocarcinoma by integrative analysis of multi-omics data. *Int. Immunopharmacol.* **2021**, *101*, 108253. [CrossRef]
31. Parra, M.; Stahl, S.; Hellmann, H. Vitamin B(6) and Its Role in Cell Metabolism and Physiology. *Cells* **2018**, *7*, 84. [CrossRef]
32. Bird, R.P. The Emerging Role of Vitamin B6 in Inflammation and Carcinogenesis. *Adv. Food Nutr. Res.* **2018**, *83*, 151–194. [PubMed]
33. Midttun, O.; Theofylaktopoulou, D.; McCann, A.; Fanidi, A.; Muller, D.C.; Meyer, K.; Ulvik, A.; Zheng, W.; Shu, X.O.; Xiang, Y.B.; et al. Circulating concentrations of biomarkers and metabolites related to vitamin status, one-carbon and the kynurenine pathways in US, Nordic, Asian, and Australian populations. *Am. J. Clin. Nutr.* **2017**, *105*, 1314–1326. [CrossRef] [PubMed]
34. Theofylaktopoulou, D.; Midttun, O.; Ueland, P.M.; Meyer, K.; Fanidi, A.; Zheng, W.; Shu, X.O.; Xiang, Y.B.; Prentice, R.; Pettinger, M.; et al. Impaired functional vitamin B6 status is associated with increased risk of lung cancer. *Int. J. Cancer* **2018**, *142*, 2425–2434. [CrossRef] [PubMed]
35. Stach, K.; Stach, W.; Augoff, K. Vitamin B6 in Health and Disease. *Nutrients* **2021**, *13*, 3229. [CrossRef]
36. Calderon-Ospina, C.A.; Nava-Mesa, M.O.; Paez-Hurtado, A.M. Update on Safety Profiles of Vitamins B1, B6, and B12: A Narrative Review. *Ther. Clin. Risk Manag.* **2020**, *16*, 1275–1288. [CrossRef]
37. Federico, A.; Morgillo, F.; Tuccillo, C.; Ciardiello, F.; Loguercio, C. Chronic inflammation and oxidative stress in human carcinogenesis. *Int. J. Cancer* **2007**, *121*, 2381–2386. [CrossRef]
38. Elinav, E.; Nowarski, R.; Thaiss, C.A.; Hu, B.; Jin, C.; Flavell, R.A. Inflammation-induced cancer: Crosstalk between tumours, immune cells and microorganisms. *Nat. Rev. Cancer* **2013**, *13*, 759–771. [CrossRef]
39. Merigliano, C.; Mascolo, E.; Burla, R.; Saggio, I.; Verni, F. The Relationship between Vitamin B6, Diabetes and Cancer. *Front. Genet.* **2018**, *9*, 388. [CrossRef]
40. Myte, R.; Gylling, B.; Haggstrom, J.; Schneede, J.; Magne Ueland, P.; Hallmans, G.; Johansson, I.; Palmqvist, R.; Van Guelpen, B. Untangling the role of one-carbon metabolism in colorectal cancer risk: A comprehensive Bayesian network analysis. *Sci. Rep.* **2017**, *7*, 43434. [CrossRef]
41. Selhub, J.; Byun, A.; Liu, Z.; Mason, J.B.; Bronson, R.T.; Crott, J.W. Dietary vitamin B6 intake modulates colonic inflammation in the IL10-/- model of inflammatory bowel disease. *J. Nutr. Biochem.* **2013**, *24*, 2138–2143. [CrossRef]
42. Quail, D.F.; Joyce, J.A. Microenvironmental regulation of tumor progression and metastasis. *Nat. Med.* **2013**, *19*, 1423–1437. [CrossRef] [PubMed]
43. Tape, C.J.; Ling, S.; Dimitriadi, M.; McMahon, K.M.; Worboys, J.D.; Leong, H.S.; Norrie, I.C.; Miller, C.J.; Poulogiannis, G.; Lauffenburger, D.A.; et al. Oncogenic KRAS Regulates Tumor Cell Signaling via Stromal Reciprocation. *Cell* **2016**, *165*, 910–920. [CrossRef]
44. Biswas, S.K. Does the Interdependence between Oxidative Stress and Inflammation Explain the Antioxidant Paradox? *Oxid. Med. Cell. Longev.* **2016**, *2016*, 5698931. [CrossRef] [PubMed]
45. Halliwell, B. The antioxidant paradox. *Lancet* **2000**, *355*, 1179–1180. [CrossRef] [PubMed]
46. Jain, S.S.; Bird, R.P. Elevated expression of tumor necrosis factor-alpha signaling molecules in colonic tumors of Zucker obese (fa/fa) rats. *Int. J. Cancer* **2010**, *127*, 2042–2050. [CrossRef] [PubMed]
47. Hu, Y.C.; Yi, Z.J.; Zhou, Y.; Li, P.Z.; Liu, Z.J.; Duan, S.G.; Gong, J.P. Overexpression of RIP140 suppresses the malignant potential of hepatocellular carcinoma by inhibiting NF-kappaB-mediated alternative polarization of macrophages. *Oncol. Rep.* **2017**, *37*, 2971–2979. [CrossRef] [PubMed]
48. Lin, C.; Zhang, J. Inflammasomes in Inflammation-Induced Cancer. *Front. Immunol.* **2017**, *8*, 271. [CrossRef] [PubMed]
49. Zhang, P.; Tsuchiya, K.; Kinoshita, T.; Kushiyama, H.; Suidasari, S.; Hatakeyama, M.; Imura, H.; Kato, N.; Suda, T. Vitamin B6 Prevents IL-1beta Protein Production by Inhibiting NLRP3 Inflammasome Activation. *J. Biol. Chem.* **2016**, *291*, 24517–24527. [CrossRef]
50. Huq, M.D.; Wei, L.N. Post-translational modification of nuclear co-repressor receptor-interacting protein 140 by acetylation. *Mol. Cell. Proteom.* **2005**, *4*, 975–983. [CrossRef]
51. Huang, S.C.; Wei, J.C.; Lin, P.T.; Wu, D.J.; Huang, Y.C. Plasma pyridoxal 5′-phosphate is not associated with inflammatory and immune responses after adjusting for serum albumin in patients with rheumatoid arthritis: A preliminary study. *Ann. Nutr. Metab.* **2012**, *60*, 83–89. [CrossRef]
52. Campbell, B.M.; Charych, E.; Lee, A.W.; Moller, T. Kynurenines in CNS disease: Regulation by inflammatory cytokines. *Front. Neurosci.* **2014**, *8*, 12. [CrossRef] [PubMed]
53. Ciorba, M.A. Kynurenine pathway metabolites: Relevant to vitamin B-6 deficiency and beyond. *Am. J. Clin. Nutr.* **2013**, *98*, 863–864. [CrossRef]

54. Di Salvo, M.L.; Safo, M.K.; Contestabile, R. Biomedical aspects of pyridoxal 5′-phosphate availability. *Front. Biosci. Elite Ed.* **2012**, *4*, 897–913. [PubMed]
55. Ueland, P.M.; Ulvik, A.; Rios-Avila, L.; Midttun, O.; Gregory, J.F. Direct and Functional Biomarkers of Vitamin B6 Status. *Ann. Rev. Nutr.* **2015**, *35*, 33–70. [CrossRef] [PubMed]
56. Ulvik, A.; Midttun, O.; Pedersen, E.R.; Eussen, S.J.; Nygard, O.; Ueland, P.M. Evidence for increased catabolism of vitamin B-6 during systemic inflammation. *Am. J. Clin. Nutr.* **2014**, *100*, 250–255. [CrossRef] [PubMed]
57. Shiels, M.S.; Katki, H.A.; Freedman, N.D.; Purdue, M.P.; Wentzensen, N.; Trabert, B.; Kitahara, C.M.; Furr, M.; Li, Y.; Kemp, T.J.; et al. Cigarette smoking and variations in systemic immune and inflammation markers. *J. Natl. Cancer Inst.* **2014**, *106*, dju294. [CrossRef]
58. Zhang, H.; Zhang, G.; Zhang, J.; Xiao, M.; Cui, S.; Wu, S.; Jin, C.; Yang, J.; Lu, X. Transcription factor SP1 and oncoprotein PPP1R13L regulate nicotine-induced epithelial-mesenchymal transition in lung adenocarcinoma via a feedback loop. *Biochem. Pharmacol.* **2022**, *206*, 115344. [CrossRef]

nutrients

MDPI

Article

EGCG Alleviates DSS-Induced Colitis by Inhibiting Ferroptosis Through the Activation of the Nrf2-GPX4 Pathway and Enhancing Iron Metabolism

Junzhou Chen [1,2,†], Conghui Yin [1,2,†], Yilong Zhang [1,2], Xin Lai [1,2], Chen Liu [1,2], Yuheng Luo [1,2], Junqiu Luo [1,2], Jun He [1,2], Bing Yu [1,2], Quyuan Wang [1,2], Huifen Wang [1,2], Daiwen Chen [1,2,*] and Aimin Wu [1,2,*]

1 Institute of Animal Nutrition, Sichuan Agricultural University, Chengdu 611130, China; chenjunzhou2023@163.com (J.C.); 18735193091@163.com (C.Y.); 18563633520@163.com (Y.Z.); xin.lai2018@gmail.com (X.L.); liuchen-ipp@hotmail.com (C.L.); luoluo212@126.com (Y.L.); 13910@sicau.edu.cn (J.L.); hejun8067@163.com (J.H.); ybingtian@163.com (B.Y.); ice_5885327@163.com (Q.W.); wanghuifen1005@163.com (H.W.)

2 Key Laboratory for Animal Disease-Resistance Nutrition, China Ministry of Education, Sichuan Agricultural University, Chengdu 611130, China

* Correspondence: dwchen@sicau.edu.cn (D.C.); wuaimin0608@163.com or wuaimin@sicau.edu.cn (A.W.)

† These authors contributed equally to this work.

Abstract: Background: Ferroptosis is a regulated cell death process linked to various diseases. This study explored whether Epigallocatechin-3-gallate (EGCG), a tea-derived antioxidant, could regulate ferroptosis to alleviate dextran sulfate sodium (DSS)-induced colitis. Methods: A DSS-induced colitis model was used to assess EGCG's effects. Ferroptosis markers, oxidative stress, and iron metabolism were evaluated, alongside Nrf2-GPX4 pathway activation and ferritin (FTH/L) expression. Results: Iron dysregulation and oxidative stress contributed to DSS-induced colitis by activating ferroptosis in colonic epithelial cells. EGCG supplementation inhibited ferroptosis, reducing oxidative damage. Mechanistically, EGCG activated the Nrf2-GPX4 pathway, enhancing antioxidant defense, and improved iron metabolism by upregulating ferritin expression. Conclusions: EGCG effectively suppressed DSS-induced ferroptosis and colitis, highlighting its potential as a ferroptosis inhibitor and therapeutic agent.

Keywords: colitis; ferroptosis; iron metabolism; Epigallocatechin-3-Gallate (EGCG); antioxidant

1. Introduction

Inflammatory bowel disease (IBD), including Crohn's disease and ulcerative colitis, is a chronic inflammatory disorder of the gastrointestinal tract that has become increasingly prevalent worldwide [1]. In recent decades, the incidence of IBD has risen significantly in developed countries and is now emerging as a major public health challenge in developing nations [2]. Patients with IBD suffer from recurring episodes of abdominal pain, diarrhea, weight loss, and malnutrition, often leading to a substantial decline in quality of life [3]. The pathogenesis of IBD is complex, involving genetic predisposition, environmental factors, gut microbiota dysbiosis, and immune system dysregulation [4]. Furthermore, IBD is associated with an elevated risk of colorectal cancer and poses a considerable burden on healthcare systems [5]. Consequently, understanding the underlying mechanisms of IBD and identifying effective therapeutic strategies remain critical areas of research.

Recent studies have highlighted the importance of oxidative stress and iron metabolism dysregulation in the pathophysiology of IBD [6,7]. Iron is an essential trace element required for numerous physiological processes, including oxygen transport, DNA synthesis, and energy metabolism [8,9]. However, disruptions in iron homeostasis, particularly the accumulation of excess-free iron, can trigger oxidative stress and lipid peroxidation through the Fenton reaction [10,11]. These processes contribute to cellular damage and death, exacerbating intestinal barrier dysfunction and inflammation.

Ferroptosis is a distinct form of regulated cell death characterized by iron-dependent lipid peroxide accumulation, which causes oxidative stress and cell membrane damage [12]. Unlike other forms of cell death such as apoptosis and necrosis, ferroptosis involves a unique biochemical pathway driven by excessive iron levels and the associated oxidative stress [13]. This process begins with the Fenton reaction, where iron catalyzes the formation of reactive oxygen species (ROS), particularly hydroxyl radicals, that attack unsaturated lipids in cell membranes, leading to lipid peroxidation [14]. This oxidative damage disrupts cell membrane integrity, ultimately resulting in cell death [14,15]. The regulation of ferroptosis involves a delicate balance between iron metabolism, antioxidant defenses, and lipid peroxidation processes [16]. Key players in this regulatory network include glutathione peroxidase 4 (GPX4), which detoxifies lipid peroxides by converting them into less harmful alcohols, and solute carrier family 7 member 11 (SLC7A11), which imports cystine to support glutathione synthesis, a critical antioxidant in cells [17]. When GPX4 is inhibited or when glutathione levels are depleted, lipid peroxides accumulate, and ferroptosis is triggered [17,18]. This process has been implicated in several pathological conditions, including cancer, neurodegenerative diseases, and inflammatory disorders like colitis [19,20]. In the context of IBD, ferroptosis is closely associated with intestinal epithelial cell damage and gut barrier dysfunction. Studies have shown that IBD patients exhibit elevated iron levels in the gut, possibly due to increased iron absorption and impaired barrier integrity [21]. Excess-free iron promotes oxidative stress, lipid peroxidation, and inflammatory responses, creating a vicious cycle of tissue damage and chronic inflammation [13,22]. Additionally, ferroptosis may disrupt the gut microenvironment, perpetuating inflammation and disease progression. These findings suggest that targeting ferroptosis could provide a novel therapeutic approach for IBD.

Epigallocatechin-3-gallate (EGCG), a major polyphenolic compound in tea leaves, has garnered significant attention for its potent antioxidant and iron-chelating properties [23]. EGCG can bind to free iron, preventing its involvement in the Fenton reaction, thereby reducing the generation of ROS and lipid peroxidation [24,25]. Additionally, EGCG modulates the expression of key ferroptosis regulators, including glutathione peroxidase 4 (GPX4) and solute carrier family 7 member 11 (SLC7A11), and it upregulates ferritin heavy chain/light chain (FTH/L), facilitating the sequestration of excess-free iron [26]. These mechanisms collectively mitigate ferroptosis and protect cells from oxidative damage [27]. Several studies have demonstrated that EGCG can alleviate inflammation and oxidative stress in colitis, highlighting its potential therapeutic benefits in inflammatory bowel disease (IBD) [28]. However, the exact mechanisms underlying these effects remain poorly understood. While prior research has largely focused on EGCG's antioxidant and anti-inflammatory properties, no studies have specifically addressed whether EGCG alleviates colitis by modulating ferroptosis, an iron-dependent form of cell death implicated in intestinal epithelial damage.

This study aims to investigate the protective effects of EGCG in DSS-induced colitis, focusing on its mechanisms in regulating ferroptosis and improving oxidative stress and iron metabolism. The results revealed that iron dysregulation and oxidative stress contributed to the activation of ferroptosis in colonic epithelial cells, which worsened colitis. EGCG supplementation suppressed ferroptosis by enhancing antioxidant defenses through the activation of the Nrf2-GPX4-signaling pathway and by improving iron metabolism via the upregulation of ferritin (FTH/L). By mitigating oxidative damage and regulating ferroptosis, EGCG effectively alleviated the symptoms of DSS-induced colitis. These findings suggest that EGCG holds promise as both a ferroptosis inhibitor and a therapeutic option for colitis.

2. Materials and Methods

2.1. Chemicals and Antibodies

EGCG (purity ≥ 98%) was provided by Teaturn Bio-pharmaceutical Co., Ltd. (Wuxi, China). Anti-TfR1, SLC40A1, FTH/L, Nrf2, pNrf2, GPX4, P62, and HO-1 were purchased from Abcam; anti-Keap1, SLC3A2, and SLC7A11 were purchased from Cell Signaling Technology; and β-actin was purchased from Santa Cruz biotechnology (Dallas, TX, USA).

2.2. Animal Experiment

The animal experimental procedure, approved by the Institutional Animal Care and Use Committee of Sichuan Agricultural University (SICAU-2023-082; date: 4 September 2023), involved 40 healthy 5-week-old C57BL/6N male mice housed in a controlled environment (24 ± 2 °C, 45–55% humidity, 12 h light/dark cycle) with ad libitum access to food and water. Mice were monitored daily for signs of distress (e.g., hunching, reduced movement, severe diarrhea), with humane endpoints defined as >20% body weight loss, severe dehydration, or persistent distress unresponsive to care. Inclusion criteria required healthy mice, while exclusion criteria involved signs of severe distress, >15% weight loss, or unrelated illness. Excluded mice were removed, and reasons were recorded.

All mice were randomly divided into a 2 × 2 factorial arrangement, fed irradiated basic diets, and gavaged with PBS or 50 mg EGCG/kg body weight per day, respectively (n = 16). The experiment lasted for 5 weeks, including a 4-week EGCG gavage and a 1-week DSS challenge period. DSS (2.5%, dextran sulfate sodium) was administered through drinking water to induce colitis. After the treatment, the animals were then anesthetized with isoflurane and subsequently euthanized (Figure 1).

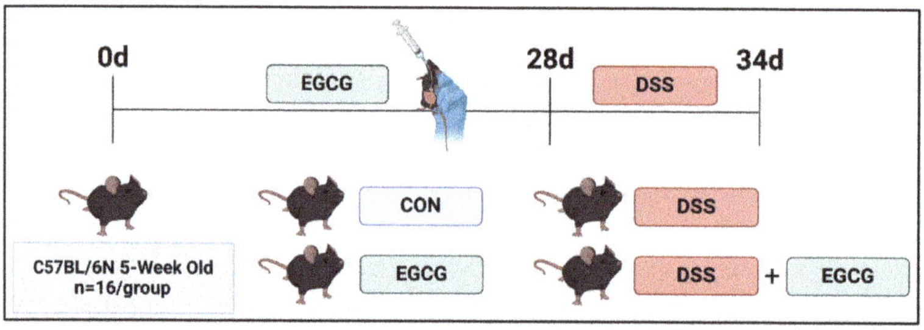

Figure 1. Timeline of the animal experiment. The test mice were divided into four groups as follows. Control group: PBS; EGCG group: 50 mg EGCG/kg body weight; DSS group: 3% DSS; DSS + EGCG group: 3% DSS + 50 mg EGCG/kg body weight. n = 16. The picture was created with BioRender.com (accessed on 10 March 2023).

To minimize potential confounders, all cages were rotated weekly within the animal housing facility to control for potential environmental effects, and feeding schedules were standardized to avoid circadian influences on metabolic outcomes.

2.3. Sample Collection

Blood was collected via cardiac puncture using anticoagulant tubes (approximately 2–3 drops). The remaining blood was transferred to 1.5 mL EP tubes and centrifuged at 4500 rpm for 10 min to collect serum. Approximately 30 mg of liver, spleen, and kidney tissues were placed into 1.5 mL EP tubes with tissue iron digestion solution for iron determination. The colon was divided into four sections, stored in separate 1.5 mL EP tubes, and used for analyses of iron content, western blot (WB), qPCR, and enzyme activity.

2.4. ROS and Lipid ROS Determination

To measure ROS, 50 μM H_2DCFDA (Sigma–Aldrich, D6883, St. Louis, MO, USA) was added to mouse colonic epithelial cells (MCEC) and incubated for 30 min at 37 °C. Lipid ROS was then detected by staining the cells with 5 μM of C11-BODIPY (Thermofisher, Waltham, MA, USA, D3861) for 30 min at 37 °C. After washing the cells three times with PBS, flow cytometry was used to analyze the results. The flow cytometric analysis was performed using a BD FACSAria III flow cytometer (BD Biosciences, Franklin Lakes, NJ, USA). The samples were analyzed under the following conditions: excitation wavelengths of 488 nm for FITC, 640 nm for PE, and 405 nm for APC channels. Emission wavelengths were set at 530/30 nm for FITC, 585/42 nm for PE, and 670/30 nm for APC. Voltage settings for forward scatter (FSC) and side scatter (SSC) were optimized for each sample to ensure accurate signal detection.

2.5. Measurement of Fe^{2+}

To measure the intracellular ferrous iron (Fe^{2+}) level, mouse colonic epithelial cells were seeded into 12-well plates. When the cells reached about 70% of the plates, they were treated with different concentrations of Fe_3S_4 nanozymes (0, 25, 50, 100 μg/mL) for 24 h and then incubated with 1 μM of Far-Red Labile Fe^{2+} dye at 37 °C for 30 min without light. After washing with PBS, the intracellular Fe^{2+} levels were analyzed by flow cytometry.

2.6. Blood Parameter Determination

The following blood parameters were measured using an automatic biochemical analyzer (Beckman Coulter, München, Germany): red blood cell count (RBC), hemoglobin (HGB), hematocrit (HCT), mean corpuscular volume (MCV), and mean corpuscular hemoglobin (MCH). Blood samples were collected via cardiac puncture on the day of sampling to ensure accuracy. All measurements were performed according to the manufacturer's instructions, and the assays were conducted in triplicate to ensure reliability.

2.7. Determination of Iron Parameters

Serum iron and non-heme iron contents in liver, spleen, and kidney tissues were determined. The measurement of liver, spleen, and kidney non-heme iron was performed as described previously by [29], with minor modifications. Briefly, tissues were homogenized in ice-cold saline, while non-heme iron was extracted using an acid digestion method and then measured by spectrophotometry. Serum iron, total iron-binding capacity (TIBC), unsaturated iron-binding capacity (UIBC), and serum transferrin (TF) were measured as described previously [30], with the addition of standard curve calibration for accurate quantification (Pointe Scientific, 416501-173). All assays were performed in triplicate.

2.8. Histological Examination of Colon

Colon tissue sections were collected from the same part (proximal colon) to minimize variability. The tissues were fixed in 4% buffered formalin at 4 °C for 24 h, then embedded in paraffin and sectioned into 4 μm-thick slices. Sections were stained with Hematoxylin and Eosin (HE) and Perls Prussian blue for evaluating tissue morphology and iron deposition, respectively. Histopathological changes were observed under a Zeiss Axioscope 5/7 Microscope.

2.9. Measurement of Malondialdehyde (MDA) and Glutathione (GSH) Levels

The levels of malondialdehyde (MDA) and glutathione (GSH) were measured using commercially available assay kits from Jiancheng Bioengineering Institute (Nanjing, China, GSH A003-1-2, MDA A003-4-1) following the manufacturer's protocol. MDA, an indicator of lipid peroxidation, was determined using the thiobarbituric acid reactive substances (TBARS) assay, and GSH levels were assessed using a colorimetric assay. All measurements were performed in triplicate, and results were expressed as nanomoles (nmol) per milligram of tissue.

2.10. qPCR and Western Blot

The extraction of hepatic and splenic total RNA was conducted by TRIzol reagent (Invitrogen, Waltham, MA, USA, 108-95-2) according to the manufacturer's specifications and diluted to 1 μg/uL. The working solution was configured in accordance with the protocols shown in the Reverse Transcription Kit (Takara, San Jose, CA, USA, RR037Q). The ΔΔCT method was used to calculate relative gene expressions by collecting the cycle threshold (Ct) and normalizing it to the housekeeping gene HPRT [31].

The isolation of colon total protein was performed with a RIPA buffer with phenylmethanesulfonylfluoride (PMSF, BeiJing, China, 1 mM). Western blotting was conducted as described previously [30]. The primary antibodies were diluted at 1:1000. CD98 (CST, 13180, Danvers, MA, USA), SLC7A11 (CST, 98051), pNRF2 (Abcam, ab76026, Cambridge, UK), NRF2 (Abcam, ab137550), HO-1 (Abcam; ab13248), P62 (Abcam, ab56416), Keap1 (Abcam, ab28913), GPX4 (Abcam, ab125066), TFR1 (Abcam, ab84036), Fpn (Abcam, ab78066), FTH/L (Abcam, ab75973). IL-6 (Abcam, ab68933), IL-1β (Abcam, ab387291), TNF-α (Abcam, ab478219), and ACSL4 (Abcam, ab512982). Secondary goat anti-mouse and anti-rabbit antibodies conjugated with HRP (Santa Cruz, Dallas, TX, USA sc-2030 and sc-2031) were diluted to a 1:3000 solution.

2.11. Enzyme-Linked Immunosorbent Assay (ELISA)

Serum IL-1β, TNF-α, and IL-8 contents were determined using the IL-1β (Jiangsu Meimian Industrial Co., Ltd., Cat#: MM-0905 M1, Nanjing, China), TNF-α (Jiangsu Meimian Industrial Co., Ltd., Cat#: MM-0132 M1), and IL-8 (Jiangsu Meimian Industrial Co., Ltd., Cat#: MM-0123 M1) ELISA kits, respectively. The actual operational steps were consistent with the instructions provided in the manual and were detailed in the Supplementary Materials.

2.12. Statistical Analysis

This study was conducted as a 2 × 2 two-factorial experiment. The results demonstrated the effects of iron overload and EGCG on mice and the interaction between high iron and EGCG in mice. All the data are expressed as the means ± standard errors (SEM) using Excel software, and we used the *t*-test and One-way/Two-way Analysis of Variance (ANOVA) to determine the relationships between groups [32]. Statistical significance levels were $p < 0.05$ (*), $p < 0.01$ (**), and $p < 0.001$ (***). All results were generated using GraphPad Prism 9 (GraphPad Software, San Diego, CA, USA).

Prior to statistical analyses, data normality and homogeneity of variance were assessed using Shapiro–Wilk and Levene's tests, respectively. In cases where assumptions were violated, appropriate non-parametric tests or data transformations were applied.

2.13. Blinding

Blinding was implemented during the outcome assessment and data analysis stages. The investigator responsible for data collection and analysis was unaware of the group allocation to prevent potential bias.

3. Results

3.1. Preventive EGCG Supplementation Alleviates DSS-Induced Colitis by Reducing Inflammation and Improving Colon Morphology

To investigate the effects of DSS-induced colitis in mice and the potential role of EGCG in mitigating these effects, we monitored the body weight of the mice over time. During the preventive EGCG gavage phase, the mice experienced an increase in body weight, but after the treatment, a significant difference was observed. The DSS group showed the lowest body weight, while EGCG treatment led to a significant recovery ($p < 0.001$) (Figure 2A). Similarly, the DSS group exhibited a significant increase in fecal occult blood index, whereas the EGCG-preventive group had a significantly lower fecal occult blood index compared to the DSS group (Figure 2B). Moreover, EGCG effectively restored the organ index disruptions caused by colitis (Figure S1).

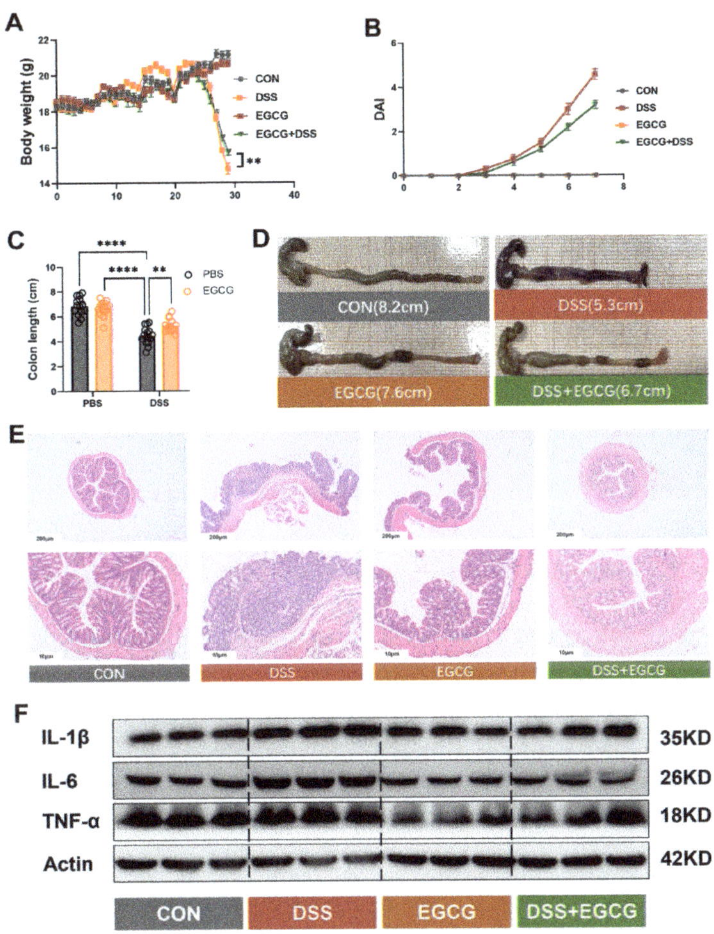

Figure 2. EGCG significantly prevents growth impairment and intestinal inflammation caused by colitis. (**A**) Body weight of mice in four groups was measured throughout the experiment. Mouse body weight was recorded every 2 days throughout the experiment (** $p < 0.01$) ($n = 16$). (**B**) The disease activity index in the last week among different treatment groups ($n = 16$). (**C**) Colon length ($n = 16$). (**D**) Measurement of colon length ($n = 16$). (**E**) Representative photographs of mice colon (scale bar = 200 μm and 50 μm) ($n = 16$). (**F**) The protein expression of IL-1β and TNF-α in colon ($n = 3$). Statistical significance is indicated as follows: ** $p < 0.01$, **** $p < 0.0001$.

In addition to body weight loss, DSS administration led to abnormalities in the colon phenotype and inflammatory response. Specifically, the DSS group exhibited a significant reduction in colon length ($p < 0.01$) (Figure 2C,D), along with pronounced inflammatory cell infiltration and increased protein expression of pro-inflammatory cytokines IL-6, IL-1β, and TNF-α ($p < 0.01$) (Figures 2E,F and S2). However, preventive supplementation with EGCG effectively alleviated these pathological changes, significantly improving colon morphology and reducing inflammatory markers.

3.2. EGCG Supplementation Improves Hematological and Iron Parameters in DSS-Induced Colitis

The blood routine parameters, including RBC, HCT, HGB, MCV, and MCH, as well as serum iron, UIBC, TIBC, and TF levels, were assessed to evaluate the impact of DSS-induced colitis and the effects of preventive EGCG supplementation (Figure 3). DSS treatment resulted in significant reductions in RBC count, HCT, and HGB levels, indicating the development of anemia, along with a decrease in serum iron, UIBC, and TF levels (Figure 3A–C,F,H,I). The decrease in these parameters reflects a disruption in iron homeostasis, which contributes to the overall inflammatory state. Furthermore, MCV was also reduced in the DSS group (Figure 3D), suggesting altered erythropoiesis and iron deficiency. Interestingly, preventive supplementation with EGCG showed a restorative effect on RBC count, HCT, HGB, serum iron, UIBC, and TF levels, demonstrating the potential of EGCG in mitigating the hematological disturbances induced by DSS-induced colitis (Figure 3A–C,F,H,I). However, no significant changes were observed in MCH and TIBC following EGCG supplementation, indicating that these two parameters may not be as responsive to EGCG intervention under the current experimental conditions (Figure 3E,G). These findings suggest that EGCG supplementation can partially reverse the hematologic and iron metabolism alterations caused by DSS-induced colitis, highlighting its potential as a therapeutic agent for inflammatory conditions associated with iron dysregulation.

3.3. Preventive EGCG Supplementation Alleviates Colitis by Regulating Tissue Iron Overload and Iron Metabolism

Analysis of tissue iron content and iron metabolism markers revealed significant changes in response to DSS-induced colitis and preventive EGCG supplementation. DSS challenge caused a notable increase in iron deposition across multiple organs, including the liver, spleen, and kidney, indicating systemic iron dysregulation. However, preventive EGCG supplementation significantly reduced iron accumulation in these organs, highlighting its role in restoring iron homeostasis. Interestingly, no significant changes were observed in colonic iron levels, potentially due to the limited capacity of the colon to sequester excess iron or its rapid utilization in local inflammatory responses.

On the molecular level, DSS treatment led to a marked upregulation of TfR1 and FTH/L at both protein and mRNA levels, consistent with increased cellular iron uptake in response to systemic iron overload. Preventive EGCG supplementation effectively reduced TfR1 and FTH/L expression, reflecting its ability to mitigate iron uptake and accumulation. Furthermore, the expression of ferroportin (Fpn, encoded by SLC40A1), the key iron-export protein, was significantly elevated in the DSS group, likely as a compensatory response to increased iron burden. EGCG supplementation normalized SLC40A1 levels, reducing the excessive iron export and contributing to systemic iron redistribution. These findings indicate that DSS-induced colitis disrupts systemic iron metabolism, leading to aberrant iron accumulation and dysregulation of key iron-related proteins. Preventive supplementation with EGCG alleviates colitis by attenuating tissue iron overload and modulating iron metabolism pathways (Figure 4).

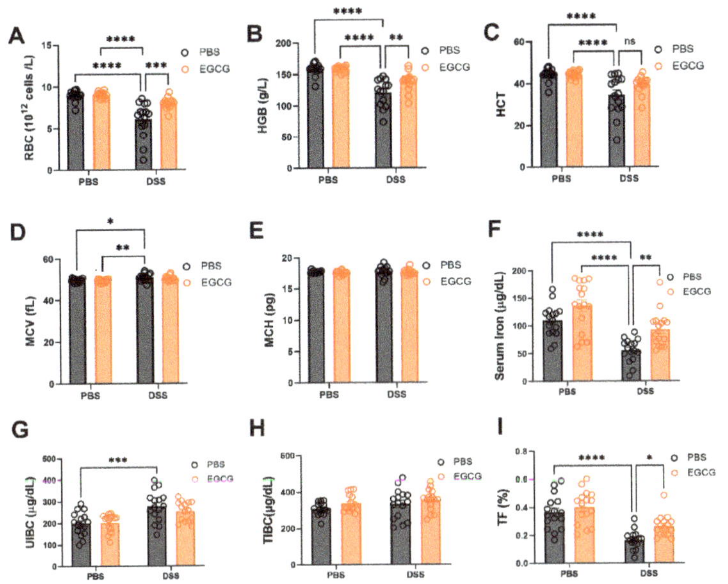

Figure 3. EGCG seems to contribute to alleviating inflammatory anemia caused by colitis. (**A**) Red blood cell count (RBC). (**B**) Hemoglobin (HGB) ($n = 16$). (**C**) Hematocrit (HCT) ($n = 16$). (**D**) Mean corpuscular volume (MCV) ($n = 16$). (**E**) Mean corpuscular hemoglobin (MCH) ($n = 16$). (**F**) Serum iron level ($n = 16$). (**G**) Unsaturated iron-binding capacity (UIBC) ($n = 16$). (**H**) Total iron-binding capacity (TIBC) ($n = 16$). (**I**) Transferrin saturation (TF) ($n = 16$). Statistical significance is indicated as follows: * $p < 0.05$, ** $p < 0.01$, *** $p < 0.001$, **** $p < 0.0001$.

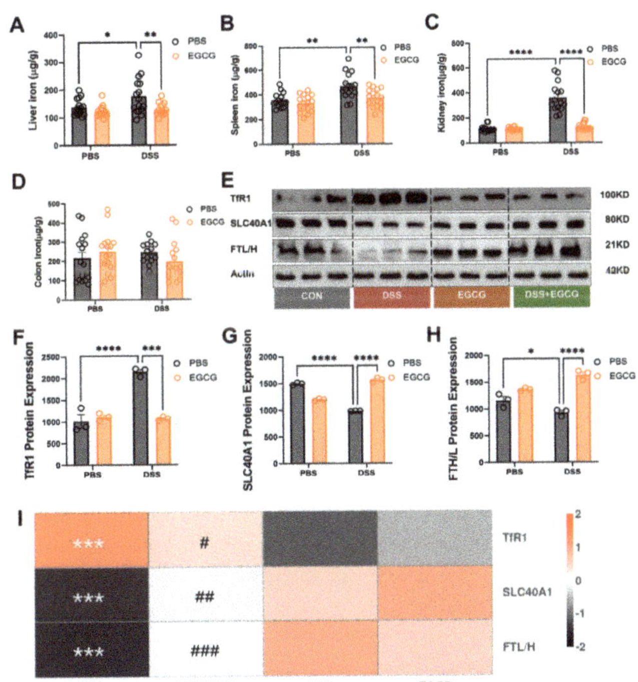

Figure 4. EGCG alleviates the disrupted iron metabolism caused by colitis. (**A**) Iron content of the liver ($n = 16$). (**B**) Iron content of the spleen ($n = 16$). (**C**) Iron content of the kidney ($n = 16$). (**D**) Iron

content of the colon (n = 16). (**E–H**) The protein expression level of TfR1, SLC40A1, and FTL in colon of mice (n = 3). (**I**) Heatmap of correlation analysis between treatment groups and proteins related to iron metabolism($^{*/\#}$ p < 0.05, $^{**/\#\#}$ p < 0.01, $^{***/\#\#\#}$ p < 0.001. * and # represent significance between different treatment groups, with * for DSS vs. CON and # for DSS+EGCG vs. DSS.). Statistical significance is indicated as follows: * $p < 0.05$, ** $p < 0.01$, *** $p < 0.001$, **** $p < 0.0001$.

3.4. EGCG Supplementation Attenuates Ferroptosis and Restores Redox Balance in DSS-Induced Colitis

Preventive EGCG supplementation demonstrated significant regulatory effects on ferroptosis markers and related proteins in DSS-induced colitis. DSS challenge led to a substantial increase in malondialdehyde (MDA), a marker of lipid peroxidation, and a marked depletion of glutathione (GSH), indicating elevated oxidative stress and ferroptosis activation. EGCG supplementation effectively reduced MDA levels and restored GSH content, alleviating oxidative damage (Figure 5A,B). At the molecular level, DSS treatment disrupted the balance of the Nrf2-signaling pathway, leading to increased expression of Nrf2, phosphorylated Nrf2 (pNRF2), and P62, along with a reduction in KEAP1 levels, a key negative regulator of Nrf2. Preventive EGCG supplementation further enhanced the activation of the Nrf2 pathway by upregulating Nrf2, pNrf2, and P62 expression while simultaneously downregulating KEAP1. This regulation contributed to the activation of the antioxidant defense system, effectively mitigating oxidative stress in DSS-induced colitis (Figure 5D,E–H). Similarly, DSS-induced colitis suppressed the expression of key ferroptosis-regulating proteins such as GPX4, SLC7A11, and SLC3A2, while elevating HO-1 levels as a compensatory response to oxidative stress. EGCG supplementation reversed these changes, significantly increasing GPX4, SLC7A11, and SLC3A2 expression and reducing HO-1 levels (Figure 5D,I–L). Furthermore, DSS treatment caused a significant upregulation of ACSL4, a critical enzyme in lipid peroxidation and ferroptosis. EGCG supplementation markedly decreased ACSL4 expression, thereby mitigating ferroptosis and lipid peroxidation (Figure 5C,D). These results highlight EGCG's therapeutic potential in alleviating ferroptosis and restoring redox homeostasis in DSS-induced colitis by modulating oxidative stress, iron metabolism, and lipid peroxidation pathways.

3.5. Preventive EGCG Supplementation Mitigates Ferroptosis and Inflammatory Responses in RSL3-Induced Cell Model

In an RSL3-induced ferroptosis model, significant cellular damage was observed, characterized by reduced cell viability and elevated ferroptosis markers. RSL3 treatment led to a marked decrease in cell viability, as assessed by CCK-8 assays (Figure 6A), accompanied by increased levels of C11-BODIPY, reactive oxygen species (ROS), and intracellular Fe^{2+}, indicating enhanced lipid peroxidation and oxidative stress (Figures 6B,C and S3A,B). Preventive EGCG supplementation effectively mitigated these effects, restoring cell viability and reducing the accumulation of ferroptosis markers. At the molecular level, RSL3 treatment induced significant inflammatory responses, as evidenced by elevated gene expression of IL-1β, IL-6, and TNF-α (Figure 6D–F). EGCG supplementation effectively suppressed these inflammatory markers, demonstrating its anti-inflammatory potential in ferroptosis-associated conditions. Furthermore, RSL3 exposure significantly increased the gene expression of PTGS2, Nrf2, pNrf2, and P62, which are associated with ferroptosis and cellular stress responses (Figure 6G,H,M,N). Simultaneously, the gene expression of ferroptosis-regulating proteins, including GPX4, SLC7A11, SLC3A2, and iron metabolism markers such as FTH, FTL, and SLC40A1, was notably downregulated, reflecting disrupted antioxidant defenses and iron homeostasis (Figure 6I–Q). EGCG supplementation reversed these changes by downregulating PTGS2, while upregulating GPX4, SLC7A11, SLC3A2, FTH, FTL, and SLC40A1 gene expression, thereby restoring redox balance and iron metabolism (Figure 6J–L,O–Q). Additionally, EGCG further increased the gene expression of P62, Nrf2, and pNrf2, while the gene expression of Keap1 continued to decrease (Figure 6H,I,M,N). These findings suggest that EGCG mitigates RSL3-induced ferroptosis by modulating oxidative stress, restoring iron metabolism, and reducing inflammatory responses, underscoring its therapeutic potential in ferroptosis-related diseases.

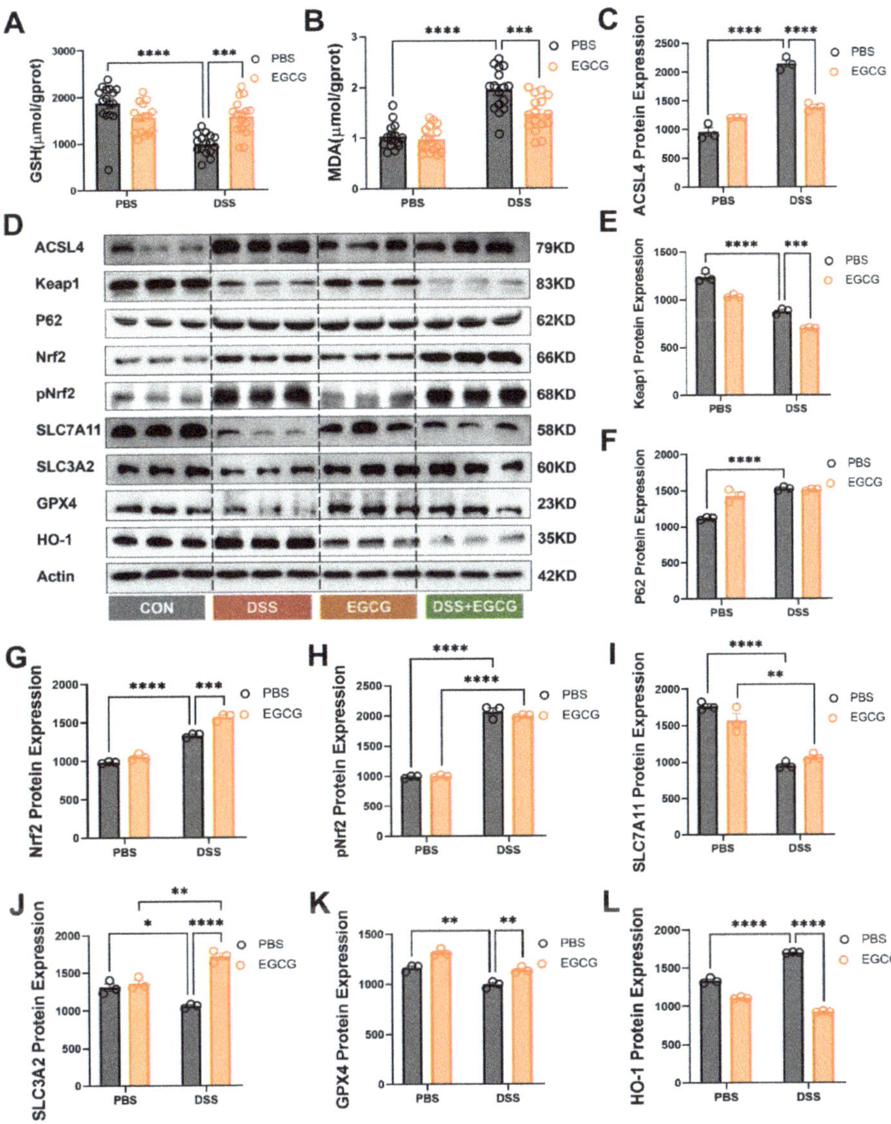

Figure 5. EGCG alleviates colitis by inhibiting the occurrence of ferroptosis in cells. (**A**) GSH level in the colon (n = 16). (**B**) MDA level in the colon (n = 16). (**C**) Quantification of ACSL4 protein expression (n = 3). (**D**) Western blot analysis of ferroptosis-related protein expression (n = 3). (**E–L**) Quantification of Keap1, P62, Nrf2, pNrf2, SLC7A11, SLC3A2, GPX4, and HO-1 protein expression (n = 3). Statistical significance is indicated as follows: * $p < 0.05$, ** $p < 0.01$, *** $p < 0.001$, **** $p < 0.0001$.

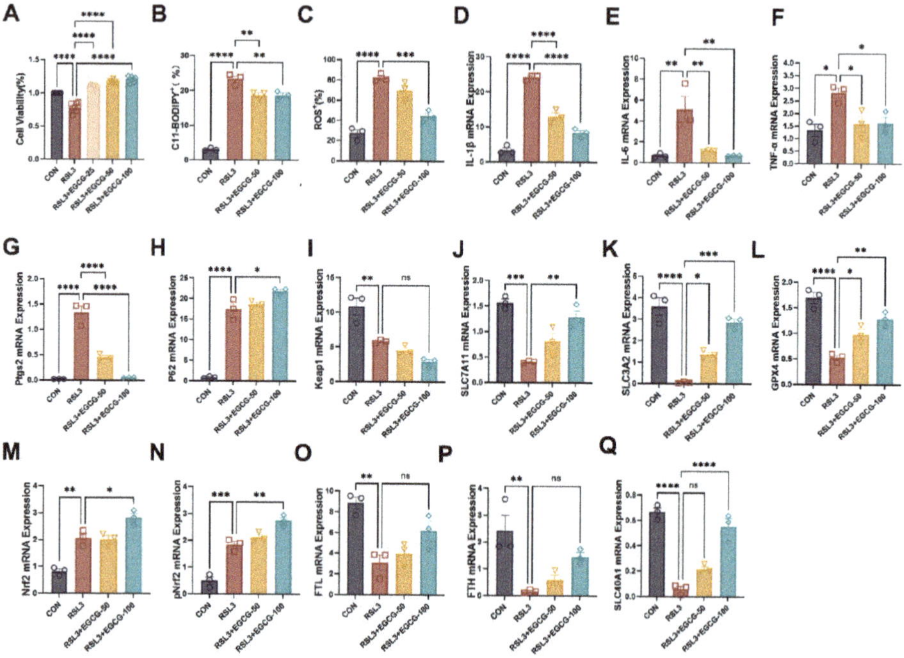

Figure 6. EGCG inhibits ferroptosis in MCEC. (**A**) Cell viability ($n = 6$). (**B**) Positive rate of lipid peroxidation in MCEC ($n = 3$). (**C**) Positive rate of total ROS in MCEC ($n = 3$). (**D–Q**) IL-1β, IL-6,TNF-α, Ptgs2, P62, Keap1, SLC7A11, SLC3A2, GPX4, Nrf2, pNrf2, FTL, FTH, and SLC40A1 mRNA expression were tested by qPCR ($n = 3$). Statistical significance is indicated as follows: ^{ns} $p < 0.1$, * $p < 0.05$, ** $p < 0.01$, *** $p < 0.001$, **** $p < 0.0001$.

4. Discussion

The present study underscores the therapeutic potential of epigallocatechin-3-gallate (EGCG) in mitigating DSS-induced colitis through its multifaceted actions on inflammation, oxidative stress, iron metabolism, and ferroptosis. Beyond its direct effects observed in our experimental models, these findings invite broader insights into the pathophysiological mechanisms of colitis and the potential applicability of EGCG in related diseases.

Colitis, a hallmark of inflammatory bowel diseases (IBD), is driven by chronic immune activation and a breakdown of intestinal barrier function [33]. Inflammatory cytokines such as IL-6, IL-1β, and TNF-α play pivotal roles in exacerbating tissue damage, and oxidative stress further aggravates the inflammatory milieu [34]. Many studies have highlighted the central role of oxidative stress in IBD pathology. For instance, Zeng et al. (2022) reported that elevated ROS levels impair epithelial integrity and activate inflammatory cascades [35]. In our study, DSS-induced colitis resulted in pronounced oxidative damage, reflected by elevated MDA levels and GSH depletion. These findings align with the established notion that oxidative stress is a driver of IBD progression, emphasizing the need for antioxidant-based interventions. EGCG's ability to restore GSH and reduce MDA levels confirms its potent antioxidant capacity, consistent with prior studies demonstrating EGCG's role in reducing oxidative stress through Nrf2 activation (Zhang et al., 2020). This suggests that EGCG may act as a dual-function agent, modulating both inflammation and oxidative stress pathways [36].

The disruption of systemic iron metabolism in colitis adds another layer of complexity to the disease mechanism [37]. Iron, a critical cofactor for cellular functions, becomes pathogenic when dysregulated, contributing to oxidative damage and ferroptosis [38]. Iron overload in the liver, spleen, and kidney observed in DSS-treated mice mirrors findings by Swanson et al. (2019), who noted that excessive iron exacerbates inflammatory responses through the Fenton reaction, leading to increased ROS production [39]. Our study demonstrated that EGCG supplementation significantly reduced iron accumulation in these tissues, possibly by regulating key mediators of iron metabolism such as TfR1 and SLC40A1. These findings align with earlier reports showing that EGCG's iron-chelating properties attenuate hepatic iron overload. Interestingly, we observed no significant changes in colonic iron levels despite systemic dysregulation. This may be attributed to the rapid utilization of free iron in local inflammatory responses, a hypothesis supported by Chen et al. (2024), who noted that colonic epithelial cells prioritize iron utilization for rapid turnover during inflammation [40,41].

One of the most intriguing aspects of this study is the interplay between ferroptosis and colitis [42]. Ferroptosis, a regulated form of cell death driven by iron-dependent lipid peroxidation, has emerged as a central mechanism in inflammatory and degenerative diseases [43]. Increased ACSL4 expression and reduced GPX4 levels observed in our study confirm ferroptosis activation in DSS-treated mice, consistent with the findings of Xu et al. (2020), who demonstrated ferroptosis as a critical contributor to epithelial cell death in IBD [44,45]. EGCG supplementation mitigated these changes, restoring GPX4 and reducing ACSL4 expression, highlighting its potential to regulate ferroptosis through both antioxidant and iron homeostasis pathways [45]. Additionally, the role of Nrf2 signaling in ferroptosis cannot be overlooked. DSS treatment disrupted the Nrf2 pathway by increasing p Nrf2 and P62 while suppressing Keap1 [46,47]. EGCG effectively restored Nrf2 pathway homeostasis, a finding consistent with Sun et al. (2021), who demonstrated that Nrf2 activation protects against ferroptosis by upregulating GPX4 and SLC7A11 [42].

From a translational perspective, the restoration of hematological parameters by EGCG highlights its potential clinical relevance. Anemia of inflammation, a common comorbidity in IBD, is characterized by impaired erythropoiesis and iron sequestration. DSS-treated mice exhibited reduced RBC, HCT, and HGB levels, reflecting these hallmarks. EGCG's ability to normalize these parameters by modulating iron homeostasis and reducing inflammatory cytokines underscores its potential to address anemia in inflammatory conditions. This is consistent with the work of Ganz (2020), who emphasized the importance of hepcidin-SLC40A1 regulation in anemia of inflammation [13]. By downregulating TfR1 and normalizing SLC40A1 expression, EGCG appears to modulate the Hamp1-SLC40A1 axis, a critical pathway in maintaining systemic iron balance.

Our findings also extend to the role of EGCG in the cellular context, as demonstrated in the RSL3-induced ferroptosis cell model. The reduction of IL-1β, IL-6, and TNF-α by EGCG reflects its anti-inflammatory properties, which are well-documented in the literature [34]. Furthermore, EGCG's regulation of ferroptosis-related proteins, such as GPX4, SLC7A11, and ACSL4, aligns with its observed effects in vivo, underscoring its dual anti-inflammatory and anti-ferroptosis mechanisms [48]. These observations highlight the potential of EGCG as a therapeutic agent for ferroptosis-related diseases, extending beyond colitis to conditions such as neurodegenerative diseases and cancer, as suggested by Tang et al. (2024) [49,50].

In conclusion, this study reveals the multifaceted mechanisms through which EGCG mitigates DSS-induced colitis, encompassing anti-inflammatory, antioxidant, and ferroptosis-regulatory pathways. Its ability to restore iron homeostasis and suppress ferroptosis highlights its therapeutic potential in inflammatory and ferroptosis-associated diseases. Future research should focus on optimizing EGCG formulations to enhance bioavailability and exploring its synergistic potential with existing therapies to fully harness its clinical utility.

5. Conclusions

This study has limitations, including the inability of the DSS-induced colitis model to fully mimic human IBD complexity and a small sample size, which may limit generalizability. Future studies with larger cohorts and alternative models are needed. Despite this, EGCG shows potential as an IBD therapy. Future research should explore its efficacy in humans, optimize dosage and bioavailability, and evaluate its combination with existing treatments. Additionally, investigating EGCG's role in other inflammatory and iron-related diseases could expand its clinical applications.

Supplementary Materials: The following supporting information can be downloaded at: https://www.mdpi.com/article/10.3390/nu17030547/s1. Figure S1. EGCG might mitigate the abnormal organ measurements linked to colitis. (A) Liver weight in different treatment groups. (B) Spleen weight in different treatment groups. (C) Kidney weight in different treatment groups. (D) Liver index (liver weight/body weight ratio). (E) Spleen index (liver weight/body weight ratio). (F) Kidney index (liver weight/body weight ratio). Statistical significance is indicated as follows: * $p < 0.05$, ** $p < 0.01$, *** $p < 0.001$, **** $p < 0.0001$. Figure S2. Effects of EGCG on Inflammatory Markers IL-6, IL-1β, and TNF-α in Colitis. (A) Serum IL-1β content. (B) Serum IL-6 content. (C) Serum TNF-α content. Statistical significance is indicated as follows: * $p < 0.05$, ** $p < 0.01$, *** $p < 0.001$, **** $p < 0.0001$. Figure S3. EGCG Inhibits ROS and Fe^{2+} to Alleviate Ferroptosis. (A) Flow cytometry images of lipid peroxidation in MCEC. The cells were stained with 5 μM C11-BODIPY, a dye used to detect lipid peroxidation. Flow cytometry analysis was performed to assess the positive rate of lipid peroxidation in MCEC after treatment with EGCG and RSL3. (B) Flow cytometry histogram of labile iron pool (LIP) in MCEC.

Author Contributions: J.C., C.Y., Y.Z., X.L., Q.W. and H.W.: performed experiments. J.C., C.Y., X.L., Y.Z., D.C. and A.W.: designed experiments. J.C., C.Y. and C.L.: wrote the paper. J.C., C.Y., Y.Z., Y.L., J.L., J.H., B.Y., D.C. and A.W.: interpreted data and modified the paper. D.C. and A.W.: funding acquisition. All authors have read and agreed to the published version of the manuscript.

Funding: This work was supported by the National Natural Science Foundation of Sichuan Province (Grant No. 2024NSFSC0297) and the Joint Funds of the National Natural Science Foundation of China (Grant No. U22A20513).

Institutional Review Board Statement: The animal study protocol was approved by the Institutional Animal Care and Use Committee of the Laboratory Animal Center at Sichuan Agricultural University (SICAU-2020-063, approval date: 4 September 2023).

Informed Consent Statement: Not applicable.

Data Availability Statement: This study was not pre-registered in a publicly accessible protocol repository, as is common in preclinical animal research. Future studies will aim to follow standardized protocol registration practices. The datasets generated and analyzed during the current study are available from the corresponding author upon reasonable request.

Acknowledgments: The authors would like to thank the Teaturn Bio-pharmaceutical Co., Ltd. (Wuxi, China) for the EGCG materials used for the experiments.

Conflicts of Interest: The authors declare that there are no conflicts of interest.

Abbreviations

Abbreviations	Full Name
ACSL4	Acyl-CoA synthetase long-chain family member 4
FAC	Ferric citrate

FTH/L	Ferritin heavy/light chain
Fpn	Ferroportin(SLC40A1)
GSH	Glutathione
GPX4	Glutathione peroxidase 4
HGB	Hemoglobin
HCT	Hematocrit
IL-6	Interleukin-6
IL-1β	Interleukin-1β
HO-1	Heme oxygenase 1
Keap1	Kelch-like ECH-associated protein 1
MCV	Mean corpuscular volume
MCH	Mean corpuscular hemoglobin
MCHC	Mean corpuscular hemoglobin concentration
MDA	Malondialdehyde
Nrf2	Nuclear factor erythroid 2-related factor 2
pNrf2	Phosphorylated Nuclear factor erythroid 2-related factor 2
P62	Sequestosome 1
RBC	Red blood cell count
ROS	Reactive oxygen species
SLC3A2	Solute carrier family 3 member 2
SLC7A11	Solute carrier family 7 member 11
TF	Transferrin saturation
TIBC	Total iron binding capacity
TfR1	Transferrin receptor 1
TNF-α	Tumor Necrosis Factor-alpha
UIBC	Unsaturated iron binding capacity

References

1. Kaplan, G.G.; Ng, S.C. Understanding and preventing the global increase of inflammatory bowel disease. *Gastroenterology* **2017**, *152*, 313–321.e312. [CrossRef] [PubMed]
2. Molodecky, N.A.; Kaplan, G.G. Environmental risk factors for inflammatory bowel disease. *Gastroenterol. Hepatol.* **2010**, *6*, 339.
3. Kobayashi, T.; Siegmund, B.; Le Berre, C.; Wei, S.C.; Ferrante, M.; Shen, B.; Bernstein, C.N.; Danese, S.; Peyrin-Biroulet, L.; Hibi, T. Ulcerative colitis (primer). *Nat. Rev. Dis. Primers* **2020**, *6*, 74. [CrossRef] [PubMed]
4. Ng, S.C.; Shi, H.Y.; Hamidi, N.; Underwood, F.E.; Tang, W.; Benchimol, E.I.; Panaccione, R.; Ghosh, S.; Wu, J.C.Y.; Chan, F.K.L.; et al. Worldwide incidence and prevalence of inflammatory bowel disease in the 21st century: A systematic review of population-based studies. *Lancet* **2017**, *390*, 2769–2778. [CrossRef]
5. Seyedian, S.S.; Nokhostin, F.; Malamir, M.D. A review of the diagnosis, prevention, and treatment methods of inflammatory bowel disease. *J. Med. Life* **2019**, *12*, 113. [CrossRef]
6. Xie, H.; Cao, C.; Shu, D.; Liu, T.; Zhang, T. The important role of ferroptosis in inflammatory bowel disease. *Front. Med.* **2024**, *11*, 1449037. [CrossRef]
7. Niu, R.; Lan, J.; Liang, D.; Xiang, L.; Wu, J.; Zhang, X.; Li, Z.; Chen, H.; Geng, L.; Xu, W.; et al. GZMA suppressed GPX4-mediated ferroptosis to improve intestinal mucosal barrier function in inflammatory bowel disease. *Cell Commun. Signal.* **2024**, *22*, 474. [CrossRef]
8. Puig, S.; Ramos-Alonso, L.; Romero, A.M.; Martínez-Pastor, M.T. The elemental role of iron in DNA synthesis and repair. *Metallomics* **2017**, *9*, 1483–1500. [CrossRef]
9. Venkataramani, V. Iron homeostasis and metabolism: Two sides of a coin. *Ferroptosis Mech. Dis.* **2021**, *1301*, 25–40.
10. Rochette, L.; Dogon, G.; Rigal, E.; Zeller, M.; Cottin, Y.; Vergely, C. Lipid peroxidation and iron metabolism: Two corner stones in the homeostasis control of ferroptosis. *Int. J. Mol. Sci.* **2022**, *24*, 449. [CrossRef]
11. Lee, J.; Hyun, D.-H. The interplay between intracellular iron homeostasis and neuroinflammation in neurodegenerative diseases. *Antioxidants* **2023**, *12*, 918. [CrossRef] [PubMed]
12. Dixon, S.J.; Lemberg, K.M.; Lamprecht, M.R.; Skouta, R.; Zaitsev, E.M.; Gleason, C.E.; Patel, D.N.; Bauer, A.J.; Cantley, A.M.; Yang, W.S.; et al. Ferroptosis: An iron-dependent form of nonapoptotic cell death. *Cell* **2012**, *149*, 1060–1072. [CrossRef] [PubMed]
13. Stockwell, B.R.; Angeli, J.P.F.; Bayir, H.; Bush, A.I.; Conrad, M.; Dixon, S.J.; Fulda, S.; Gascón, S.; Hatzios, S.K.; Kagan, V.E.; et al. Ferroptosis: A regulated cell death nexus linking metabolism, redox biology, and disease. *Cell* **2017**, *171*, 273–285. [CrossRef]

14. Yang, W.S.; SriRamaratnam, R.; Welsch, M.E.; Shimada, K.; Skouta, R.; Viswanathan, V.S.; Cheah, J.H.; Clemons, P.A.; Shamji, A.F.; Clish, C.B.; et al. Regulation of ferroptotic cancer cell death by GPX4. *Cell* **2014**, *156*, 317–331. [CrossRef]
15. Doll, S.; Freitas, F.P.; Shah, R.; Aldrovandi, M.; da Silva, M.C.; Ingold, I.; Grocin, A.G.; da Silva, T.N.X.; Panzilius, E.; Scheel, C.H.; et al. FSP1 is a glutathione-independent ferroptosis suppressor. *Nature* **2019**, *575*, 693–698. [CrossRef]
16. Friedmann Angeli, J.P.; Schneider, M.; Proneth, B.; Tyurina, Y.Y.; Tyurin, V.A.; Hammond, V.J.; Herbach, N.; Aichler, M.; Walch, A.; Eggenhofer, E.; et al. Inactivation of the ferroptosis regulator Gpx4 triggers acute renal failure in mice. *Nat. Cell Biol.* **2014**, *16*, 1180–1191. [CrossRef]
17. Zou, Y.; Palte, M.J.; Deik, A.A.; Li, H.; Eaton, J.K.; Wang, W.; Tseng, Y.-Y.; Deasy, R.; Kost-Alimova, M.; Dančík, V.; et al. A GPX4-dependent cancer cell state underlies the clear-cell morphology and confers sensitivity to ferroptosis. *Nat. Commun.* **2019**, *10*, 1617. [CrossRef]
18. Yang, W.S.; Kim, K.J.; Gaschler, M.M.; Patel, M.; Shchepinov, M.S.; Stockwell, B.R. Peroxidation of polyunsaturated fatty acids by lipoxygenases drives ferroptosis. *Proc. Natl. Acad. Sci. USA* **2016**, *113*, E4966–E4975. [CrossRef]
19. Chen, X.; Kang, R.; Kroemer, G.; Tang, D. Broadening horizons: The role of ferroptosis in cancer. *Nat. Rev. Clin. Oncol.* **2021**, *18*, 280–296. [CrossRef]
20. Osterholm, E.A.; Georgieff, M.K. Chronic inflammation and iron metabolism. *J. Pediatr.* **2015**, *166*, 1351–1357.e1351. [CrossRef]
21. Sun, Y.; Chen, P.; Zhai, B.; Zhang, M.; Xiang, Y.; Fang, J.; Xu, S.; Gao, Y.; Chen, X.; Sui, X.; et al. The emerging role of ferroptosis in inflammation. *Biomed. Pharmacother.* **2020**, *127*, 110108. [CrossRef] [PubMed]
22. Wan, Y.; Yang, L.; Jiang, S.; Qian, D.; Duan, J. Excessive apoptosis in ulcerative colitis: Crosstalk between apoptosis, ROS, ER stress, and intestinal homeostasis. *Inflamm. Bowel Dis.* **2022**, *28*, 639–648. [CrossRef] [PubMed]
23. Yang, C.; Wu, A.; Tan, L.; Tang, D.; Chen, W.; Lai, X.; Gu, K.; Chen, J.; Chen, D.; Tang, Q. Epigallocatechin-3-Gallate alleviates liver oxidative damage caused by Iron overload in mice through inhibiting Ferroptosis. *Nutrients* **2023**, *15*, 1993. [CrossRef] [PubMed]
24. Bao, G.-H.; Xu, J.; Hu, F.-L.; Wan, X.-C.; Deng, S.-X.; Barasch, J. EGCG inhibit chemical reactivity of iron through forming an Ngal–EGCG–iron complex. *Biometals* **2013**, *26*, 1041–1050. [CrossRef]
25. Muro, P.; Zhang, L.; Li, S.; Zhao, Z.; Jin, T.; Mao, F.; Mao, Z. The emerging role of oxidative stress in inflammatory bowel disease. *Front. Endocrinol.* **2024**, *15*, 1390351. [CrossRef]
26. Xu, S.; He, Y.; Lin, L.; Chen, P.; Chen, M.; Zhang, S. The emerging role of ferroptosis in intestinal disease. *Cell Death Dis.* **2021**, *12*, 289. [CrossRef]
27. Li, L.; Peng, P.; Ding, N.; Jia, W.; Huang, C.; Tang, Y. Oxidative stress, inflammation, gut dysbiosis: What can polyphenols do in inflammatory bowel disease? *Antioxidants* **2023**, *12*, 967. [CrossRef]
28. Inoue, H.; Akiyama, S.; Maeda-Yamamoto, M.; Nesumi, A.; Tanaka, T.; Murakami, A. High-dose green tea polyphenols induce nephrotoxicity in dextran sulfate sodium-induced colitis mice by down-regulation of antioxidant enzymes and heat-shock protein expressions. *Cell Stress Chaperones* **2011**, *16*, 653–662. [CrossRef]
29. Yamanishi, H.; Iyama, S.; Yamaguchi, Y.; Kanakura, Y.; Iwatani, Y. Total iron-binding capacity calculated from serum transferrin concentration or serum iron concentration and unsaturated iron-binding capacity. *Clin. Chem.* **2003**, *49*, 175–178. [CrossRef]
30. Chezmar, J.L.; Nelson, R.C.; Malko, J.A.; Bernardino, M.E. Hepatic iron overload: Diagnosis and quantification by noninvasive imaging. *Gastrointest. Radiol.* **1990**, *15*, 27–31. [CrossRef]
31. Lai, X.; Wu, A.; Bing, Y.; Liu, Y.; Luo, J.; Yan, H.; Zheng, P.; Yu, J.; Chen, D. Retinoic acid protects against lipopolysaccharide-induced ferroptotic liver injury and iron disorders by regulating Nrf2/HO-1 and RARβ signaling. *Free Radic. Biol. Med.* **2023**, *205*, 202–213. [CrossRef] [PubMed]
32. Festing, M.F. Design and statistical methods in studies using animal models of development. *Ilar J.* **2006**, *47*, 5–14. [CrossRef] [PubMed]
33. Piechota-Polanczyk, A.; Fichna, J. The role of oxidative stress in pathogenesis and treatment of inflammatory bowel diseases. *Naunyn-Schmiedeberg's Arch. Pharmacol.* **2014**, *387*, 605–620. [CrossRef]
34. Mokra, D.; Joskova, M.; Mokry, J. Therapeutic effects of green tea polyphenol (−)-Epigallocatechin-3-Gallate (EGCG) in relation to molecular pathways controlling inflammation, oxidative stress, and apoptosis. *Int. J. Mol. Sci.* **2022**, *24*, 340. [CrossRef]
35. Zeng, F.; Shi, Y.; Wu, C.; Liang, J.; Zhong, Q.; Briley, K.; Xu, B.; Huang, Y.; Long, M.; Wang, C.; et al. A drug-free nanozyme for mitigating oxidative stress and inflammatory bowel disease. *J. Nanobiotechnol.* **2022**, *20*, 107. [CrossRef]
36. Wang, J.; Jia, R.; Celi, P.; Ding, X.; Bai, S.; Zeng, Q.; Mao, X.; Xu, S.; Zhang, K. Green tea polyphenol epigallocatechin-3-gallate improves the antioxidant capacity of eggs. *Food Funct.* **2020**, *11*, 534–543. [CrossRef]
37. Walker, E.M.; Walker, S.M. Effects of iron overload on the immune system. *Ann. Clin. Lab. Sci.* **2000**, *30*, 354–365.
38. Simmen, S.; Cosin-Roger, J.; Melhem, H.; Maliachovas, N.; Maane, M.; Baebler, K.; Weder, B.; Maeyashiki, C.; Spanaus, K.; Scharl, M.; et al. Iron prevents hypoxia-associated inflammation through the regulation of nuclear factor-κB in the intestinal epithelium. *Cell. Mol. Gastroenterol. Hepatol.* **2019**, *7*, 339–355. [CrossRef]
39. Swanson, K.V.; Deng, M.; Ting, J.P.-Y. The NLRP3 inflammasome: Molecular activation and regulation to therapeutics. *Nat. Rev. Immunol.* **2019**, *19*, 477–489. [CrossRef]

40. Chen, H.; Li, Y.-Y.; Nio, K.; Tang, H. Unveiling the Impact of BMP9 in Liver Diseases: Insights into Pathogenesis and Therapeutic Potential. *Biomolecules* **2024**, *14*, 1013. [CrossRef]
41. Weiss, G.; Ganz, T.; Goodnough, L.T. Anemia of inflammation. *Blood J. Am. Soc. Hematol.* **2019**, *133*, 40–50. [CrossRef] [PubMed]
42. Sun, Y.; He, L.; Wang, T.; Hua, W.; Qin, H.; Wang, J.; Wang, L.; Gu, W.; Li, T.; Li, N.; et al. Activation of p62-Keap1-Nrf2 pathway protects 6-hydroxydopamine-induced ferroptosis in dopaminergic cells. *Mol. Neurobiol.* **2020**, *57*, 4628–4641. [CrossRef] [PubMed]
43. Wang, S.; Wang, R.; Hu, D.; Zhang, C.; Cao, P.; Huang, J.; Wang, B. Epigallocatechin gallate modulates ferroptosis through downregulation of tsRNA-13502 in non-small cell lung cancer. *Cancer Cell Int.* **2024**, *24*, 200. [CrossRef] [PubMed]
44. Xu, M.; Tao, J.; Yang, Y.; Tan, S.; Liu, H.; Jiang, J.; Zheng, F.; Wu, B. Ferroptosis involves in intestinal epithelial cell death in ulcerative colitis. *Cell Death Dis.* **2020**, *11*, 86. [CrossRef]
45. Moerke, C.; Theilig, F.; Kunzendorf, U.; Krautwald, S. ACSL4 as the first reliable biomarker of ferroptosis under pathophysiological conditions. *Ferroptosis Health Dis.* **2019**, 111–123. [CrossRef]
46. Han, H.; Zhang, G.; Zhang, X.; Zhao, Q. Nrf2-mediated ferroptosis inhibition: A novel approach for managing inflammatory diseases. *Inflammopharmacology* **2024**, *32*, 2961–2986. [CrossRef]
47. Zhou, X.; Liang, L.; Zhao, Y.; Zhang, H. Epigallocatechin-3-gallate ameliorates angiotensin II-induced oxidative stress and apoptosis in human umbilical vein endothelial cells through the activation of Nrf2/caspase-3 signaling. *J. Vasc. Res.* **2017**, *54*, 299–308. [CrossRef]
48. Yue, L.; Yang, Y.-R.; Ma, W.-X.; Wang, H.-Y.; Fan, Q.-W.; Wang, Y.-Y.; Li, C.; Wang, J.; Hu, Z.-M.; Wang, X.-F.; et al. Epigallocatechin gallate attenuates gentamicin-induced nephrotoxicity by suppressing apoptosis and ferroptosis. *Molecules* **2022**, *27*, 8564. [CrossRef]
49. Tang, S.; Zhang, Y.; Botchway, B.O.; Wang, X.; Huang, M.; Liu, X. Epigallocatechin-3-Gallate Inhibits Oxidative Stress Through the Keap1/Nrf2 Signaling Pathway to Improve Alzheimer Disease. *Mol. Neurobiol.* **2024**, 1–15. [CrossRef]
50. Wheeler, D.S.; Catravas, J.D.; Odoms, K.; Denenberg, A.; Malhotra, V.; Wong, H.R. Epigallocatechin-3-gallate, a green tea–derived polyphenol, inhibits IL-1β-dependent proinflammatory signal transduction in cultured respiratory epithelial cells. *J. Nutr.* **2004**, *134*, 1039–1044. [CrossRef]

nutrients

MDPI

Article

Unveiling the Anti-Aging Potential of 3HB: Lifespan Extension and Cellular Senescence Delay

Yongpan An [1,2], Qian Wang [1], Panshuang Qiao [2], Jihan Liu [2], Ang Ma [3], Yutong Chen [1], Daqian Yang [1], Yi Ying [2], Nannan Li [2], Feng Lu [2], Hang Zhang [2], Guoqiang Chen [4], Yinhua Zhu [3], Baoxue Yang [2,*] and Zhengwei Xie [1,2,5,6,*]

[1] Peking University International Cancer Institute, Health Science Center, Peking University, 38 Xueyuan Lu, Haidian District, Beijing 100191, China; anyongpan123@163.com (Y.A.); 2211110101@stu.pku.edu.cn (Q.W.); cyt18304335821@163.com (Y.C.); yangdaqian9206@163.com (D.Y.)

[2] Department of Pharmacology, School of Basic Medical Sciences, Peking University, 38 Xueyuan Lu, Haidian District, Beijing 100191, China; panshuangqiao@bjmu.edu.cn (P.Q.); liujihan@stu.pku.edu.cn (J.L.); yingyi1125@163.com (Y.Y.); 1610305107@pku.edu.cn (N.L.); fenglu202110@163.com (F.L.); hangzhang@bjmu.edu.cn (H.Z.)

[3] State Key Laboratory for Quality Ensurance and Sustainable Use of Dao-di Herbs, Artemisinin Research Center, Institute of Chinese Materia Medica, China Academy of Chinese Medical Sciences, Beijing 100700, China; ama@icmm.ac.cn (A.M.); zhuyinhua@cau.edu.cn (Y.Z.)

[4] School of Life Sciences, Tsinghua University, Beijing 100084, China; chengq@tsinghua.edu.cn

[5] State Key Laboratory of Natural and Biomimetic Drugs, Department of Molecular and Cellular Pharmacology, School of Pharmaceutical Sciences, Peking University Health Science Center, 38 Xueyuan Lu, Haidian District, Beijing 100191, China

[6] Peking University—Yunnan Baiyao International Medical Research Center, Peking University Health Science Center, Peking University, 38 Xueyuan Lu, Haidian District, Beijing 100191, China

* Correspondence: baoxue@bjmu.edu.cn (B.Y.); xiezhengwei@hsc.pku.edu.cn (Z.X.)

Abstract: Background/Objective: Aging is a significant risk factor for chronic diseases and disability, yet effective anti-aging interventions remain elusive. We explored the potential of 3-hydroxybutyrate (3HB), an endogenous metabolite with established safety, to modulate longevity in mice. Methods: In this study, we employed 2BS and WI-38 cell models, a yeast model, and naturally aging mouse models to investigate the effects of 3HB on aging in various systems. Additionally, we utilized RNA sequencing and metabolomics technologies to explore the potential mechanisms underlying the action of 3HB. Results: Our findings demonstrate that 3HB supplementation effectively delays cellular senescence, extending yeast lifespan by 51.3% and the median lifespan of naturally senescent mice by 21.0%. Notably, 3HB prolonged healthy lifespan in mice while mitigating age-related tissue morphology changes and organ senescence. Mechanistically, we identified that 3HB's anti-aging properties are mediated through its ability to delay cellular senescence and metabolic reprogramming, while promoting the production of beneficial metabolites like trigoneline and isoguvacine. Conclusions: These findings highlight the promising therapeutic potential of 3HB as an anti-aging intervention and provide novel insights into its underlying mechanisms.

Keywords: 3HB; aging; cellular senescence; metabolism

1. Introduction

Human aging, a complex biological tapestry woven from declining physiological function, diminished resilience, and heightened susceptibility to disease, poses a growing challenge as our population ages rapidly. Globally, the over 65 demographic outpaces all others, with the United Nations predicting one in six people will exceed 65 by 2050, while the over 80 population triples. This demographic shift intensifies the urgency of unraveling

https://doi.org/10.3390/nu17101647

aging's intricate mechanisms, as its shadow looms large over chronic diseases like cardiovascular pathologies, cancer, and neurodegenerative disorders [1,2]. Understanding how to decelerate aging and compress its associated maladies thus emerges as a pivotal quest for our society.

Driven by the desire to extend lifespans and curb the tide of age-related diseases, the past decade has witnessed a surge in anti-aging strategies. From regenerative medicine and gene therapy to dietary tweaks, like ketogenic diets and calorie restriction, the scientific community has explored diverse avenues. However, while dietary and lifestyle interventions face challenges in adherence and long-term sustainability, more invasive approaches, like regenerative medicine and gene therapy, remain largely experimental and ethically complex. This has thrust the development of aging intervention drugs to the forefront, offering a potentially less intrusive and scalable solution. Anti-aging drug candidates, like dasatinib + quercetin [3], β-nicotinamide mononucleotide (NMN) [4], metformin [5,6], oridonin [7], Alpha-Ketoglutarate [8], berberine [9], and rapamycin [10,11], have shown promise, yet their clinical translation requires extensive research and rigorous safety assessments. The need for safer, easier-to-apply compounds with comparable efficacy remains, calling for continued innovation in this burgeoning field.

Emerging as a promising candidate in the anti-aging arsenal is 3-hydroxybutyrate (3HB), a naturally occurring metabolite with a favorable safety profile. Derived from human ketone bodies, 3HB boasts a wide range of safe doses. Its precursor, 1,3-butanediol (1,3-BDO), readily converts to 3HB in the liver, fueling bodily functions and holding a recognized status as a safe food additive [12]. Beyond its established uses, compelling evidence points towards 3HB's therapeutic potential in diverse age-related ailments, like atherosclerosis [13], diabetes [12], muscular dystrophy [14], colitis [15], and kidney-related diseases [16]. 3HB's influence extends beyond specific diseases, impacting vascular aging and even demonstrating lifespan extension in fruit flies and nematodes [17–19]. Intriguingly, the ketogenic diet, known to elevate 3HB levels, also exhibits lifespan-extending effects in mice, suggesting a potential link between 3HB and the diet's longevity benefits [20,21]. However, a crucial question remains: can direct 3HB supplementation replicate these lifespan-extending effects in mammals and enhance their healthy lifespan?

Cellular senescence and metabolic dysregulation are hallmarks of aging, making their modulation key targets for anti-aging interventions. As an endogenous metabolite with established safety due to its precursor's use as a food additive, 3HB holds promise. Studies have shown its ability to improve metabolic health in mice alongside a ketogenic diet. However, its impact on cellular senescence and specific lifespan-extending metabolite changes remained unclear.

We addressed these crucial gaps by demonstrating that 3HB directly delays cellular senescence, extends lifespans in both yeast and mice (including healthy lifespan), and mitigates age-related tissue and organ decline. Mechanistically, this anti-aging effect appears to involve both senescence delay and the promotion of beneficial metabolites like trigoneline and isoguvacine. Notably, 3HB also presents cost advantages due to its availability from microbial poly-(3-hydroxybutyrate) [22]. These findings establish 3HB as a promising anti-aging candidate with a well-tolerated precursor, providing both practical and theoretical value for future research and potential applications.

2. Materials and Methods

2.1. Drug Source

Since 3HB is stably preserved as 3HB-Na, in this experiment, we all utilized 3HB-Na for the experiments, which was obtained from Chen lab Tsinghua University, Beijing, China. Trigonelline and isoguvacine were all purchased from TargetMol, Boston, MA, USA.

2.2. Cell Lines and Cell Culture

WI-38 and 2BS cells were provided by the National Institutes for Food and Drug Control. We counted the cells and inoculated each passage at the same density, supplemented with 10% FBS in an incubator at 37 °C and 5% CO_2 (Gibco, London, UK) in MEM (Gibco).

2.3. Cell Viability Test and Growth Analysis

The cell viability was evaluated by the CCK-8 detection kit (Dojindo, Kumamoto, Japan). The 2BS or WI-38 cells were seeded into 96-well plates (5000/well) and then treated with drugs for 24 h. A 1:10 diluted CCK-8 solution was added to the culture medium and incubated for 1 h at 37 °C. Then a microplate reader (Biotek, Winooski, VT, USA, MQX200) was used to measure the absorbance at 450 nm.

$$\text{Cell survival rate (\%)} = (\text{OD treatment} - \text{OD}_{\text{blank}})/(\text{OD}_{\text{control}} - \text{OD}_{\text{blank}}) \times 100\%$$

The CCK-8 kit is also used as a method for assessing cell proliferation by plating cells (2000/well) in 96-well plates. Then the cells were treated with drugs for 1 week. We refreshed the medium every day with fresh drugs or DMSO. At an appropriate time point, we treated them with CCK-8 solution for 1 h as described above, and measured the absorbance at 450 nm.

2.4. Senescence-Associated β-Galactosidase (SA-β-Gal) Staining

We washed the cells in PBS, then fixed them with 4% formaldehyde at room temperature for 5 min, and then washed them again. Then cells were stained with a buffer (1 mg/mL 5-bromo-4-chloro-3-indolyl-β-d-galactopyranoside (X-gal), 40 mM citric acid at 37 °C/Sodium phosphate, pH 6.0) Stain overnight, 5 mM potassium ferrocyanide, 5 mM potassium ferricyanide, 150 mM NaCl, 2 mM $MgCl_2$). The cells were then analyzed according to the instructions provided (CST, Danvers, MA, USA, 9860S).

2.5. Yeast Mutant Generation

Wild-type yeast all came from the library from Krogen lab (UCSF), San Francisco, CA, USA. Standard SD medium (1% yeast extract, 1% bacterial protein, 2% glucose) was used for routine growth of all yeast strains on a rotary shaker at 250 rpm at 30 °C. The experiments designed to assess the lifespan of the yeast were carried out with the yeast in the logarithmic growth phase by culturing the yeast overnight and then diluting it 4 h before use.

2.6. Yeast Replication Lifespan Test

As mentioned in previous reports, we derived a modified U-shape. Due to our work on berberine [9], we used a high-pressure microfluidic chip, which resulted in a slightly shorter yeast lifespan, but the effects of lifespan extension in yeast, lifespan extension in human senescent cells, and lifespan extension in mice treated with various compounds were all consistent. We observed mother cells for two days using time-lapse microscopy. This method relies on U-shaped wells in a microfluidic system to keep the mother cells in place while allowing the flowing medium to carry away the daughter cells. Survival curves were plotted based on data collected from multiple experiments. We plotted survival curves and cell cycle curves using Matlab 2018a.

2.7. Animals and Survival Curve

All young and naturally aged mice were purchased from SPF Biotechnology Co., Ltd., Beijing, China. The mice were kept in an environment with minimum pressure and standard conditions (constant temperature and light/dark at 12:12 h). The cage size was

325 mm × 210 mm × 150 mm. The cages were made of plastic and were lined with corn cob bedding. Each cage housed four mice. Animals were randomly assigned to control and treatment groups. We purchased 8 ICR mice at the age of 2 months, with an average weight of 35 g. We purchased 69 ICR mice at the age of 11 months, with an average weight of 47 g.

Survival curves: Before grouping, the weight of each mouse was measured, and they were randomly divided into groups according to their weight. All mice were included in the experiment, with no mice excluded. We selected 11-month-old male ICR mice, dissolved 3HB-Na in drinking water (1 g/L), and administered 3HB-Na to 11-month-old mice in drinking water until the mice died naturally, and recorded the body weights and survival conditions.

2.8. Grip Test

The mice were placed on top of the grid strength meter, so they grabbed the grid with all four paws. The grip strength of 5 trials was recorded, and the final data were taken as the maximum grip strength (g).

2.9. Physical Appearance and Posture Score

Physical appearance and posture scores were performed on 2- and 20-month-old ICR mice [23]. Physical appearance: 0-normal, 1-lack of grooming, 2-rough hair coat, 3-very rough hair coat. Posture: 0-normal, 1-sitting in hunched position, 4-hunched posture, head resting on floor, 6-lying prone on cage floor/unable to maintain upright posture. The score is the sum of the two.

2.10. Tissue Morphology Staining and Statistics

Male ICR mice were studied in a young control group (2 months of age), an old control group, and an old treatment group (20 months of age), and 3HB (1 g/L) was administered in the form of drinking water from 11 months of age. The mice were euthanized by cervical dislocation performed by personnel who had undergone professional training. The hearts, livers, kidneys, and muscles of the mice were taken.

Masson's trichrome stain: To test fibrosis of heart tissue, Masson's trichrome stain kit (Solarbio, Beijing, China, G1340) was used. The tissue was fixed with 4% formaldehyde, followed by paraffin embedding and sectioning. The sections were then stained according to the manufacturer's instructions. The slices were quickly dehydrated with 95% alcohol and 100% alcohol, cleaned with xylene, and then covered with a coverslip. Images were collected using a strong light microscope (20× magnification objective lens) (OLYMPUS, Tokyo, Japan, BX43) and analyzed by ImageJ 1.53a software (NIH, Bethesda, MD, USA) to measure the fibrosis area and the total area. Each organization used 5 different areas for measurement.

H & E staining: To test the morphological changes of tissues. The kidney, liver, brain, and muscle were fixed with 4% formaldehyde, followed by paraffin embedding and sectioning. The sections were stained with H & E for morphological analysis.

For renal tissue, when the tubular brush border was lost, the lumen was dilated, and the epithelial cells were flattened and atrophied, the damaged tubules were counted. The percentage of injured tubules to total tubules was calculated and scored according to the following criteria: 0 = normal: 1 $\leq$ 20%; 2 = 20% to 40%; 3 = 40% to 60%; 4 = 60% to 80%; and 5 $\geq$ 80%. For the liver, the Knodell Histological Activity Index (HAI) was utilized for scoring. The system uses four independent criteria for scoring: (1) peripheral fragmentation necrosis (PN) with or without bridging necrosis (BN) in the confluent area (0–10 points), (2) hepatocellular degeneration and focal necrosis in the lobules (0~4 points), (3) inflammation in the confluent area (0~4 points), and (4) fibrosis (0~4 points), and the sum of the scores of each of the four indexes is the total score. For muscle, 100 muscle fibers were randomly selected from each mouse and muscle fiber area and feret were detected using imageJ.

2.11. RNA Extraction and qPCR

TRIzol was used to lyse cells, and then isopropanol and chloroform were used to extract RNA. Using cDNA synthesis kit, a total of 1 μg RNA was used for cDNA reverse transcription (Abmgood, Richmond, BC, Canada). Real-time qPCR was used to evaluate the target gene's expression, and the expression level was normalized to ACTIN. Supplementary Table S1 lists all primers.

2.12. RNA-Seq

For animal handling, see tissue morphology staining. We performed RNA extraction and RNA-seq detection with ICR mice muscle tissue. Total RNA was extracted from the tissue using TRIzol® Reagent according to the manufacturer's instructions (Invitrogen, Waltham, MA, USA) and genomic DNA was removed using DNase I (TaKara, San Jose, CA, USA). Then, RNA quality was determined with a 2100 Bioanalyser (Agilent, Santa Clara, CA, USA) and quantified using the ND-2000 (NanoDrop Technologies, Wilmington, DE, USA). Only the high-quality RNA sample (OD260/280 = 1.8~2.2, OD260/230 $\geq$ 2.0, RIN $\geq$ 6.5, 28S:18S $\geq$ 1.0, >2 μg) was used to construct the sequencing library. After quantification with TBS380, the paired-end RNA-seq sequencing library was sequenced with the Illumina HiSeq xten/NovaSeq 6000 sequencer (2 $\times$ 150 bp read length). RNA sequencing and raw data quality control were performed by Shanghai Majorbio Bio-pharm Technology Co., Ltd., Shanghai, China.

2.13. Echocardiographic Measurements

We performed cardiac ultrasound in 2-month-old, 20-month-old, and 3HB-intervention 20-month-old male ICR mice. To measure cardiac physiological functions, an ultrasound cardiotachograph (VINNO 6 VET, VINNO, Suzhou, China) was used for the detection and analysis of echocardiography. B-mode ultrasonography was applied in seeking the long axis of left ventricular, then 2-dimensional M-mode was transferred for data acquisition. Left ventricle internal dimension diastole (LVIDd), left ventricle internal dimension systole (LVIDs), and ejection fraction (EF), among others, were directly measured by using M-modeanalysis. Fractional shortening (FS) was calculated by LVIDd and LVIDs.

2.14. Tissue SA-β-Gal Staining

Male ICR mice were studied in an old control group and an old treatment group (20 months of age), and 3HB (1 g/L) was administered in the form of drinking water from 11 months of age. The mice were euthanized by cervical dislocation performed by personnel who had undergone professional training. The hearts, livers, kidneys, and colons of the mice were taken, and frozen sections were prepared by liquid nitrogen flash freezing. Frozen sections were first rewarmed, washed with PBS 3 times (for at least 5 min each time), and fixed with an appropriate volume of β-galactosidase staining fixative to cover the tissue adequately (fixed for at least 15 min at room temperature). Wash the tissues with PBS immersion 3 times for at least 5 min each time. Aspirate the PBS and add an appropriate volume of staining work. Incubate overnight at 37 °C. The tissues were washed three times with PBS, stained with nuclear solid red for 1 min, and washed in water $\rightarrow$ anhydrous ethanol $\rightarrow$ xylene. Three randomly selected fields of view were photographed for each mouse and the blue area was counted using ImageJ 1.53a.

2.15. Serological Testing

For animal handling, see tissue morphology staining and statistics. For serum biochemical analysis, blood samples were collected, coagulated at room temperature for 2 h, or overnight at 4 °C, and then centrifuged (1000× *g*, 10 min) to obtain serum. A 200 μL aliquot of serum was taken and analyzed with a chemical analyzer (Mindray, Mahwah, NJ, USA, BS-350E) for uric acid (UA), blood urea nitrogen (BUN), alanine aminotransferase (ALT), aspartate aminotransferase (AST), creatine kinase isoenzymes (CK-MB), triglyceride (TG), total cholesterol (TCHO), High-Density Lipoprotein (HDL), and Low-Density Lipoprotein (LDL).

2.16. Metabolomics Assay

Feces were collected from 2-month-old, 20-month-old, and 3HB-intervention 20-month-old male ICR mice. Around 8 p.m., we placed the mouse on a sterile aluminum foil and allowed it to defecate naturally. We transferred the fecal pellets to a labeled sterile centrifuge tube using sterile forceps and then froze them rapidly in liquid nitrogen for storage at −80 °C. Samples were weighed before the extraction of metabolites and dried lyophilized were ground in a 2 mL Eppendorf tube containing a 5 mm tungsten bead for 1 min at 65 Hz in a Grinding Mill. Metabolites were extracted using 1 mL precooled mixtures of methanol, acetonitrile, and water (*v*/*v*/*v*, 2:2:1) and then placed for 1 h ultrasonic shaking in ice baths. Subsequently, the mixture was placed at −20 °C for 1 h and centrifuged at 14,000× *g* for 20 min at 4 °C. The supernatants were recovered and concentrated to dryness in vacuum.

UHPLC-MS/MS analysis: Metabolomics profiling was analyzed using a UPLC-ESI-Q-Orbitrap-MS system (UHPLC, Shimadzu Nexera X2 LC-30AD: Shimadzu, Japan) coupled with Q-Exactive Plus (Thermo Scientific, San Jose, CA, USA). For liquid chromatography (LC) separation, samples were analyzed using a ACQUITY UPLC® HSS T3 column (2.1 × 100 mm, 1.8 μm) (Waters, Milford, MA, USA). The flow rate was 0.3 mL/min and the mobile phase contained the following: A, 0.1% FA in water and B, 100% acetonitrile (ACN). The gradient was 0% buffer B for 2 min and was linearly increased to 48% in 4 min, and then up to 100% in 4 min and maintained for 2 min, and then decreased to 0% buffer B in 0.1 min, with a 3 min re-equilibration period employed.

Data preprocessing and filtering: The raw MS data were processed using MS-DIAL for peak alignment, retention time correction, and peak area extraction. The metabolites were identified by accuracy mass (mass tolerance < 10 ppm) and MS/MS data (mass tolerance < 0.02 Da), which were matched with HMDB, massbank and other public databases and our self-built metabolite standard library. In the extracted-ion features, only the variables having more than 50% of the nonzero measurement values in at least one group were kept. Multivariate statistical analysis: R (version:4.0.3) and R packages were used for all multivariate data analyses and modeling. Data were mean-centered using Pareto scaling. Models were built on principal component analysis (PCA), orthogonal partial least-square discriminant analysis (PLS-DA), and partial least-square discriminant analysis (OPLS-DA). All the models evaluated were tested for over fitting with methods of permutation tests.

KEGG Enrichment analysis: To identify the perturbed biological pathways, the differential metabolite data performed the KEGG pathway analysis using the KEGG database (http://www.kegg.jp, accessed on 20 June 2022). KEGG enrichment analyses were carried out with the Fisher's exact test, and FDR correction for multiple testing was performed. Enriched KEGG pathways were nominally statistically significant at the $p < 0.05$ level.

2.17. Statistics

Results were assessed by two-tailed Student's t tests or ANOVAs to compare two and more than two samples, respectively. Data with means $\pm$ sem $p < 0.05$ was the significance threshold. * $p < 0.05$, ** $p < 0.01$, *** $p < 0.001$. Ns, not significant. Unless otherwise stated, the results are based on the results of at least three independent experiments. Unless otherwise stated, GraphPad Prism (Version 8.0.2) was used for statistics.

3. Results

3.1. 3HB Delays Cellular Senescence and Extends the Lifespan of Yeast

To investigate if 3HB can delay cellular senescence in human cell lines, we treated both senescent human embryonic lung fibroblasts WI-38 and 2BS (PD45) with different concentrations of 3HB. 3HB significantly increased the viability of senescent cells in both cell lines in a dose-dependent manner (Figure 1A,B). Importantly, 3HB treatment not only enhanced cell viability but also alleviated morphological hallmarks of senescence, such as granular cytoplasm and inclusion body accumulation. Consistent with these observations, SA-β-gal staining, a marker of senescence, was significantly reduced in 3HB-treated 2BS cells compared to aged controls (38.8% reduction, Figure 1C,D). Simultaneously, the intervention of 3HB reduced the expression levels of p53, p21, IL-6, IL-1β, and CXCL2 in senescent 2BS cells (Figure S1A). Altogether, these findings suggest that 3HB effectively maintains the viability of senescent cells, slows down the replicative senescence process, and holds promise as a potential anti-aging intervention.

While developing anti-aging drugs is notoriously difficult, long-term lifespan testing in model organisms remains crucial for identifying promising candidates. Saccharomyces cerevisiae, a single-celled fungus commonly used in aging research, provides a valuable window into human aging due to its highly conserved aging mechanisms with mammals [24]. To accurately assess the replicative lifespan of yeast in this study, we utilized an automated device based on a microfluidic chip [25], capable of measuring lifespan within 3 days. Yeast incubated in SD medium for 20 h were then collected and loaded onto the chip. Lifespan was monitored at 3HB concentrations ranging from 0 to 80 μM. Our results demonstrated a dose-dependent prolongation of the replicative lifespan of the BY4741 strain compared to the control, with 10 μM of 3HB leading to a remarkable 51.3% extension (Figure 1E). Notably, 3HB treatment also significantly reduced cell cycle duration (Figures 1F–J and S1B,C), reducing its heterogeneity and further contributing to chronological lifespan extension. These findings strongly suggest 3HB's potential as a promising anti-aging intervention.

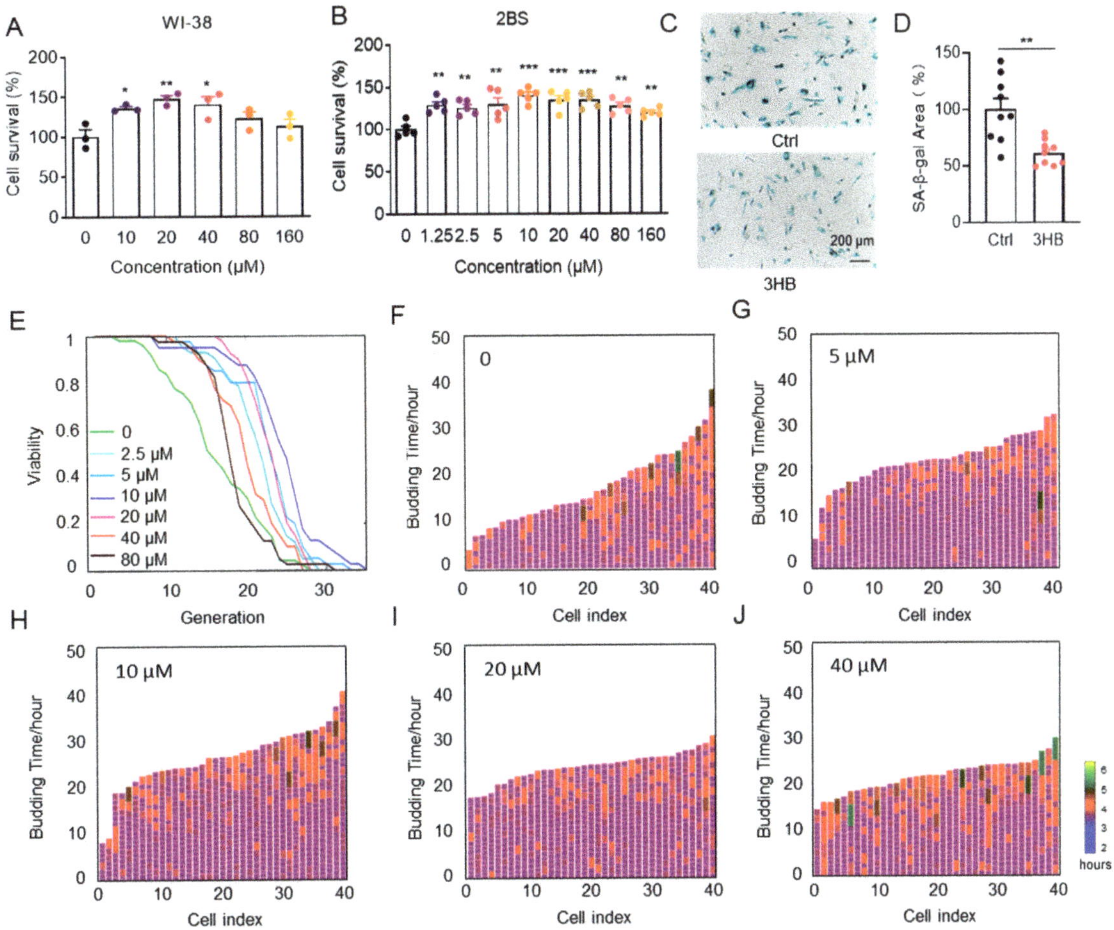

Figure 1. 3HB delays cellular senescence and extends the lifespan of yeast. (**A**) The effect of different concentrations of 3HB on the proliferation of replicatively senescent WI-38 cells was measured by the CCK-8 assay. (**B**) The effect of different concentrations of 3HB on the proliferation of replicatively senescent 2BS cells was measured by the CCK-8 assay. (**C**) SA-β-gal staining of replicatively senescent 2BS cells treated with 10 μM 3HB or DMSO for 48 h. (**D**) Quantification of the rate of SA-β-gal positive cells in replicatively senescent 2BS cells. (**E**) 3HB extends the replication lifespan of yeast. (**F–J**) Germination diagrams of wild-type and 3HB-treated mother cells show cell cycle duration and heterogeneity (n = 40 for each group). (See index color scale. Duration is 1.4 h or less. Cell cycle is colored in the color purple). The x-axis shows a single parent cell as a vertical bar, while budding events are shown as white horizontal partitions. Data represent the mean ± SEM. p values were determined by one-way ANOVA, two-way ANOVA, or Student's t-test. (* $p < 0.05$, ** $p < 0.01$, *** $p < 0.001$).

3.2. Treatment with 3HB Significantly Extended Lifespan by 123 Days and Improved Healthspan as Measured by Increased Physical Activity

Based on the aforementioned observations, we posit that 3HB has the potential to extend the lifespan of mice. To verify this hypothesis, we designed an in vivo experiment where 11-month-old ICR male mice were divided equally into two groups: a control group and a 3HB-treated group. We ensured that there was no significant difference in initial body weight and grip strength between the two groups (Figure S2A,B). Over the course of the experiment, we observed a remarkable extension in the median lifespan of the 3HB-treated group compared to the control group. The median (mean) lifespan of the 3HB-treated mice was extended by 123 (52) days (approximately 21.0% (8.4%)), increasing from 587 (618) days to 710 (670) days (Figure 2A).

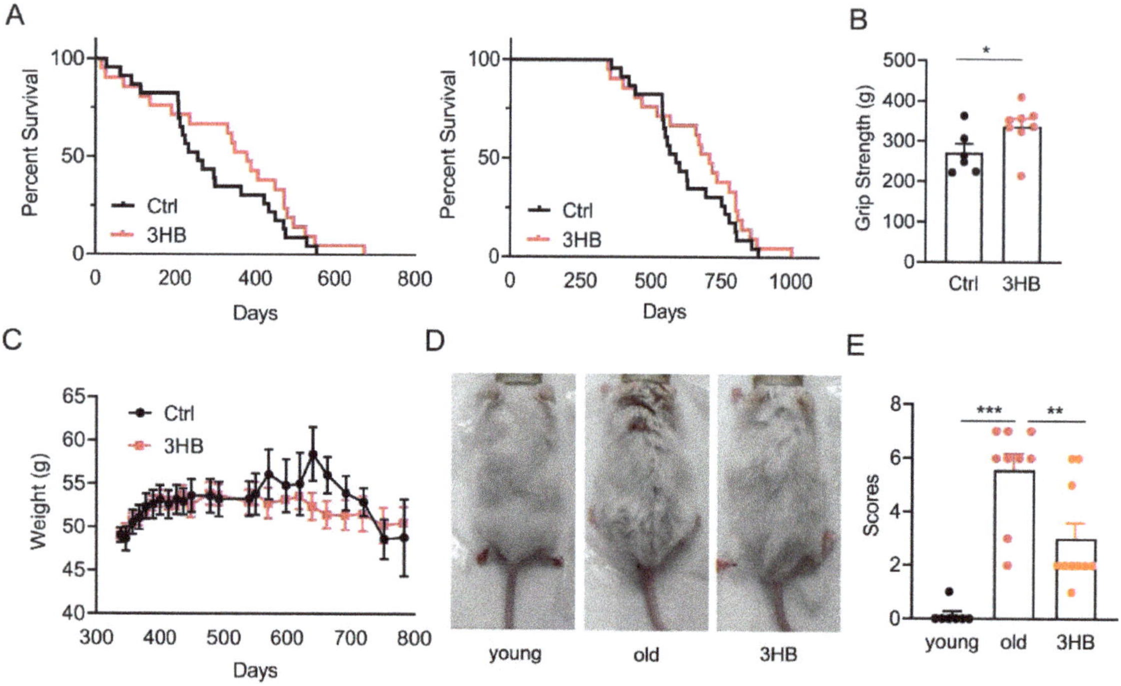

Figure 2. 3HB extends the lifespan of mice. (**A**) Lifespan curves of 11-month-old ICR mice under 3HB intervention from the beginning of treatment (left) and from birth (right) (Ctrl $n = 23$, 3HB $n = 21$). (**B**) Effect of 3HB on grip strength of 20-month-old ICR male mice ($n \geq 6$). (**C**) Changes in body weight of ICR mice under 3HB intervention ($n \geq 6$). (**D**,**E**) Effects of 3HB on hair and body size of 20-month-old male ICR mice and statistics ($n \geq 6$). Data represent the mean ± SEM. p values were determined by one-way ANOVA, two-way ANOVA, or Student's t-test. (* $p < 0.05$, ** $p < 0.01$, *** $p < 0.001$).

Functional tests revealed that 3HB treatment significantly improved the grip strength (Figure 2B) and clinical scores (Figure 2D,E) of the aged mice compared to the control group. Notably, 3HB intervention also influenced the age-induced body weight changes. While the control group mice experienced an increase followed by a decrease in body weight as they aged, the 3HB-treated group displayed a more stable body weight pattern with a reduced amplitude of change (Figure 2C). Interestingly, there was no significant difference in dietary intake between the two groups (Figure S2C), suggesting that the observed effects were not due to differences in food consumption. The results of the cardiac ultrasound showed that 3HB had a tendency to improve all cardiac indices in aging mice, but there was no statistical difference (Figure S2D–L). Collectively, these findings strongly suggest that 3HB can extend the lifespan and improve the healthy lifespan of naturally aging mice.

3.3. 3HB Has the Potential to Improve Age-Related Histomorphometric Changes in Kidney and Muscle

During aging, the senescence of individual cells leads to reduced tissue and organ function as well as morphological changes [26]. To investigate how 3HB might counteract these declines, we analyzed major organs in young (2-month-old), aged (20-month-old), and aged mice treated with 3HB (20-month-old with 3HB intervention). We found that 3HB treatment notably ameliorated age-related changes in kidney function, including improved renal indices (Figure 3A) and trends towards better kidney function parameters like uric acid (UA), urea nitrogen (BUN), and increased muscle weight (Figures 3B and S3A,B). We performed HE staining analysis on the kidney tissues of aged mice and 3HB-treated aged mice. The results showed that the glomerular structure was restored and glomerular atrophy was reduced in the mice treated with 3HB (Figure 3C,D). This suggests 3HB protects against aging-related kidney damage.

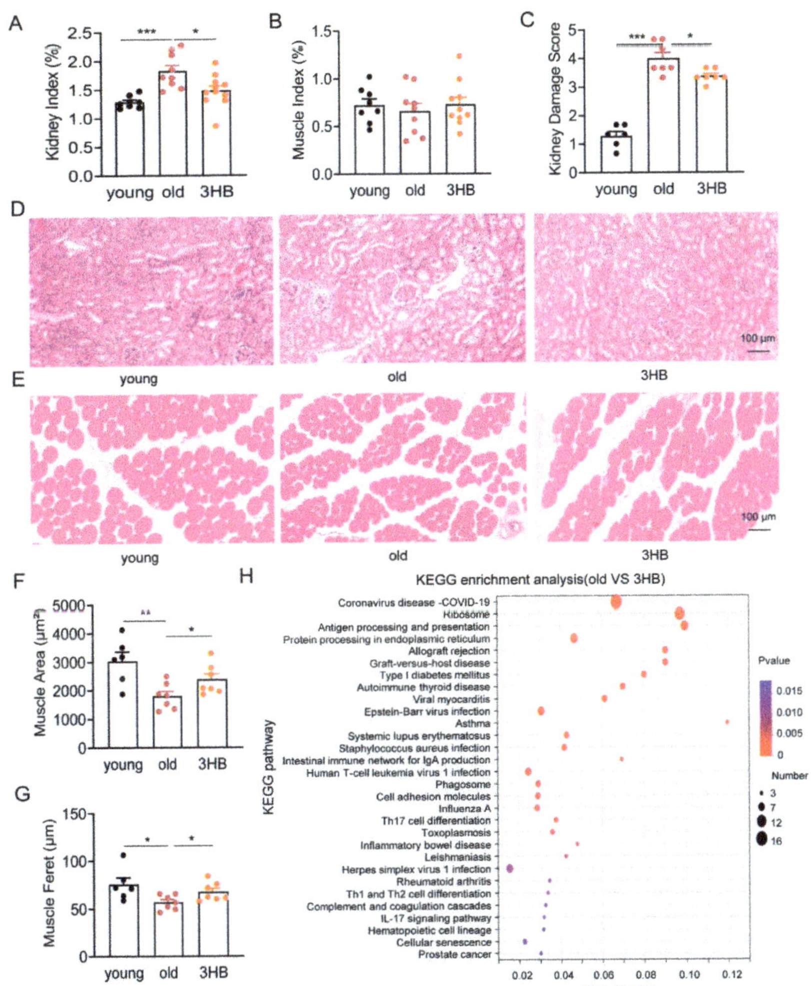

Figure 3. *Cont.*

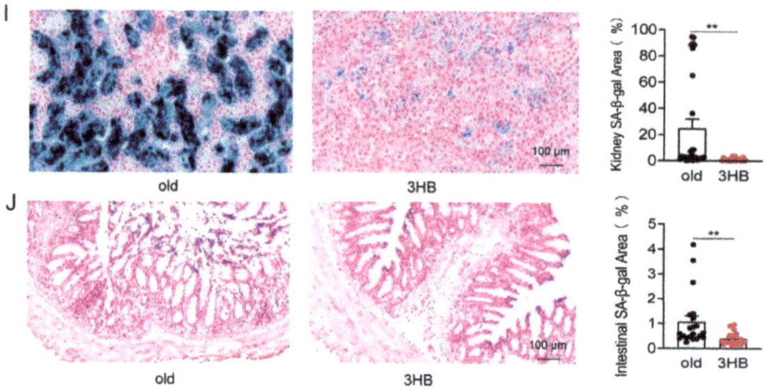

Figure 3. Effects of 3HB intervention on morphological changes and cellular senescence in mouse organ tissues. (**A**,**B**) Kidney and muscle organ index of male ICR mice at 2 months (young), 20 months (old), and 20 months treated with 3HB (3HB) (Organ weight/body weight * 100%). (**C**,**D**) HE staining to detect the histomorphology of kidney of male ICR mice at 2 months (young), 20 months (old), and 20 months treated with 3HB (3HB), and their quantitative statistics. (**E–G**) HE staining to detect the histomorphology of muscle of male ICR mice at 2 months (young), 20 months (old), and 20 months treated with 3HB (3HB), and muscle fiber area and feret statistics. (**H**) KEGG enrichment analysis (kidney tissue) of signaling pathway changes due to 3HB intervention. (**I**) SA-β-Gal staining to detect the effect of 3HB intervention on the cellular senescence of kidney tissues in 20-month-old male ICR mice and statistics. (**J**) SA-β-Gal staining to detect the effect of 3HB intervention on the cellular senescence of colon tissue in 20-month-old male ICR mice and statistics. Data represent the mean ± SEM ($n \geq 6$). p values were determined by one-way ANOVA, two-way ANOVA, or Student's t-test. (* $p < 0.05$, ** $p < 0.01$, *** $p < 0.001$).

3HB also counteracted age-induced muscle changes, characterized by increased muscle fiber area and feret diameter (Figure 3E–G), indicating restored muscle health. While 3HB showed positive effects on kidney and muscle, it did not significantly impact liver, brain, heart, spleen, or thymus function or morphology (Figure S3C–N).

These findings suggest that 3HB has the potential to improve age-related histomorphometric changes in specific tissues, like kidney and muscle, warranting further research into its potential as an anti-aging intervention.

3.4. 3HB Combats Aging by Targeting Cellular Senescence in Kidney and Colon

To understand how 3HB exerts its lifespan and healthspan-promoting effects, we delved into gene expression changes in mouse kidneys. We performed RNA sequencing on kidney tissues from young (2-month-old), aged (20-month-old), and aged mice treated with 3HB (20-month-old with 3HB intervention). Analyzing differentially expressed genes between aged and 3HB-treated aged mice, as well as those intersecting with differentially expressed genes from young mice, revealed an enrichment of cellular senescence signaling pathways in both groups (Figures 3H and S4A). This suggests that 3HB might act by influencing senescence processes. Focusing on senescence markers in various organs, we found that 3HB delayed cellular senescence in kidney and colon tissues (Figure 3I,J). However, 3HB did not show significant effects on cellular senescence in liver and heart tissues (Figure S4B–E).

3.5. 3HB Modulated Lipid Metabolism and Reversed Some Age-Related Metabolic Changes

Delving deeper into mechanisms, we performed GO and KEGG analyses on gene expression data, revealing a significant enrichment of metabolism-related signaling pathways across different groups (Figure 4A–C). This suggests 3HB might influence metabolic processes during its lifespan-extending effects. Focusing on lipid metabolism, we observed that 3HB reversed age-related increases in triglycerides and total cholesterol in mice (Figure 4D,E), potentially contributing to its health benefits. Notably, low-density lipoprotein (LDL) and high-density lipoprotein (HDL) levels remained unaffected (Figure S5A,B).

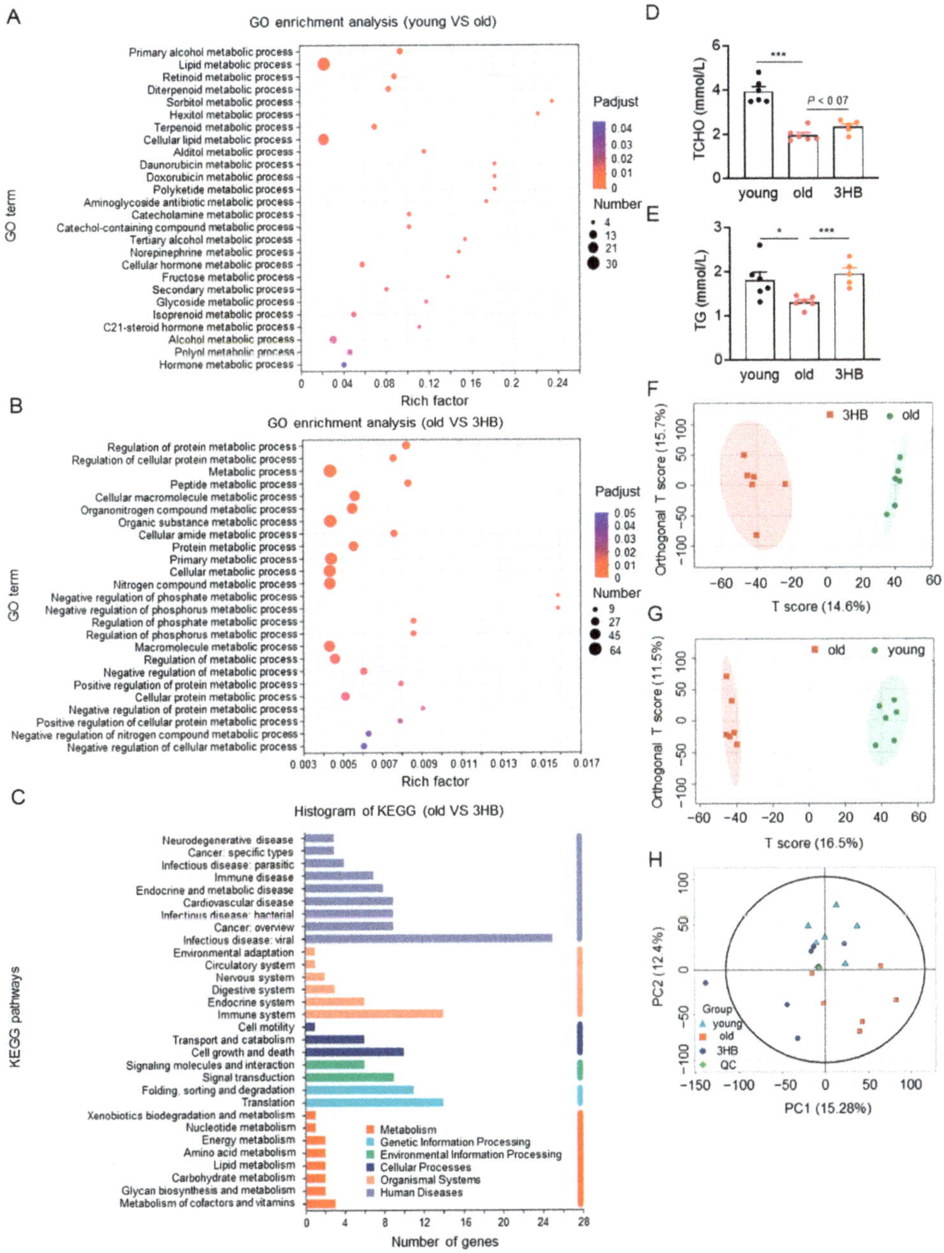

Figure 4. The influence of 3HB on metabolic changes of aged mice. (**A**) GO enrichment analysis (kidney tissue) of changes in metabolic signaling pathways due to 3HB intervention ($n = 3$). (**B**) GO enrichment analysis of genes for differences between the 3 groups (2-month-old, 20-month-old, and

20-month-old mice with 3HB intervention) demonstrated changes in metabolism-related signaling pathways ($n = 3$). (**C**) KEGG annotation analysis (kidney tissue) of changes in signaling pathways due to 3HB intervention ($n = 3$). (**D**,**E**) Blood biochemistry for total cholesterol (TCHO) and triglycerides (TG) in male ICR mice at 2 months (young), 20 months (old), and 20 months treated with 3HB (3HB). Metabolomics of feces from 20-month-old ICR mice at 2 months, 20 months (old), and 20 months treated with 3HB (3HB) ($n \geq 6$). (**F**) PCA analysis (NEG) of differential metabolites in the aged and 3HB-intervened aged groups. (**G**) PCA analysis (NEG) of differential metabolites between the younger and older groups ($n \geq 6$). (**H**) PCA analysis of differential metabolites between the three groups (NEG) ($n \geq 6$). Data represent the mean ± SEM. p values were determined by one-way ANOVA, two-way ANOVA, or Student's t-test. (* $p < 0.05$, *** $p < 0.001$).

To gain further insights into metabolic changes, we performed metabolomic sequencing on fecal samples from young, aged, and 3HB-treated aged mice. Principal component analysis (PCA) revealed distinct metabolic profiles for each group and highlighted the impact of both aging and 3HB intervention (Figures 4F,G and S5C,D). Additionally, PCA within the 3 groups showed that 3HB treatment shifted some aged mice closer to the young mouse metabolic profile (Figures 4H and S5E–G).

These combined findings suggest that 3HB exerts its lifespan-extending effects through diverse metabolic pathways, with a notable modulation of lipid metabolism and a potential reversal of some age-related metabolic changes.

3.6. Trigonelline and Isoguvacine Might Contribute to 3HB's Anti-Aging Effects by Reducing Cellular Senescence

To delve deeper into 3HB's metabolic influence, we analyzed differential metabolites between young and aged mice, revealing over 50 significantly altered compounds, including histidine, trigonelline, and taurocholic acid (Figure 5A). KEGG enrichment analysis linked these changes to pathways, like taurine and hypotaurine metabolism, carbohydrate digestion, and lipolysis regulation, suggesting broad metabolic reprogramming during aging (Figure S6A).

Similarly, comparing aged and 3HB-treated mice identified over 30 differentially expressed metabolites, including valine betaine and cocaine (Figure 5B). KEGG analysis linked these changes to similar pathways, like taurine metabolism and lipolysis regulation, but also highlighted cholesterol metabolism and central carbon metabolism (Figure S6B). This suggests 3HB might specifically target aspects of lipid metabolism alongside broader metabolic modulation.

Zooming in further, we focused on metabolites reversed by 3HB treatment in aged mice. Twelve compounds showed significant changes, including trigonelline and isoguvacine (Figure 5C). Notably, both trigonelline and isoguvacine are down-regulated in aged mice and up-regulated in young and 3HB-treated mice. Investigating their impact on cellular senescence, we found that both compounds reduced SA-β-gal positive cells, suggesting anti-senescence potential (Figure 5D,E).

Overall, this deep dive into differential metabolites reveals that 3HB induces broad metabolic changes in aged mice, potentially targeting lipolysis and cholesterol metabolism. Furthermore, specific metabolites, like trigonelline and isoguvacine, might contribute to 3HB's anti-aging effects by reducing cellular senescence.

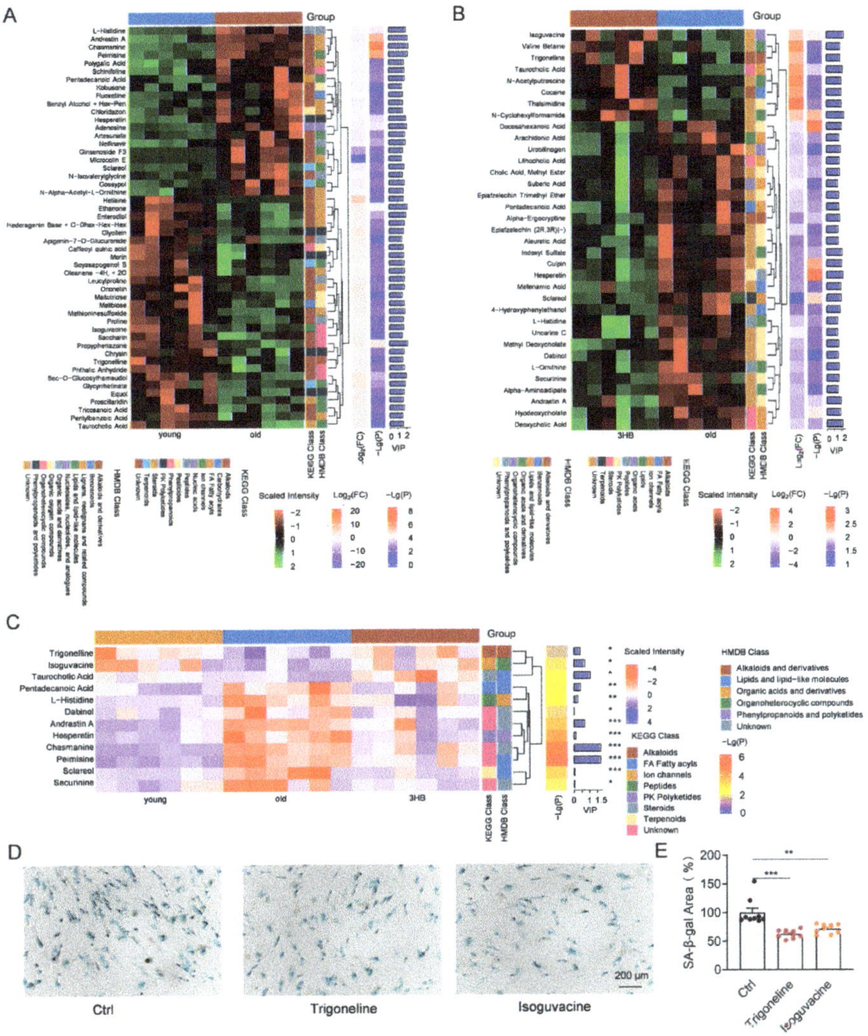

Figure 5. 3HB affects cellular senescence by altering metabolites in mice. (**A**) Heatmap analysis of metabolite changes in young and senescent mice ($n \geq 6$). (**B**) Heatmap analysis of changes in metabolites due to 3HB intervention ($n \geq 6$). (**C**) Heatmap analysis of differential metabolites between 3 groups (2-month-old, 20-month-old, and 20-month-old male ICR mice with 3HB intervention) ($n \geq 6$). (**D**) SA-β-gal staining of replicatively senescent 2BS cells treated with trigoneline (10 μM), Isoguvacine (10 μM) or DMSO for 48 h. (**E**) Quantification of the rate of SA-β-gal positive cells in replicatively senescent 2BS cells. Data represent the mean ± SEM. *p* values were determined by one-way ANOVA, two-way ANOVA, or Student's *t*-test. (* $p < 0.05$, ** $p < 0.01$, *** $p < 0.001$).

4. Discussion

This study unveils the promising anti-aging potential of 3HB, an endogenous metabolite. We observed remarkable benefits in aged mice: improved senescent cell viability, delayed cellular senescence, extended lifespan and healthspan, and restored health markers in kidney and muscle tissues. Notably, 3HB specifically countered senescence in the kidney and colon, further supporting its rejuvenating effects.

Delving deeper, our analyses suggest two key mechanisms: combating cellular senescence and modulating metabolic pathways. Sequencing data revealed that 3HB upregulated metabolites, like trigonelline and isoguvacine, potentially contributing to its lifespan-extending effects. These intriguing findings provide novel evidence for 3HB's application in promoting healthy aging and warrant further investigation into its precise mechanisms of action.

While promising anti-aging candidates, like senolytics and mTOR inhibitors, exist, concerns regarding safety and clinical translation due to side effects remain [27–29]. Endogenous metabolites, like 3HB, offer a safer alternative due to their natural presence in the body. In this study, we found that 3HB intervention extended the median lifespan of mice by 21% (123 days) and the mean lifespan by 8.4% (52 days) throughout their entire life cycle (as shown in Figure 2A). We then compared 3HB with other known compounds that delay aging. Our findings revealed that metformin can extend the mean lifespan of mice by 4.15% from the start of the intervention [6]; NMN/NR can extend the mean lifespan of mice by 30.2% from the start of the intervention, and the mean lifespan throughout the entire life cycle can be extended by 4.7% [4]; rapamycin can extend the mean lifespan throughout the entire life cycle by 7% to 16% [10,11]; dasatinib + quercetin can extend the mean lifespan of mice by 36% from the start of the intervention [3]. From these studies, we can see that the anti-aging effects of 3HB are comparable to or even more outstanding than those of these well-known anti-aging compounds. Its established production process and the safe use history as a food additive (through its precursor) further solidify its potential. 3HB stands out with its unique combination of safety, efficacy, and applicability.

Beyond lifespan extension, 3HB ameliorated aging-related damage in the kidney and muscle, suggesting it improves healthy lifespan alongside longevity. This raises the possibility of using 3HB to treat age-related diseases like atherosclerosis [13,30], diabetes [31], and muscle loss [32]. While the ketogenic diet offers similar benefits, its dietary challenges limit its clinical practicality [33]. Direct 3HB supplementation may be a more viable option. This study adds to the growing evidence for 3HB's role in treating age-related diseases.

In addition, we observed that 3HB improved cellular senescence in kidney and intestinal tissues but had no effect on cellular senescence in liver and heart tissues. Previous studies have indicated that the liver is the primary site for the synthesis of 3HB, but the liver itself utilizes relatively little 3HB. 3HB can cross the blood–brain barrier and be used by the brain as an energy source, especially during fasting or low-carbohydrate diets, when 3HB becomes an important alternative energy source for the brain. Moreover, 3HB is utilized by the heart and muscle tissues as an energy source, particularly during fasting or prolonged exercise. The kidneys can reabsorb 3HB from the bloodstream and use it as an energy source in the renal tubules [34]. Our results also showed that, compared to liver and heart tissues, the kidney and intestinal tissues of 18-month-old ICR mice exhibited more pronounced signs of aging. This may also be an important reason why 3HB did not exert effects in liver and heart tissues. These findings also provide a reference for the timing of tissue aging within the body.

Cellular senescence and metabolic changes are key drivers of aging [2,35–37]. We found that 3HB delays aging by improving both. It ameliorates organ senescence and influences metabolic pathways associated with taurine and hypotaurine metabolism, lipolysis regulation, and central carbon metabolism. Additionally, 3HB reverses age-induced changes in amino acid metabolism, lipid metabolism, and various organ systems. These findings support a new mechanism for 3HB's anti-aging effects while also providing valuable data on metabolic changes in aging.

Our study identified trigonelline and isoguvacine as metabolites impacted by 3HB and capable of delaying cellular senescence. Trigonelline has previously been shown to extend lifespan and delay age-related diseases in *C. elegans* [38] and improve cognitive function in mice [39]. These findings further support the notion that 3HB delays aging by altering specific metabolites. Our work not only reveals a new mechanism for 3HB but also lays the groundwork for discovering more age-delaying molecules.

However, there are still some limitations in this study. We only used male ICR mice for validation. In the future, we will repeat lifespan studies in female mice and other strains of mice (such as C57BL/6) to assess the variability of genetics and gender. Meanwhile, previous studies have shown that 3HB mimics caloric restriction and fasting and exerts other effects through pathways such as AKT and FOXO [14,40]. This is similar to the mechanisms by which most compounds delay aging. It has also been found that Trigonelline is an NAD precursor [41]. Therefore, the mechanism by which 3HB delays aging may not include killing old cells, and the combination of dasatinib + quercetin may play a role in delaying aging through multiple mechanisms.

5. Conclusions

This study reveals the anti-aging potential of 3-hydroxybutyrate (3HB), an endogenous metabolite. The results show that 3HB can delay cellular senescence and extend yeast lifespan, and it also increases the median lifespan of mice by 21.0%, while alleviating age-related tissue and organ decline. Mechanistically, we found that the anti-aging properties of 3HB are mediated by its ability to delay cellular senescence and reprogram metabolism, while also promoting the production of beneficial metabolites such as trigonelline and isoguvacine. Additionally, 3HB has advantages in terms of cost and safety, as it can be obtained from microbial poly-(3-hydroxybutyrate) and is an endogenous metabolite. These findings highlight the promising therapeutic potential of 3HB as an anti-aging intervention and provide new insights into its underlying mechanisms.

Supplementary Materials: The following supporting information can be downloaded at: https://www.mdpi.com/article/10.3390/nu17101647/s1, Figure S1. 3HB delays cellular senescence and extends the lifespan of yeast; Figure S2. Effect of 3HB on mouse cardiac function; Figure S3. The influence of 3HB on tissues of aged mice; Figure S4. The influence of 3HB intervention on tissue cell senescence in mice; Figure S5. The influence of 3HB on metabolic changes of aged mice; Figure S6. The influence of 3HB on metabolic changes of aged mice; Table S1.

Author Contributions: Conceptualization, Y.A. and Z.X.; data curation, Y.A.; formal analysis, Y.A. and Z.X.; funding acquisition, B.Y. and Z.X.; investigation, Y.A., Q.W., G.C., and Z.X.; methodology, Y.A. and Z.X., resources, G.C., Z.X., and B.Y.; software, Q.W., P.Q., J.L., Y.C., D.Y., Y.Y., N.L., F.L., H.Z., A.M., and Y.Z.; supervision, Y.A., Q.W., P.Q., J.L., Y.C., D.Y., Y.Y., N.L., F.L., A.M., Y.Z., H.Z., B.Y., and Z.X.; validation, Y.A., Q.W., P.Q., J.L., Y.C., D.Y., Y.Y., N.L., F.L., A.M., Y.Z., and H.Z.; visualization, Y.A., Q.W., P.Q., J.L., Y.C., D.Y., Y.Y., N.L., F.L., H.Z., A.M., Y.Z., B.Y., and Z.X.; writing—original draft, Y.A.; writing—review and editing, Y.A., B.Y., and Z.X. All authors have read and agreed to the published version of the manuscript.

Funding: This work was supported by the National key R&D program of China (2023YFF1205103, 2018YFA0900200), NSFC (32170756, 81903539).

Institutional Review Board Statement: This study was conducted according to the recommendations in the Guide for the Care and Use of Laboratory Animals of China Association for Laboratory Animal Science and approved by the Institutional Animal Care and Use Committee at the Peking University Health Science Center (Beijing, China, LA2018189). The approval date is 1 March 2018. The duration is six years.

Informed Consent Statement: This research did not involve human participants.

Data Availability Statement: RNA-seq data from kidneys of mice treated with 3HB and control mice (GSE262770). Any additional information required to re-analyze the data reported in this paper is available from the lead contact upon request.

Acknowledgments: The authors would like to thank Hong Zhou and Min Li for their kind discussion and suggestions.

Conflicts of Interest: The authors declare no competing interests.

References

1. Kennedy, B.K.; Berger, S.L.; Brunet, A.; Campisi, J.; Cuervo, A.M.; Epel, E.S.; Franceschi, C.; Lithgow, G.J.; Morimoto, R.I.; Pessin, J.E.; et al. Geroscience: Linking aging to chronic disease. *Cell* **2014**, *159*, 709–713. [CrossRef] [PubMed]
2. Lopez-Otin, C.; Blasco, M.A.; Partridge, L.; Serrano, M.; Kroemer, G. Hallmarks of aging: An expanding universe. *Cell* **2023**, *186*, 243–278. [CrossRef] [PubMed]
3. Xu, M.; Pirtskhalava, T.; Farr, J.N.; Weigand, B.M.; Palmer, A.K.; Weivoda, M.M.; Inman, C.L.; Ogrodnik, M.B.; Hachfeld, C.M.; Fraser, D.G.; et al. Senolytics improve physical function and increase lifespan in old age. *Nat. Med.* **2018**, *24*, 1246–1256. [CrossRef]
4. Zhang, H.; Ryu, D.; Wu, Y.; Gariani, K.; Wang, X.; Luan, P.; D'Amico, D.; Ropelle, E.R.; Lutolf, M.P.; Aebersold, R.; et al. NAD(+) repletion improves mitochondrial and stem cell function and enhances life span in mice. *Science* **2016**, *352*, 1436–1443. [CrossRef] [PubMed]
5. Barzilai, N.; Crandall, J.P.; Kritchevsky, S.B.; Espeland, M.A. Metformin as a Tool to Target Aging. *Cell Metab.* **2016**, *23*, 1060–1065. [CrossRef]
6. Martin-Montalvo, A.; Mercken, E.M.; Mitchell, S.J.; Palacios, H.H.; Mote, P.L.; Scheibye-Knudsen, M.; Gomes, A.P.; Ward, T.M.; Minor, R.K.; Blouin, M.J.; et al. Metformin improves healthspan and lifespan in mice. *Nat. Commun.* **2013**, *4*, 2192. [CrossRef]
7. An, Y.; Zhu, J.; Wang, X.; Sun, X.; Luo, C.; Zhang, Y.; Ye, Y.; Li, X.; Abulizi, A.; Huang, Z.; et al. Oridonin Delays Aging Through the AKT Signaling Pathway. *Front. Pharmacol.* **2022**, *13*, 888247. [CrossRef]
8. Asadi Shahmirzadi, A.; Edgar, D.; Liao, C.Y.; Hsu, Y.M.; Lucanic, M.; Asadi Shahmirzadi, A.; Wiley, C.D.; Gan, G.; Kim, D.E.; Kasler, H.G.; et al. Alpha-Ketoglutarate, an Endogenous Metabolite, Extends Lifespan and Compresses Morbidity in Aging Mice. *Cell Metab.* **2020**, *32*, 447–456.e446. [CrossRef]
9. Dang, Y.; An, Y.; He, J.; Huang, B.; Zhu, J.; Gao, M.; Zhang, S.; Wang, X.; Yang, B.; Xie, Z. Berberine ameliorates cellular senescence and extends the lifespan of mice via regulating p16 and cyclin protein expression. *Aging Cell* **2020**, *19*, e13060. [CrossRef]
10. Harrison, D.E.; Strong, R.; Sharp, Z.D.; Nelson, J.F.; Astle, C.M.; Flurkey, K.; Nadon, N.L.; Wilkinson, J.E.; Frenkel, K.; Carter, C.S.; et al. Rapamycin fed late in life extends lifespan in genetically heterogeneous mice. *Nature* **2009**, *460*, 392–395. [CrossRef]
11. Li, J.; Kim, S.G.; Blenis, J. Rapamycin: One drug, many effects. *Cell Metab.* **2014**, *19*, 373–379. [CrossRef] [PubMed]
12. Zhang, Y.; Li, Z.; Liu, X.; Chen, X.; Zhang, S.; Chen, Y.; Chen, J.; Chen, J.; Wu, F.; Chen, G.Q. 3-Hydroxybutyrate ameliorates insulin resistance by inhibiting PPARgamma Ser273 phosphorylation in type 2 diabetic mice. *Signal Transduct. Target. Ther.* **2023**, *8*, 190. [CrossRef] [PubMed]
13. Zhang, S.J.; Li, Z.H.; Zhang, Y.D.; Chen, J.; Li, Y.; Wu, F.Q.; Wang, W.; Cui, Z.J.; Chen, G.Q. Ketone Body 3-Hydroxybutyrate Ameliorates Atherosclerosis via Receptor Gpr109a-Mediated Calcium Influx. *Adv. Sci.* **2021**, *8*, 2003410. [CrossRef] [PubMed]
14. Chen, J.; Li, Z.; Zhang, Y.; Zhang, X.; Zhang, S.; Liu, Z.; Yuan, H.; Pang, X.; Liu, Y.; Tao, W.; et al. Mechanism of reduced muscle atrophy via ketone body (D)-3-hydroxybutyrate. *Cell Biosci.* **2022**, *12*, 94. [CrossRef]
15. Qiu, X.; Zou, Z.; Lin, T.; Guo, C.; Lin, D. Engineered Lactobacillus rhamnosus Producing 3-Hydroxybutyrate: A Dual-Action Therapeutic Strategy for Colon Cancer Cachexia. *Biotechnol. Bioeng.* **2025**. [CrossRef]
16. Tomita, I.; Kume, S.; Sugahara, S.; Osawa, N.; Yamahara, K.; Yasuda-Yamahara, M.; Takeda, N.; Chin-Kanasaki, M.; Kaneko, T.; Mayoux, E.; et al. SGLT2 Inhibition Mediates Protection from Diabetic Kidney Disease by Promoting Ketone Body-Induced mTORC1 Inhibition. *Cell Metab.* **2020**, *32*, 404–419.e406. [CrossRef]
17. Han, Y.M.; Bedarida, T.; Ding, Y.; Somba, B.K.; Lu, Q.; Wang, Q.; Song, P.; Zou, M.H. beta-Hydroxybutyrate Prevents Vascular Senescence through hnRNP A1-Mediated Upregulation of Oct4. *Mol. Cell* **2018**, *71*, 1064–1078.e1065. [CrossRef]
18. Edwards, C.; Canfield, J.; Copes, N.; Rehan, M.; Lipps, D.; Bradshaw, P.C. D-beta-hydroxybutyrate extends lifespan in C. elegans. *Aging* **2014**, *6*, 621–644. [CrossRef]
19. Fan, S.Z.; Lin, C.S.; Wei, Y.W.; Yeh, S.R.; Tsai, Y.H.; Lee, A.C.; Lin, W.S.; Wang, P.Y. Dietary citrate supplementation enhances longevity, metabolic health, and memory performance through promoting ketogenesis. *Aging Cell* **2021**, *20*, e13510. [CrossRef]
20. Newman, J.C.; Covarrubias, A.J.; Zhao, M.; Yu, X.; Gut, P.; Ng, C.P.; Huang, Y.; Haldar, S.; Verdin, E. Ketogenic Diet Reduces Midlife Mortality and Improves Memory in Aging Mice. *Cell Metab.* **2017**, *26*, 547–557.e548. [CrossRef]
21. Roberts, M.N.; Wallace, M.A.; Tomilov, A.A.; Zhou, Z.; Marcotte, G.R.; Tran, D.; Perez, G.; Gutierrez-Casado, E.; Koike, S.; Knotts, T.A.; et al. A Ketogenic Diet Extends Longevity and Healthspan in Adult Mice. *Cell Metab.* **2017**, *26*, 539–546.e535. [CrossRef] [PubMed]

22. Zhao, K.; Deng, Y.; Chun Chen, J.; Chen, G.Q. Polyhydroxyalkanoate (PHA) scaffolds with good mechanical properties and biocompatibility. *Biomaterials* **2003**, *24*, 1041–1045. [CrossRef] [PubMed]
23. Guo, H.; Chou, W.C.; Lai, Y.; Liang, K.; Tam, J.W.; Brickey, W.J.; Chen, L.; Montgomery, N.D.; Li, X.; Bohannon, L.M.; et al. Multi-omics analyses of radiation survivors identify radioprotective microbes and metabolites. *Science* **2020**, *370*, 549. [CrossRef] [PubMed]
24. Gershon, H.; Gershon, D. The budding yeast, Saccharomyces cerevisiae, as a model for aging research: A critical review. *Mech. Ageing Dev.* **2000**, *120*, 1–22. [CrossRef]
25. Jo, M.C.; Liu, W.; Gu, L.; Dang, W.; Qin, L. High-throughput analysis of yeast replicative aging using a microfluidic system. *Proc. Natl. Acad. Sci. USA* **2015**, *112*, 9364–9369. [CrossRef]
26. Zhou, W.; Cao, J. The Genomics of Aging at the Single-Cell Scale. *Annu. Rev. Genomics. Hum. Genet.* **2025**, *26*. [CrossRef]
27. Augustine, J.J.; Bodziak, K.A.; Hricik, D.E. Use of sirolimus in solid organ transplantation. *Drugs* **2007**, *67*, 369–391. [CrossRef]
28. McNeil, J.J.; Wolfe, R.; Woods, R.L.; Tonkin, A.M.; Donnan, G.A.; Nelson, M.R.; Reid, C.M.; Lockery, J.E.; Kirpach, B.; Storey, E.; et al. Effect of Aspirin on Cardiovascular Events and Bleeding in the Healthy Elderly. *N. Engl. J. Med.* **2018**, *379*, 1509–1518. [CrossRef]
29. Magkouta, S.; Veroutis, D.; Papaspyropoulos, A.; Georgiou, M.; Lougiakis, N.; Pippa, N.; Havaki, S.; Palaiologou, A.; Thanos, D.F.; Kambas, K.; et al. Author Correction: Generation of a selective senolytic platform using a micelle-encapsulated Sudan Black B conjugated analog. *Nat. Aging* **2025**, *5*, 528. [CrossRef]
30. Deng, Y.; Xie, M.; Li, Q.; Xu, X.; Ou, W.; Zhang, Y.; Xiao, H.; Yu, H.; Zheng, Y.; Liang, Y.; et al. Targeting Mitochondria-Inflammation Circuit by beta-Hydroxybutyrate Mitigates HFpEF. *Circ. Res.* **2021**, *128*, 232–245. [CrossRef]
31. Wu, X.; Miao, D.; Liu, Z.; Liu, K.; Zhang, B.; Li, J.; Li, Y.; Qi, J. beta-hydroxybutyrate antagonizes aortic endothelial injury by promoting generation of VEGF in diabetic rats. *Tissue Cell* **2020**, *64*, 101345. [CrossRef] [PubMed]
32. Wallace, M.A.; Aguirre, N.W.; Marcotte, G.R.; Marshall, A.G.; Baehr, L.M.; Hughes, D.C.; Hamilton, K.L.; Roberts, M.N.; Lopez-Dominguez, J.A.; Miller, B.F.; et al. The ketogenic diet preserves skeletal muscle with aging in mice. *Aging Cell* **2021**, *20*, e13322. [CrossRef] [PubMed]
33. Olson, C.A.; Iniguez, A.J.; Yang, G.E.; Fang, P.; Pronovost, G.N.; Jameson, K.G.; Rendon, T.K.; Paramo, J.; Barlow, J.T.; Ismagilov, R.F.; et al. Alterations in the gut microbiota contribute to cognitive impairment induced by the ketogenic diet and hypoxia. *Cell Host Microbe* **2021**, *29*, 1378–1392.e1376. [CrossRef]
34. Mierziak, J.; Burgberger, M.; Wojtasik, W. 3-Hydroxybutyrate as a Metabolite and a Signal Molecule Regulating Processes of Living Organisms. *Biomolecules* **2021**, *11*, 402. [CrossRef]
35. Sharma, R.; Diwan, B. A Cellular Senescence-Centric Integrated Approach to Understanding Organismal Aging. *Curr. Aging Sci.* **2023**, *16*, 12–24. [CrossRef]
36. Palmer, A.K.; Jensen, M.D. Metabolic changes in aging humans: Current evidence and therapeutic strategies. *J. Clin. Investig.* **2022**, *132*, e158451. [CrossRef]
37. Catic, A. Cellular Metabolism and Aging. *Prog. Mol. Biol. Transl. Sci.* **2018**, *155*, 85–107. [CrossRef]
38. Zeng, W.Y.; Tan, L.; Han, C.; Zheng, Z.Y.; Wu, G.S.; Luo, H.R.; Li, S.L. Trigonelline Extends the Lifespan of C. Elegans and Delays the Progression of Age-Related Diseases by Activating AMPK, DAF-16, and HSF-1. *Oxid. Med. Cell Longev.* **2021**, *2021*, 7656834. [CrossRef]
39. Aktar, S.; Ferdousi, F.; Kondo, S.; Kagawa, T.; Isoda, H. Transcriptomics and biochemical evidence of trigonelline ameliorating learning and memory decline in the senescence-accelerated mouse prone 8 (SAMP8) model by suppressing proinflammatory cytokines and elevating neurotransmitter release. *Geroscience* **2023**, *46*, 1671–1691. [CrossRef]
40. Izuta, Y.; Imada, T.; Hisamura, R.; Oonishi, E.; Nakamura, S.; Inagaki, E.; Ito, M.; Soga, T.; Tsubota, K. Ketone body 3-hydroxybutyrate mimics calorie restriction via the Nrf2 activator, fumarate, in the retina. *Aging Cell* **2018**, *17*, e12699. [CrossRef]
41. Membrez, M.; Migliavacca, E.; Christen, S.; Yaku, K.; Trieu, J.; Lee, A.K.; Morandini, F.; Giner, M.P.; Stiner, J.; Makarov, M.V.; et al. Trigonelline is an NAD(+) precursor that improves muscle function during ageing and is reduced in human sarcopenia. *Nat. Metab.* **2024**, *6*, 433–447. [CrossRef] [PubMed]

MDPI AG
Grosspeteranlage 5
4052 Basel
Switzerland
Tel.: +41 61 683 77 34

Nutrients Editorial Office
E-mail: nutrients@mdpi.com
www.mdpi.com/journal/nutrients

www.ingramcontent.com/pod-product-compliance
Lightning Source LLC
Chambersburg PA
CBHW061612210926
51850CB00009B/2301
* 9 7 8 3 7 2 5 8 4 9 1 9 2 *